Equine Science

Equine Science

Zoe Davies

Third Edition

WILEY Blackwell

Registered Offices
John Wiley & Sons, Inc., 111 River Street, Hoboken, NJ 07030, USA
John Wiley & Sons Ltd, The Atrium, Southern Gate, Chichester, West Sussex, PO19 8SQ, UK

Editorial Office
9600 Garsington Road, Oxford, OX4 2DQ, UK

For details of our global editorial offices, customer services, and more information about Wiley products visit us at www.wiley.com.

Wiley also publishes its books in a variety of electronic formats and by print-on-demand. Some content that appears in standard print versions of this book may not be available in other formats.

Library of Congress Cataloging-in-Publication Data

Names: Davies, Zoe, author.
Title: Equine science / Zoe Davies.
Description: Third edition. | Hoboken, NJ : John Wiley & Sons, 2017. |
    Includes index. |
Identifiers: LCCN 2017020437 (print) | LCCN 2017035568 (ebook) | ISBN
    9781118741177 (pdf) | ISBN 9781118741160 (epub) | ISBN 9781118741184 (pbk.)
Subjects: LCSH: Horses. | Horses–Health.
Classification: LCC SF285.3 (ebook) | LCC SF285.3 .P54 2017 (print) | DDC
    636.1–dc23
LC record available at https://lccn.loc.gov/2017020437

Cover image: Courtesy of Eva-Maria Broomer
Cover design by Wiley

Set in 10/12pt WarnockPro by SPi Global, Chennai, India
Printed and bound by CPI Group (UK) Ltd, Croydon, CR0 4YY

C9781118741184_191023

This book is dedicated to my lovely family, Ian, Sophie and Katie, and to all the horses I have owned or helped as part of my work that have inspired me to write it.

Contents

Preface

Horses are integral to our culture, and they continue to be used for work, leisure and competition throughout the world. Knowledge of this magnificent animal is continually improving as science delves deeper, uncovering new information that helps us to understand how the horse functions.

This edition of *Equine Science* has been rewritten and expanded to provide more detailed and up-to-date information for those studying equine courses at higher academic levels or more knowledgeable horse owners keen to understand the inner workings of horses in their care. The systems of the horse are covered extensively with new and expanded information, with full colour artwork and photographs to assist the reader in understanding its scientific content.

Knowledge of equine science for all involved with horses results in higher standards of management and welfare, particularly for those working or competing, no matter what the discipline.

Zoe Davies, MSc., R.Nutr.

Acknowledgement

I would like to thank Sarah Pilliner for her important contributions to some chapters of this new edition and Julie Musk for her editing skills and support during the production process. I would also like to thank Harthill Stud and all the other contributors for supplying many of the photographs.

1

The Biochemical Nature of Cells

Biochemistry is the study of chemicals within biology. A knowledge of biological molecules and their structure and function is essential for a full understanding of the nature, performance and behaviour of horses. There are approximately one hundred elements that exist on Earth; of these, 16 are essential for life and only four make up 95% of all living matter, namely carbon, hydrogen, oxygen and nitrogen.

The combination of carbon with other elements creates a huge variety of organic molecules, and all organic compounds therefore contain a carbon backbone. The four main classes of organic molecules are proteins, carbohydrates, lipids and nucleic acids. In addition, a relatively small number of inorganic ions such as sodium and potassium are essential for life, as components of larger molecules or extracellular fluids. Table 1.1 shows examples of organic and inorganic molecules.

Horses therefore contain water plus a huge number of macromolecules which have been built up from smaller simpler ones. These molecules are also involved in the basic structure and function of all cells (Figure 1.1). These simple building blocks are similar in all organisms, suggesting a common origin for all life forms.

Metabolism

All chemical reactions that take place within the horse are collectively known as 'metabolism'. Metabolic reactions can be anabolic (building up large molecules from smaller ones) or catabolic (breaking down larger molecules into smaller ones). Anabolic reactions usually involve removal of water molecules and are known as condensation reactions, such as when glycogen is built up from glucose molecules. Catabolic reactions are the reverse and usually involve larger molecules being split when reacting with water. These are known as hydrolysis reactions, for example digestion of proteins in the digestive system.

Horses must have a supply of energy to fuel energy-requiring processes, such as sustaining life and movement. This is obtained from cellular respiration – the oxidation of organic molecules such as glucose into simpler molecules namely carbon dioxide and water.

Water

All life on Earth began in water and water is the main component of all organisms, including horses, providing an environment in which metabolic reactions can occur. Approximately 65–70% of the bodyweight (bwt) of the horse on a fat-free basis is made up of water and newborn foals may contain as much as 90% water. Male horses contain slightly more water than females.

Fluids are present in the body in two main compartments: inside cells and outside cells. Approximately two-thirds of water is found within cells and this is known as intracellular fluid (ICF). The remainder (one-third) is

Table 1.1 Examples of organic and inorganic compounds in the horse's body.

Organic compounds	Inorganic compounds
Glucose ($C_6H_{12}O_6$)	Water (H_2O)
Ethane (C_2H_6)	Ammonia (NH_3)
Glycine (amino acid) ($C_2H_5NO_2$)	Carbon dioxide (CO_2)
Cytosine (nucleotide base) ($C_4H_5N_3O$)	Nitrate ion (NO_{3-})

outside cells and is called extracellular fluid (ECF). From this, roughly 80% of ECF is found in interstitial fluid, that is, bathing and surrounding cells in tissues, and about 20% in blood plasma. Interstitial fluid encompasses lymph, cerebrospinal fluid, synovial fluid, and pleural, pericardial and peritoneal fluids, to name but a few.

The horse's body also naturally generates metabolic water as a result of breaking down protein, carbohydrates and fat, mostly from condensation reactions. This does not provide a large amount of water, but does contribute to the daily water balance and may change the horse's need for water. Diet will also affect water requirements. Horses grazing on pasture which has a low dry matter will sometimes drink little or no additional water compared to those on a mostly dry forage diet such as hay. Voluntary water intake by resting horses in a moderate temperature environment is roughly 25–70 ml/kg bwt/day. For a 500-kg horse this equates to 12.5–35 litres per day. Obviously this depends upon water intake such as from feed and drinking and water losses. High-protein feeds such as alfalfa will need more water to help remove excess nitrogen.

Water intake is regulated by the thirst centre in the hypothalamus. Water loss greater than gain (from intake and metabolic water) leads to dehydration. This leads to an increased osmotic pressure of body fluids and

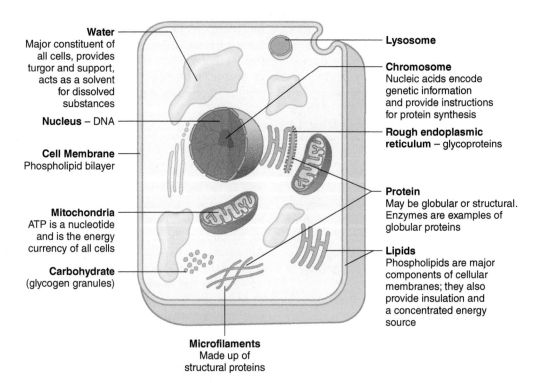

Water
Major constituent of all cells, provides turgor and support, acts as a solvent for dissolved substances

Nucleus – DNA

Cell Membrane
Phospholipid bilayer

Mitochondria
ATP is a nucleotide and is the energy currency of all cells

Carbohydrate
(glycogen granules)

Lysosome

Chromosome
Nucleic acids encode genetic information and provide instructions for protein synthesis

Rough endoplasmic reticulum – glycoproteins

Protein
May be globular or structural. Enzymes are examples of globular proteins

Lipids
Phospholipids are major components of cellular membranes; they also provide insulation and a concentrated energy source

Microfilaments
Made up of structural proteins

Figure 1.1 The biochemical nature of cells.

Figure 1.2 Structure of water.

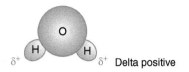

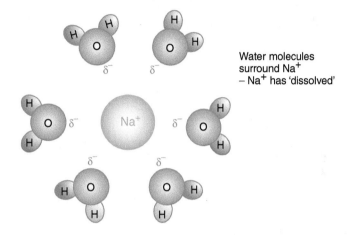

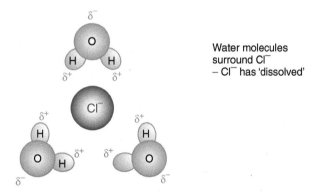

decrease in volume leading to stimulation of thirst.

Water is liquid at room temperature and many substances dissolve in it due to its weak polar nature. This means that water molecules have a weak attraction for each other, and other inorganic ions which form large numbers of weak hydrogen bonds. This gives water its unique properties, including acting as a universal solvent and a low viscosity material (Figure 1.2).

The chemical behaviour of water is a result of its dipolar nature having a small negative charge on the oxygen and two small positive charges on the hydrogen atoms. This means water molecules tend to stick together, allowing water to flow, and this is ideal for transport of substances around the body.

To change state from solid to liquid to gas, water requires a substantial amount of energy, which makes water a thermally stable compound. Water evaporates when the hydrogen bonds in water are broken, allowing the surface water molecules to escape as gas and evaporate. It takes a large amount of heat energy to break the hydrogen bonds and this uses up a substantial amount of energy; water therefore has a high latent heat of evaporation. When 1 g of water changes from liquid to vapour, it takes up 580 calories of heat. To put this in perspective, heating 1 g of water from freezing to boiling requires only 117 calories. Sweating causes rapid cooling as water carries away heat energy when it evaporates from the horse's skin.

Important Properties of Water

- High specific heat capacity – prevents rapid temperature changes and therefore creates a stable chemical environment for the horse's body.
- High latent heat of evaporation – creates rapid cooling.
- Good solvent – can take up minerals into the body and transport.
- Cohesive – water molecules stick together.
- Lubricant properties – synovial fluid in joints, pleural fluid in lungs and mucus.
- Support – amniotic fluid supporting and protecting the growing foetus.

Proteins

Proteins play a vital role in virtually all biological processes in horses (Figure 1.3).

They make up more than 50% of the dry weight of equine cells. It is also estimated that mammals have the ability to generate approximately two million different types of proteins, coded by genes, each with a specific function and shape.

Proteins consist of basic units or amino acids. Plants make all the amino acids they need from smaller molecules, whereas horses (as all animals) must obtain many amino acids from their diet. These are called essential amino acids as they cannot be made in the horse's body. Others can be made in the body and are called non-essential amino acids; however, the division is not clear, as some amino acids can be used to make others and some can be converted to others via the urea cycle. Table 1.2 lists the essential and non-essential amino acids.

Basic Structure of Amino Acids

Although there are more than 150 amino acids found in cells, only 20 commonly occur in proteins. The remaining non-protein amino acids have roles in metabolic reactions or as hormones and neurotransmitters. A new 21st amino acid has been found, named selenocysteine (SeC), which can be used to make proteins. It has properties making it

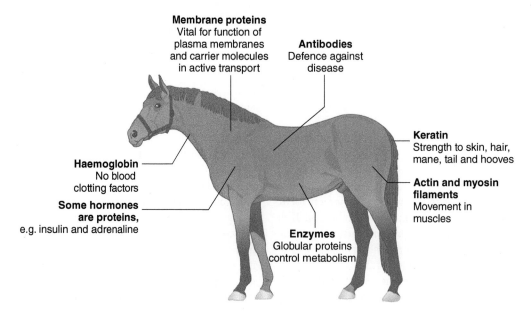

Membrane proteins
Vital for function of plasma membranes and carrier molecules in active transport

Antibodies
Defence against disease

Keratin
Strength to skin, hair, mane, tail and hooves

Haemoglobin
No blood clotting factors

Some hormones are proteins,
e.g. insulin and adrenaline

Actin and myosin filaments
Movement in muscles

Enzymes
Globular proteins control metabolism

Figure 1.3 Importance of proteins in the horse's body.

Table 1.2 Essential and non-essential amino acids.

Essential amino acids	Non-essential amino acids
Lysine	Alanine
Methionine (contains sulphur)	Arginine
Tryptophan	Asparagine
Leucine	Aspartic acid
Isoleucine	Cysteine (contains sulphur)
Phenylalanine	Glutamine
Threonine	Glutamic acid
Valine	Glycine
	Histidine
	Proline
	Serine
	Tyrosine
	Selenocysteine

very suitable in proteins that are involved in antioxidant activity. It is not universal in all organisms. Again, unlike the other amino acids, no free pool of selenocysteine exists in cells because its high reactivity would cause damage. Instead, cells store selenium in the less reactive selenide form.

All amino acids have a common structure (Figure 1.4). The R groups are varied and give the amino acids different chemical properties (Figure 1.5). Disulphide bridges in the amino acid cysteine allow cross-linkages with other cysteine molecules in a polypeptide chain. Amino acids are linked together in long chains, sometimes up to several hundred amino acid units long, to form polypeptides. Some polypeptides will be functional themselves, whereas others will be joined to other polypeptide chains before they become functional.

The simplest amino acid is glycine. All the rest are optical isomers. This means that they can result in two different arrangements of the four available bonding sites on the carbon atoms. This gives the 'D' and 'L' forms, but only the L forms (remember L for living) are found in living organisms such as horses.

Polypeptides

Polypeptide chains are chains of amino acids joined together by peptide bonds. A typical polypeptide contains 100–300 amino acids. The building of long polypeptide chains uses condensation reactions, that is, removal of water to join two amino acids together to form a peptide bond. The splitting or removal of amino acids from a polypeptide, such as occurs during digestion, uses hydrolysis, that is, the addition of water via a hydrogen (H) and hydroxyl (OH) group. Figure 1.6 shows the formation of a dipeptide.

Levels of Protein Structure

Because proteins are such large complex molecules their structures are often described by considering four different levels: primary, secondary, tertiary and quaternary.

Figure 1.4 Structure of an amino acid.

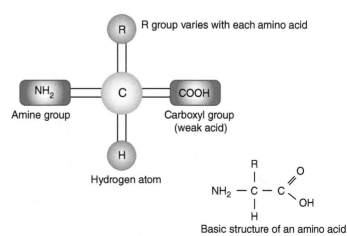

R group varies with each amino acid

Amine group

Carboxyl group (weak acid)

Hydrogen atom

Basic structure of an amino acid

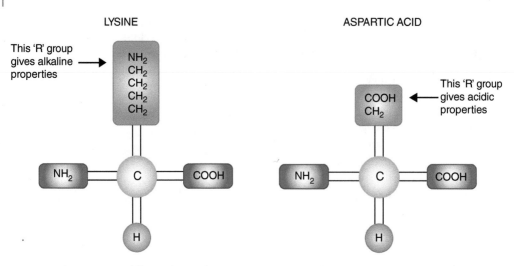

Figure 1.5 R groups give different chemical properties to amino acids.

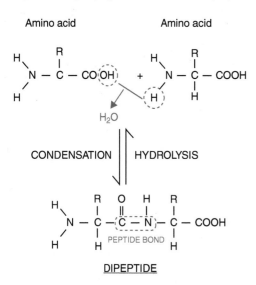

Figure 1.6 Formation of a dipeptide.

Primary Structure of Proteins (Amino Acid Sequence)

The primary structure refers to the sequence of amino acids in the protein chain. A simple primary structure of a small protein could be shown as:

Phenylalanine – Glutamine – Tyrosine –

    Serine – Isoleucine – Methionine –

    Alanine

The hormone insulin, for example, consists of a chain of 51 amino acids. The code for the primary structure of all proteins is contained in the gene or genes that code for that specific protein and this determines the precise order that the chain is built or assembled within the cell. The order also determines the way the chain will twist and turn to make up its three-dimensional (3D) shape which allows it to carry out its specific function within the horse's body.

Secondary Structure of Proteins (Alpha Helix or Beta Pleated Sheet)

The secondary structure refers to the first level of 3D twisting. These twists occur as the amino acids twist to find the most stable arrangement of their hydrogen bonds within the chain. The main secondary structures are the alpha helix spiral or beta pleated sheet. The structure depends upon the amino acids that make up the chain. The alpha helix spiral is the most common, where amino acids twist on their axes, each forming a hydrogen bond with another amino acid four units along. This stabilises the alpha helix shape.

The beta pleated sheet is a flat structure consisting of two or more amino acid chains running parallel, linked together by hydrogen bonds. Some amino acids tend to produce sharp bends in the chain, allowing the structure to bend backwards upon itself.

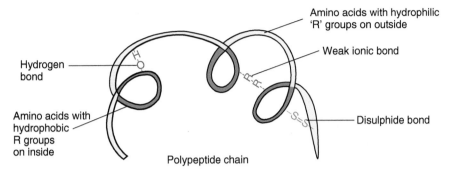

Amino acids with hydrophilic 'R' groups on outside

Weak ionic bond

Hydrogen bond

Amino acids with hydrophobic R groups on inside

Disulphide bond

Polypeptide chain

Figure 1.7 Bonding examples in the tertiary structure of proteins.

Tertiary Structure of Proteins (3D Shape/Folding)

The tertiary structure refers to the overall 3D shape and depends upon several factors: first, the exact sequence of amino acids that produces either the alpha helix or beta pleated shapes at particular points on the long amino acid chain; and second, the hydrophobic side chains on globular proteins (which are surrounded by water) that tend to point inwards, and also any weak ionic bonds or hydrogen bonds (Figure 1.7). The strongest links are found when neighbouring cysteine amino acids form disulphide bridges. These bridges occur most commonly in structural proteins, contributing to their strength. Some proteins are complete and function with a tertiary structure only, such as enzymes.

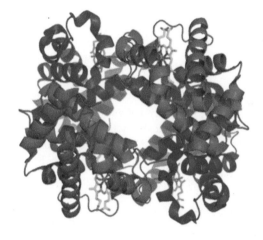

Figure 1.8 Model of haemoglobin. *Source*: Zephryis, https://en.wikipedia.org/wiki/Hemoglobin#/media/File:1GZX_Haemoglobin.png. CC-BY-SA 3.0.

Quaternary Structure of Proteins (Aggregations of Polypeptide Chains)

Many complex proteins are made up of one or more than one polypeptide chain and sometimes have additional non-protein prosthetic groups usually vital to the function of that protein, for example, the 'haem' group in haemoglobin (Hb). The arrangement of these polypeptide chains is known as the quaternary structure. Hb is a globular protein composed of four polypeptide units joined together: two identical alpha chains and two identical beta chains (Figure 1.8).

Each has the haem group at the centre of the chain which binds oxygen, that is, the Hb molecule contains just four Fe^{2+} (iron) atoms.

When one molecule of oxygen binds to Hb, it changes its shape, encouraging more oxygen molecules to bind. This is called cooperative binding. The chemical formula of Haemoglobin is $C_{2952}H_{4664}O_{832}N_{812}S_8Fe_4$. Proteins containing non-protein parts are known as conjugated proteins.

Classification of Proteins

Table 1.3 shows the structural classification of proteins. The final 3D structure results in two main classes of protein:

- Globular – large individual molecules which are round and compact in shape with complex tertiary and quaternary

Table 1.3 Structural classification of proteins.

Globular proteins	Fibrous proteins
Soluble in water, easily transported in fluids	Insoluble in water
Tertiary structure determines function of protein	Tough structurally, may be elastic
Folded into compact spherical or globular shape	Parallel polypeptide chains forming sheets or long fibres
Examples	**Examples**
Enzymes	Collagen
Haemoglobin	Cartilage
Antibodies	Tendons
Hormones	Bones
	Walls of blood vessels

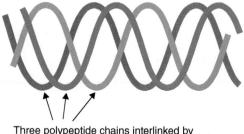

Three polypeptide chains interlinked by strong covalent bonds

Figure 1.9 Structure of collagen.

structures, mostly soluble in water, with mostly biochemical functions.
- Fibrous – tough and rope shaped, containing polypeptides bound together in long sheets or fibres.

Structure of Collagen

Collagen is an important fibrous protein which provides structure and support to tissues. It is strong and flexible. Collagen is made up of three polypeptide chains that are tightly coiled into a triple helix formation (Figure 1.9). The polypeptide chains are connected by strong interlinks formed from covalent bonds. Minerals may be added to the triple helix to increase its rigidity, such as found in bone.

Modification of Proteins

After production by ribosomes, many proteins may be passed to the inside of rough endoplasmic reticulum (ER) where they are modified by the addition of carbohydrates to produce glycoproteins. These appear to be markers to determine the destination of the protein. Proteins made by free ribosomes in the cytosol do not have added carbohydrate. Some proteins may have fatty acids added,

producing lipoproteins that help transport lipids round the horse's body.

Denaturation of Proteins

Denaturation results in the breakdown of the 3D structure of proteins and therefore, most often, their biological function. Denaturation occurs due to breakdown of the bonds holding the 3D structure in place, while the amino acid sequence usually remains unchanged. Denaturation can be caused by heat (such as raised body temperature), heavy metals, strong acids and alkalis, some solvents and detergents.

Carbohydrates

Carbohydrates are required to provide energy for fuel for cellular metabolism, that is, for life. Carbohydrates are a group of molecules consisting of carbon, hydrogen and oxygen with the general formula $(CH_2O)x$. One of the most common of all carbohydrates is glucose. Glucose is essential for nerve cells including the brain, as the brain cannot use any other form of fuel.

Monosaccharides (one) and disaccharides (two) are classed as sugars and usually end in -ose (e.g. glucose, lactose). All monosaccharides are reducing sugars in that they can be used in reduction reactions. Glucose is a very important monosaccharide (i.e. a single sugar molecule) as it is required for energy for all plants and animals. It is soluble and so easily transported. The

Table 1.4 Common carbohydrates – disaccharides, monosaccharides and polysaccharides.

Common disaccharides (double sugars)	Constituent monosaccharides
Sucrose (table sugar)	Alpha glucose + beta fructose (found in sap of plants)
Maltose	Alpha glucose + alpha glucose (found in germinating seeds)
Lactose (milk sugar)	Beta glucose + beta galactose (found in milk)
No. of carbon atoms in monosaccharide	**Type of sugar and examples**
3	Triose – glyceraldehyde
5	Pentose – ribose, deoxyribose
6	Hexose – glucose, fructose (fruit sugar), galactose (milk sugar)
Common polysaccharides	**Constituent monosaccharide**
Starch (plants – storage)	Glucose
Glycogen (animals – storage)	Glucose
Cellulose (plant cell walls)	Glucose

chemical bonds within glucose contain a large amount of energy that can be released in the mitochondria via cellular respiration. Glucose is a six-carbon sugar known as a hexose sugar and these sugars occur most frequently, whereas five-carbon sugars are known as pentose sugars. Three-carbon sugars are termed triose sugars. Lactose is the primary carbohydrate source for suckling foals. Common carbohydrates are shown in Table 1.4.

Carbohydrates also exist as isomers, having the same chemical formula with a different structural formula. This results in different properties such as taste and digestibility. Glucose exists as alpha and beta glucose (Figure 1.10). Starch and glycogen are polymers consisting of long chains of alpha glucose, whereas cellulose is a polymer of beta glucose.

Monosaccharides are joined together by glycosidic bonds to form disaccharides and polysaccharides. This is a condensation reaction, with the resultant removal of a water molecule (similar to polypeptides). When polysaccharides are broken down, the glycosidic bonds are broken by hydrolysis, that is, by the addition of a water molecule. The disaccharide maltose, for example, is built up from two alpha glucose molecules by a condensation reaction (Figure 1.11).

Fructans

Fructans are polysaccharides consisting mainly of fructose, with sometimes glucose present too. Fructans are important for storage of carbohydrates in the stems of many species of grasses and confer a degree of freezing tolerance and possibly drought tolerance as well. Fructans may be very large

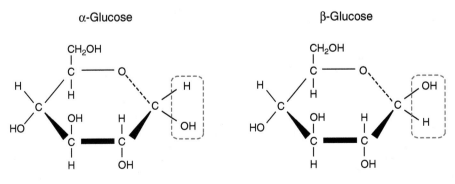

Figure 1.10 Alpha and beta structure of glucose.

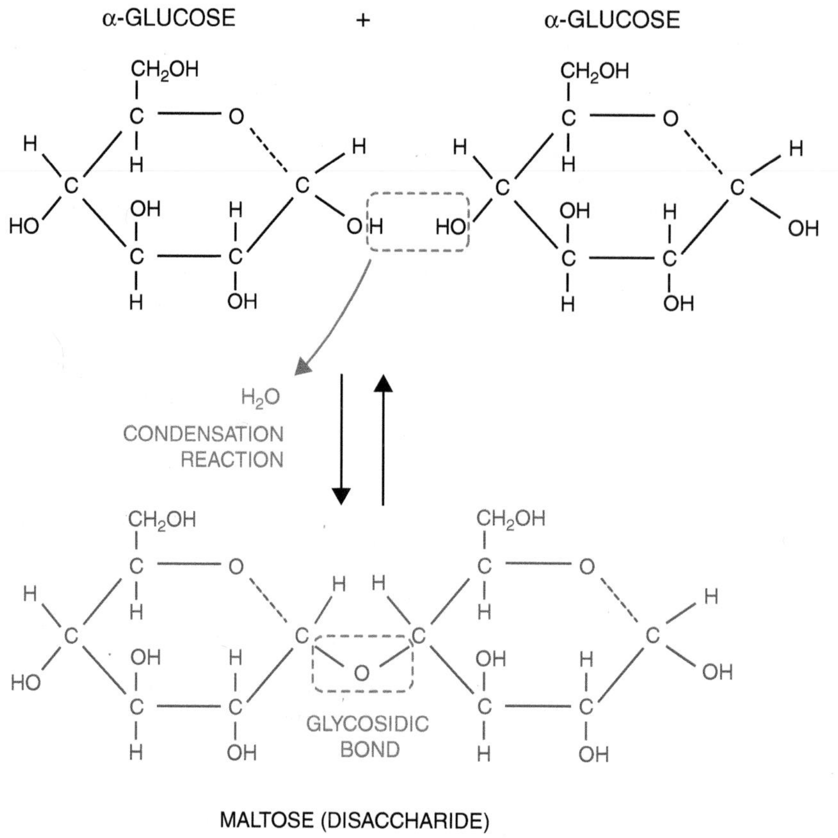

Figure 1.11 Structure of maltose from two alpha glucose molecules.

3D-structured molecules, of which there are many different ones. They have a highly complicated nomenclature based on the type and site of chemical linkages. Fructans in grass are called levans or phleins, with 2,6 linkages, whereas fructans from broad-leaved plants are mainly inulin with 2,1 linkages. Not all grasses make fructans and some have their own individual type. Fructans are important in equine nutrition as horses do not possess the enzymes to break them down in the small intestine and they therefore pass undigested into the hindgut where they become a substrate for microbes.

Starch

Starch is the main energy storage material of plants including grasses and cereals. It is also the major component of cereal grains traditionally used to feed horses, such as oats, barley and maize, which therefore contain high levels of starch. Plant cells make glucose via photosynthesis and store excess glucose primarily as starch. Starch is insoluble in water so it does not affect osmosis. Because there are few 'ends' within the starch molecule, there are fewer points for enzymic breakdown, and therefore starch is an excellent long-term storage compound for plants. Starch is a mixture of two polysaccharides of alpha glucose, namely:

- Amylose – consisting of a long unbranched chain with a coiled structure for easy storage. Makes up 25–30% of the starch molecule, linked by alpha 1,4 glycosidic bonds.
- Amylopectin – consisting of a long branched chain containing up to 1500

glucose units in which alpha 1,4 chains are cross-linked by alpha 1,6 glycosidic bonds, giving side branches for easy enzymic breakdown to glucose. Makes up 70–75% of the starch molecule, with alpha 1,6 glycosidic bonds every 24–30 glucose units.

Cellulose

Cellulose is the most common molecule on earth. It is the major structural component of plant cell walls, made up of long straight unbranched chains of beta glucose held together by 1,4 glycosidic bonds. Cellulose gives plants structure and strength. As many as 10,000 glucose molecules may be linked together in the chain. The parallel cellulose chains are cross-linked together by hydrogen bonds which form strong fibres known as microfibrils. This provides the plant cells with firm structural support for the cells and plants as a whole. The cross-linking prevents access by water, so that cellulose is very resistant to hydrolysis and is therefore an excellent structural molecule for plants (Figure 1.12).

Glycogen

Glycogen is the main energy storage form of all animals including horses and is similar to starch. It is a branched chain polysaccharide like amylopectin, being composed of alpha glucose molecules but with more alpha 1,6 glycosidic bonds mixed with alpha 1,4 glycosidic bonds, that is, more branches (Figure 1.13). This means it can be broken down quickly by enzymic hydrolysis when glucose is required for energy. Glycogen is also more water soluble than starch. Glycogen is mainly found within the horse's muscle and liver cells.

Lipids/Fats

Lipids are not the same as carbohydrates and proteins as they are not made up of long chains of monomer units. Lipids include fats and oils and have an oily or fatty consistency; they are insoluble in water but soluble in alcohol and ether, except for phospholipids which have polar heads, that is, they are hydrophilic or 'water loving'.

Lipids are varied and contain carbon, hydrogen and oxygen, and sometimes phosphorus and nitrogen. They are intermediate-size molecules. Lipids are important as fuel, and for important chemicals such as hormones, fat-soluble vitamins and structural phospholipids in plasma membranes. Carbohydrates and proteins may be converted to fats by enzymes for storage in times when food is plentiful. When food is scarce, these fat stores can be used as fuel sources. Fats are an economical way for horses to store fuel, as they yield more than twice as much

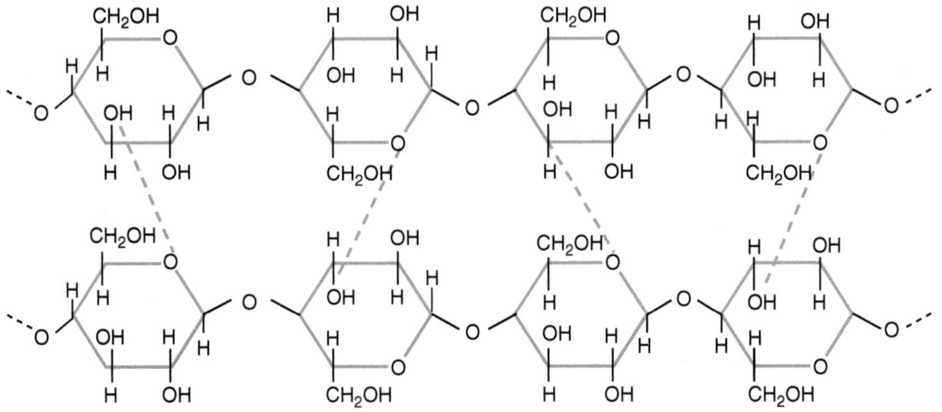

Figure 1.12 Structure of cellulose.

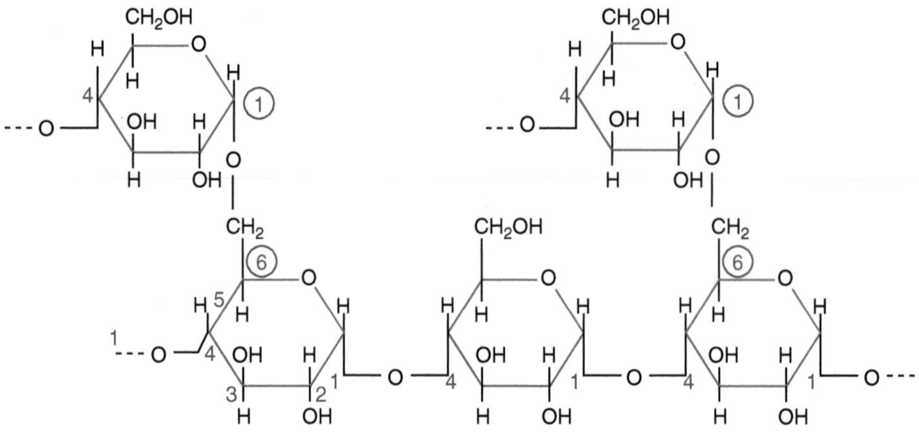

Figure 1.13 Structure of glycogen.

energy as the same amount of carbohydrate. Horses have a limited ability to store excess energy as carbohydrate per se and so convert it mostly to fat for storage. The disadvantage of this is that oxygen is required to release this energy in fat stores. So, during anaerobic respiration, such as in sprinting racehorses or horses escaping from danger, where skeletal muscle is rapidly contracting, the muscle cells must retain the potential to oxidise carbohydrate as well as more energy-dense fat. Lipids contain hydrocarbons and there are two types of lipid important in the horse's body: triglycerides and phospholipids.

Triglycerides

Triglycerides are the most common lipids in nature and are classified as fats or oils. In horses, triglycerides occur mainly in adipose or fat tissue under the skin, particularly of the neck and rump, and around the internal organs. Adipose tissue insulates against cold and protects organs against physical damage. It also contributes to the shape or 'top line' of horses.

Fat cells are an important tissue, helping to regulate the metabolism of horses, and they can also produce a wide range of proteins that act upon other cells. Triglycerides consist of one molecule of glycerol with three fatty acids (Figure 1.14). There are about 70 different fatty acids which may be condensed with glycerol, producing a wide range of triglycerides. The four components are joined together in an 'E'-shape by condensation reactions which form ester bonds. Fatty acids have long tails made up of hydrocarbons and these tails are hydrophobic 'water hating'. The tails make triglycerides insoluble in water.

Fatty acids may be saturated or unsaturated. Saturated fats do not have any double bonds between the carbon atoms, that is, the fatty acid is 'saturated' with hydrogen and there is no room for additions. Unsaturated fats have at least one double bond and this can cause the chain to kink. Most animal fats are saturated as they have no double bonds, whereas plant fats tend to be unsaturated. Saturated fats tend to be solid, such as butter and suet. Unsaturation reduces the melting point, and therefore plant fats tend to be liquid at room temperature, that is, in oil form. About 30 different fatty acids are found in animal or equine lipids.

Essential Fatty Acids

Table 1.5 lists some common fatty acids. Linolenic (omega 3) and linoleic (omega 6) fatty acids are essential – that is, they must be provided in the diet of horses – and the optimum ratio is approximately 3:1, respectively.

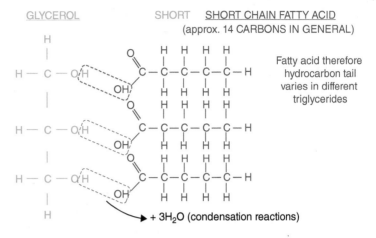

Figure 1.14 Structure of triglycerides.

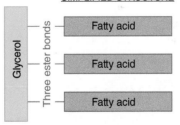

Both acids have very different metabolic pathways within the horse's body:

Omega 6 (linoleic acid)

→ Gamma linolenic acid (GLA)

→ Arachidonic acid

Omega 3 (linolenic acid)

→ Eicosapentaenoic acid (EPA)

→ Docosahexaenoic acid (DHA).

Of these, DHA and EPA are particularly vital and have important roles, providing protection against degenerative disease and illness. DHA and EPA are thought to reduce inflammation and thereby assist in joint and respiratory function and also aid fertility in the mare and stallion.

Phospholipids

Phospholipids are the main component of all biological membranes, including cells and their organelles, and are similar to triglycerides but consist of a glycerol molecule with two fatty acid chains instead of three and

Table 1.5 Some common fatty acids.

Fatty acid	No. of carbon atoms	No. of double bonds	Function
Oleic acid	18	1	Found in micro-organisms
Linoleic acid	18	2	Major fatty acid in plant lipids. In animals it is derived mainly from dietary plant oils
EPA (eicosapentaenoic acid)	20	5	Protects genes and the cell cycle, as well as regulating the stress response
DHA (docosahexaenoic acid)	22	6	Found in high concentrations, especially in phospholipids within the brain, retina and testes
Arachidonic acid	20	4	Major component of membrane phospholipids
Linolenic acid	18	3	Alpha-linolenic acid is found in higher plants (soyabean oil and rape seed)

(a)

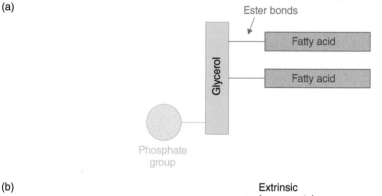

(b)

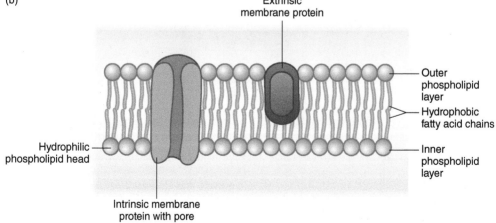

Figure 1.15 Phospholipids are the main component of all biological membranes, including cells and their organelles, and are similar to triglycerides but consist of a glycerol molecule with two fatty acid chains instead of three and a phosphate group attached (a). The phosphate group at one end is attracted to water (hydrophilic), whereas the fatty acid tail is repelled by water (hydrophobic). The hydrophobic end therefore turns inward in the phospholipid bilayer (b) and the hydrophilic phosphate end turns outward.

a phosphate group attached (Figure 1.15a). The phosphate group at one end is attracted to water (hydrophilic), whereas the fatty acid tail is repelled by water (hydrophobic). The hydrophobic end therefore turns inward in the phospholipid bilayer (Figure 1.15b) and the hydrophilic phosphate end turns outward.

Cholesterol

Cholesterol is a normal constituent of the horse's body. While not a steroid itself, cholesterol is a sterol lipid and is a precursor to several steroid hormones including testosterone, oestrogen and progesterone. It is also present in the plasma membrane, where it regulates the fluidity of the membrane, stopping phospholipids packing too closely together. Cholesterol helps to stabilise the outer surface of the plasma membrane and reduces its permeability to smaller water-soluble molecules.

Nucleic Acids

Nucleic acids are the largest molecules made by horses and are a specialised group of compounds which are concerned with transmission of inherited information in cells. Nucleic acids are slightly acidic molecules that store the information that controls activities of the cell. There are two types of nucleic acids: deoxyribonucleic acid (DNA) (double strand) and ribonucleic acid (RNA) (single strand) (Table 1.6). Both contain the elements carbon, hydrogen, oxygen, nitrogen and phosphorus.

Nucleic acids are made up of repeating units called nucleotides and are known as polynucleotides. These are linked together in long chains or strands. The strands vary in the sequence of bases found on each of the nucleotides. DNA is a large molecule containing over 300 million nucleotides. RNA is much smaller, containing a few hundred only. Certain nucleotides are important as energy suppliers, namely adenosine triphosphate (ATP) and adenosine diphosphate

(ADP), or as electron carriers in respiration, namely nicotinamide adenine dinucleotide (NAD), nicotinamide adenine dinucleotide phosphate (NADP) and flavin adenine dinucleotide (FAD).

Each nucleotide consists of three units: (i) a sugar (ribose in RNA or deoxyribose in DNA); (ii) a phosphate group; and (iii) a nitrogen-containing base. Figure 1.16 shows the structure of a nucleotide.

Deoxyribonucleic Acid (DNA)

In the 1950s Watson and Crick published the DNA model of an ordered and regular double helix. DNA is a major component of chromosomes and is found mostly in the nucleus cells, although a small amount is also found in mitochondria. One strand of DNA unravelled is several centimetres in length and contains around 4000 genes, and there is thought to be a total of around 1.8 m (6 ft) of DNA in every cell. The DNA of the horse contains all the genetic information or genetic code for making proteins in cells and is required for the horse to grow from a fertilised egg to an adult horse.

DNA has two important characteristics:

- It stores genetic information, that is, it carries the genetic code.
- It has the ability to copy or replicate itself exactly, time after time.

The structure of DNA is shown in Figure 1.17.

Horses start life as a zygote (single fertilised cell) which has a complete set of genes. The cells then divide by mitosis (see Chapter 2), copying exactly the complete set of genes, but some of these cells differentiate into nervous tissue, whereas others may turn into skin cells or muscle. This is achieved by a process known as gene expression. Gene expression is when different genes are switched 'on' or 'off' in different cells. At any time, an equine cell is probably using only 1% of its genes. For example, genes used to make insulin are only expressed in the beta cells of the islets of Langerhans in the pancreas.

Table 1.6 Comparison of RNA and DNA.

RNA	DNA
Single strand	Double strand, double helix structure
Ribose sugar	Deoxyribose sugar
Bases A, U, C, G	Bases A ,T, C, G
Smaller molecule, a few hundred nucleotides	Large molecule, 300 million nucleotides

A good example of the power of gene expression can be found in the butterfly. The eggs of the butterfly contain a complete set of genes which are still there in the adult. However, from the egg to the caterpillar to the pupa and finally the adult, different sets of genes are activated. All stages of the butterfly's metamorphosis look completely different.

This sequence of bases within DNA chains provides the genetic code for the cell. The genetic code is therefore an alphabet of just four letters: A, G, C and T. It is known as the four-letter alphabet and should not be confused with the triplet codon. A, G, C and T stand for:

- adenine
- guanine
- cytosine
- thymine.

This is the code used to make all living things, be it human, fly or horse. DNA has regularity and stability, perfect for holding important genetic information. DNA tells every cell within the horse what it is to be and when and where it is required.

Genes code for proteins. It was previously thought that genes were specific sections of DNA which encoded all proteins including enzymes. This theory is now revised to the **one gene/one polypeptide** hypothesis. Genes also encode for functional RNAs (i.e. areas of non-protein coding DNA) that have specific regulatory functions in the cell. This refers to the previously thought 'junk' DNA.

A gene codes for a functional protein where the nucleotides are read as triplets

equivalent to codons on mRNA (see discussion on codons in 'The Genetic Code'). Punctuation or stop codons mark the start and end points of the gene. The genes needed to form a functional protein are collectively called a transcription unit. Adenine and guanine are purines and have a double ring structure, whereas cytosine and thymine are pyrimidines and have a single ring structure.

In DNA, adenine always pairs with thymine and guanine with cytosine: that is, A = T and G = C. The base pairs are held together by hydrogen bonds: three between C and G and two between A and T, or A and U in RNA (see 'Ribonucleic acid (RNA)'). Bases in nucleotides pair in a specific way due to the shapes of the ring structures of the bases.

The shape of DNA is similar to a very long ladder, with two complementary strands that each twists on its axis and the base pairs positioned like rungs. Each base pair causes a small twist to create a part of the double helix structure, causing a complete 360° turn every ten base pairs. Helical structures coil and supercoil, showing phases of extension and condensation, allowing gene activity and being important for cell division. Nucleotide sequences are the genetic code.

When DNA replicates itself, it unravels and adds two new copy strands by adding nucleotides that have been made by the cell and which are available within the cytoplasm. This process is known as semi-conservative replication of DNA (Figure 1.18). In fact, this is a complicated process requiring several enzymes. Two helicases using energy from ATP separate the part of the DNA strand that is being copied. DNA binding proteins keep the strands separate. DNA polymerase then moves along the exposed separated strands, making new strands often in short segments. Finally, DNA ligase joins these segments together, completing the new strand or part strand.

Ribonucleic Acid (RNA)

RNA is involved in the 'reading' of the DNA code for the copying process. In RNA, the

Figure 1.16 Structure of a nucleotide.

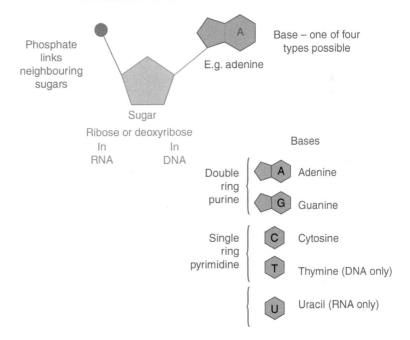

SYMBOLIC FORM OF A NUCLEOTIDE

DNA base thymine (T) is replaced by uracil (U), a fifth nucleotide which is almost chemically identical to thymine, but lacks its 5′ methyl group (see Figure 1.17). RNA adenine always pairs with uracil and guanine with cytosine, that is, A = U and G = C.

The cell contains three types of RNA each with a different function, namely:

- messenger RNA (mRNA)
- transfer RNA (tRNA)
- ribosomal RNA (rRNA).

Messenger RNA (mRNA)

mRNA could be described as a mobile copy of the gene. It carries the genetic information copied from DNA in the form of a series of three-base code 'words,' each of which specifies a particular amino acid (Table 1.7). This is the same code for all organisms, including horses. When the gene has been copied it moves from the nucleus to the ribosome in the cell where the protein is made according to the genetic code carried within the mRNA but copied from the DNA.

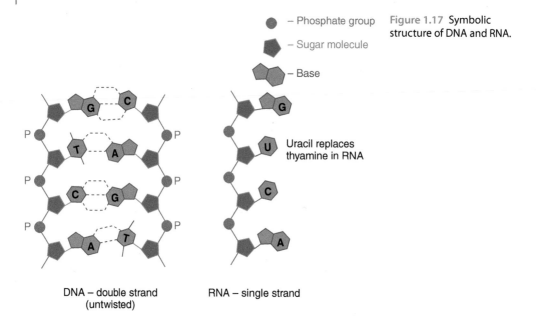

- Phosphate group
- Sugar molecule
- Base

Figure 1.17 Symbolic structure of DNA and RNA.

Uracil replaces thyamine in RNA

DNA – double strand
(untwisted)

RNA – single strand

Transfer RNA (tRNA)

tRNA could be described as a carrier molecule bringing individual amino acids from the cytoplasm to the ribosome for assembly into a protein or polypeptide chain according to the instructions carried on the mRNA (i.e. the mRNA code). Each type of amino acid has its own type of tRNA, which binds the amino acid and carries it from the cytoplasm to the ribosome to the growing end of a polypeptide chain as the next code word on mRNA calls for it. tRNA molecules have an anticodon on one end that binds to the mRNA and an amino acid binding site on the other. There are 61 different codons and three stop codons, making 64 in total (see Table 1.7).

Ribosomal RNA (rRNA)

rRNA associates with a set of proteins to form ribosomes. These complex structures, which physically move along an mRNA molecule, organise the assembly of amino acids into protein chains. They also bind tRNAs and various accessory molecules necessary for protein synthesis. Ribosomes are composed of large and small subunits, each of which contains its own rRNA molecule or molecules.

Protein Synthesis

The genetic code is read from a very small part of only one strand of DNA. Protein and amino acid synthesis can be divided into two parts, namely transcription and translation.

Transcription

DNA does not leave the nucleus and therefore must send information out of the nucleus to make proteins. It does this by transferring the genetic code to a smaller more mobile molecule – mRNA – which can then migrate to the ribosomes in the cytoplasm to act as a template for protein synthesis (Figure 1.19). mRNA is effectively a mobile copy of the gene.

The important point is that the genetic information is carried on only one of the two strands of the DNA. This is known as the coding strand, whereas the other strand is known as the template strand. These two strands are often given other names as well, which can be confusing. The two terms 'coding' and 'template' are commonly used.

The information in a gene on the coding strand is read in the direction from the 5′ end to the 3′ end (Figure 1.20). The 5′ end is the

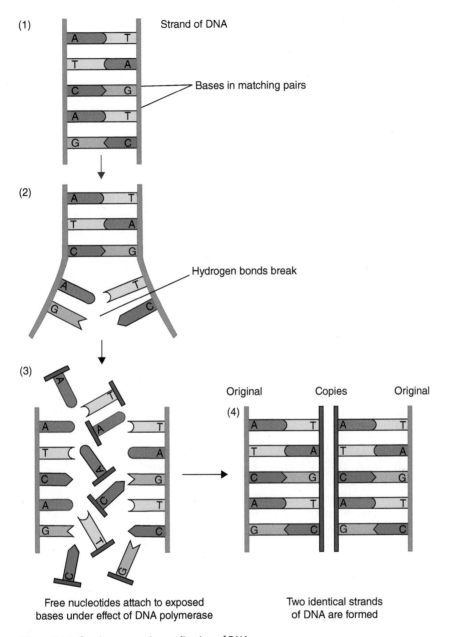

(1) Strand of DNA

Bases in matching pairs

(2)

Hydrogen bonds break

(3)

Original   Copies   Original

(4)

Free nucleotides attach to exposed
bases under effect of DNA polymerase

Two identical strands
of DNA are formed

Figure 1.18 Semi-conservative replication of DNA.

end that has the phosphate group attached to the 5′ carbon atom. The 3′ end is the end where the phosphate is attached to a 3′ carbon atom, or if it is at the very end of the DNA chain it has a free –OH group on the 3′ carbon.

Transcription is the process by which a particular segment of DNA, that is, the gene for a specific protein, is copied into mRNA by the enzyme RNA polymerase. During transcription, a DNA sequence is read by enzymes called RNA polymerases, which produce a copy mRNA strand, called a primary transcript. During this step, mRNA goes through different maturation processes, including splicing when the non-coding sequences are

Table 1.7 The genetic code – mRNA/amino acids (64 codons).

First base	Second base				Third base
G	G	A	C	U	G
	GGG GLYCINE	GAG GLUTAMIC ACID	GCG ALANINE	GUG VALINE	
	GGA GLYCINE	GAA GLUTAMIC ACID	GCA ALANINE	GUA VALINE	A
	GGC GLYCINE	GAC ASPARTIC ACID	GCC ALANINE	GUC VALINE	C
	GGU GLYCINE	GAU ASPARTIC ACID	GCU ALANINE	GUG VALINE	U
A	AGG ARGININE	AAG LYSINE	ACG THREONINE	AUG METHIONINE	G
	AGA ARGININE	AAA LYSINE	ACA THREONINE	AUA ISOLEUCINE	A
	AGC SERINE	AAC ASPARAGINE	ACC THREONINE	AUC ISOLEUCINE	C
	AGU SERINE	AAU ASPARAGINE	ACU THREONINE	AUU ISOLEUCINE	U
C	CGG ARGININE	CAG GLUTAMINE	CCG PROLINE	CUG LEUCINE	G
	CGA ARGININE	CAA GLUTAMINE	CCA PROLINE	CUA LEUCINE	A
	CGC ARGININE	CAC HISTIDINE	CCC PROLINE	CUC LEUCINE	C
	CGU ARGININE	CAU HISTIDINE	CCU PROLINE	CUU LEUCINE	U
U	UGG TRYPTOPHAN	UAG *STOP*	UCG SERINE	UUG LEUCINE	G
	UGA *STOP*	UAA *STOP*	UCA SERINE	UUA LEUCINE	A
	UGC CYSTEINE	UAC TYROSINE	UCC SERINE	UUC PHENYLALANINE	C
	UGU CYSTEINE	UAU TYROSINE	UCU SERINE	UUU PHENYLALANINE	U

eliminated. Opposite to DNA replication, transcription results in mRNA that includes the nucleotide uracil (U) in all instances where thymine (T) would have occurred in a DNA copy, that is, as would be the case in cell division. The coding mRNA is described as a unit of three nucleotides, that is, a codon (see 'The Genetic Code').

At the beginning of the process, DNA must unwind or 'unzip' to expose the base sequence of the required sequence (or rungs of the ladder) for copying. Once unzipped, RNA polymerase starts at the beginning of the required sequence and attaches to the DNA at the initiation site, that is, the start of the sequence. The enzyme then moves along the gene assembling mRNA by the addition of matching nucleotides, again in sequence. Once copied, the mRNA peels away from the DNA and the double helix rewinds. The mRNA then leaves the nucleus and travels to the ribosomes with the information or code (Figures 1.19 and 1.21).

Translation

Translation occurs on ribosomes and is the whole process by which the base sequence of an mRNA is used to order amino acids in the cytoplasm and then join them to the amino acids in the ribosomes to make a polypeptide. The code contained in the mRNA is used to translate into a polypeptide (Figures 1.19 and 1.22).

The three types of RNA participate in this essential protein building pathway in all cells. mRNA attaches to the ribosome at the point of attachment, and two tRNA molecules bring the required amino acids as

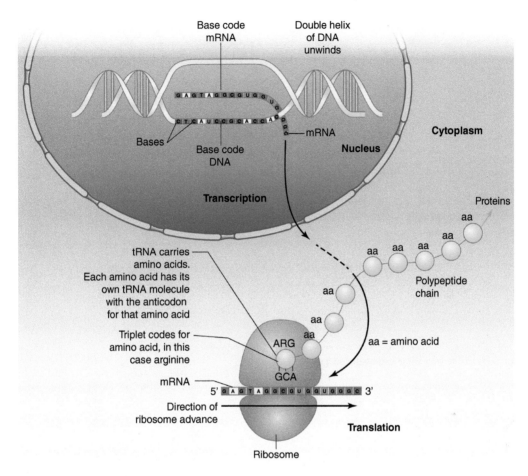

Figure 1.19 Transcription.

per instructions and fix them in position so they can be added to the polypeptide chain. The ribosome initially binds to mRNA at the start codon (ARG) which is only recognised by tRNA. The ribosome then moves from codon to codon along the mRNA, and amino acids are added one at a time, translated into polypeptide sequences as dictated originally by DNA. The process carries on until a stop codon which has no tRNA molecule moves into the ribosomes first binding site or start position, at which point all components separate, thereby releasing the completed polypeptide from the ribosome. This process effectively turns the DNA sequence into an amino acid sequence, that is, a polypeptide or protein.

The Genetic Code

Along the DNA molecule the base sequence is continuous. The four nucleotides in DNA are needed to make the 20 amino acids required for all cell functions. Because the four nucleotides, taken individually, could represent only four of the 20 possible amino acids required, a group of nucleotides is required to represent each amino acid. If

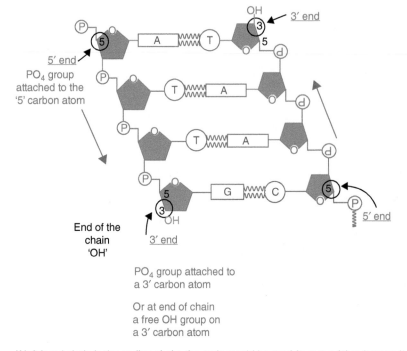

3′ end

5′ end
PO₄ group
attached to the
'5' carbon atom

End of the
chain
'OH'

3′ end

PO₄ group attached to
a 3′ carbon atom

Or at end of chain
a free OH group on
a 3′ carbon atom

If left-hand chain is the coding chain, the code would be read from top (5) to bottom (3).
The code in this very small segment would be 'A TT G'

Figure 1.20 Information in a gene on the coding strand is read in the direction from the 5′ end to the 3′ end.

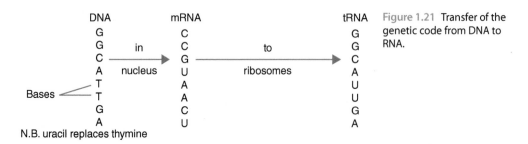

DNA		mRNA		tRNA
G		C		G
G	in	C	to	G
C		G		C
A	nucleus	U	ribosomes	A
T		A		U
T		A		U
G		C		G
A		U		A

Bases

N.B. uracil replaces thymine

Figure 1.21 Transfer of the genetic code from DNA to RNA.

two nucleotide bases were used to code for an amino acid, then only 16 different codes could be formed, which would be an insufficient number. However, if a group of three nucleotides (triplet) is used for each code word, then 64 code words can be formed (see Table 1.7). Any code using groups of three or more nucleotides will have more than enough units to encode the 20 amino acids required. This genetic code used by all cells is called a triplet code, with every three nucleotides

being 'read' from a specified starting point in the mRNA. Each triplet is called a codon and each codon codes for a specific amino acid. There are special codons which are known as stop codons which effectively cause a full stop at the end of the synthesised protein. Codons in a row between the stops are called genes.

Unlike other amino acids present in biological proteins, the recently found 21st amino acid selenocysteine is not coded for directly in the genetic code. Instead, it is encoded

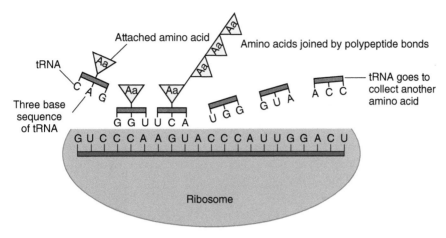

Figure 1.22 Translation takes place on the ribosomes.

in a special way by a UGA codon, which is normally a stop codon. Such a mechanism is called translational recoding.

The genetic code is universal for all living organisms and includes viruses, bacteria, plants and fungi. The code is 'degenerate' in that for each amino acid there may be more than one codon. For example, the codons for the amino acid alanine include GCU, GCC, GCA and GCG: that is, four codons code for alanine (ala) and six codons code for arginine (arg), namely CGU, CGC, CGA, CGG, AGA and AGG.

Reading the Genetic Code

Table 1.7 can be used to decode the genetic sequence as a sequence of amino acids in a polypeptide chain as instructed by a given mRNA sequence that has originated from DNA (see 'Protein Synthesis'). To find out which amino acid is coded for, look at the first letter of the codon in a row label on the left-hand side of the table. Then look for the column that intersects the same row from above that matches the second base. Finally, use the right-hand side matching the codon for the third base.

Table 1.8 shows amino acids and their codons. For example, determine the amino acid for the codon CAG: C is on the left row, A is along the top column and G is the third letter on the right-hand side. This shows the

amino acid glutamine. Therefore CAG = glutamine.

Enzymes

Enzymes are proteins that catalyse or speed up chemical reactions within the horse's body. Enzymes speed up chemical reactions without being used up in the reaction itself. They are essential for life and speed up metabolic reactions such as digestion and within cellular respiration. Enzymes may be:

- intracellular – occur within cells;
- extracellular – occur outside cells.

Enzymes are globular proteins which have a specific shape from their tertiary structure (see 'Levels of Protein Structure') and an active site. It was thought that the active site binds to the substrate molecules similar to a lock and key – the lock and key hypothesis. Enzymes are very specific to individual substrates and if the substrate did not fit the active site (i.e. the key does not fit the lock) then the reaction would not be catalysed. More recently, scientists have found that the enzyme substrate complex changes shape slightly to complete the fit, locking the substrate more tightly into the enzyme. This is known as the 'induced fit' model as opposed to the lock and key model (Figure 1.23).

Table 1.8 Amino acids and their codons.

Amino acid (aa)	Codons for this specific aa	No. of codons
Ala – alanine	GCU,GCC,GCA,GCC	4
Arg – arginine	CGU,CGC,CGA,CGG,AGA,AGG	6
Asn – asparagine	AAU,AAC	2
Asp – aspartic acid	GAU,GAC	2
Cys – cysteine	UGU,UGC	2
Gln – glutamine	CAA,CAG	2
Glu – glutamic acid	GAA,GAG	2
Gly – glycine	GGU,GGC,GGA,GGG	4
His – histidine	CAU,CAC	2
Iso – isoleucine	AUU,AUC,AUA	3
Leu – leucine	CUU,CUC,CUA,CUG	4
Lys – lysine	AAA,AAG	2
Met – methionine	AUG	1
Phe – phenylalanine	UUU,UUC	2
Pro – proline	CCU,CCC,CCA,CCG	4
Ser – serine	UCU,UCC,UCA,UCG	4
Thr – threonine	ACU,ACC,ACA,ACG	4
Try – tryptophan	UGG	1
Tyr – tyrosine	UAU,UAC	2
Val – valine	GUU,GUC,GUA,GUG	4
SeC – selenocysteine	UGA	1

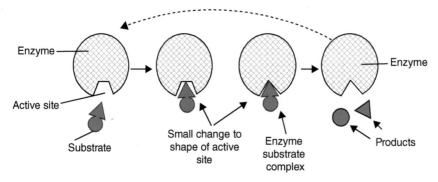

Figure 1.23 Induced fit model of enzyme action.

Enzymes speed up reactions by reducing the amount of activation energy required to start the chemical reaction. Enzymes often help chemical reactions occur at lower temperatures than they would without the enzyme and this speeds up the rate of the reaction. This activation energy is often provided in the form of heat.

Once the substrate has bound to the active site, it forms an enzyme–substrate complex. This lowers the activation energy and therefore speeds up the rate of the reaction as follows:

- If the reaction involves joining two substrate molecules together, such as amino acids forming polypeptides, the enzyme holds them closer together once attached, reducing any repulsion between the molecules.

- If the reaction is breaking down the substrate, such as glycogen to glucose, then fitting the substrate into the enzyme puts strain on the bonds within the substrate, making it easier to break them.

Factors that Affect the Activity of Enzymes

The effectiveness of enzymes in catalysing reactions is affected by several factors.

Temperature

The rate of chemical reactions increases with temperature due to the increase in heat energy which helps molecules move faster. This makes it easier for faster moving substrate molecules to 'bump into' or attach to the enzyme active site. There is an optimum temperature at which the speed of the substrate molecules makes it most likely to initiate a reaction with the enzyme attached. However, if the temperature increases even further, then the enzyme vibrates more, and the weak hydrogen bonds within the enzyme's tertiary structure (protein) holding it in shape break. At this point the enzyme is denatured and no longer fits the substrate or catalyses the reaction. There is an optimum temperature within the horse's body that allows enzymes to work at their optimal rate. The horse's normal body temperature is 37.5–38.5°C.

pH

Enzymes also have an optimal pH at which the rate of enzyme-controlled reaction is at its fastest. Most equine enzymes work best at pH 7, that is, neutral, except for some digestive enzymes, such as pepsin which acts in an acidic environment of the stomach at pH 2. If the pH is too high or too low then the ionic and hydrogen bonds that hold the tertiary structure together break down and the shape of the enzyme is altered so that the active site is changed in shape and the enzyme is denatured.

Enzyme Concentration

The more enzymes there are, the more likely a substrate will attach, so this increases the rate of reaction. If the amount of substrate does not also increase then there will be a limiting point where adding further enzymes will have no further effect as all enzyme-active sites are filled. Substrate concentration becomes the limiting factor for the reaction.

Substrate Concentration

The higher the amount of substrate, the faster the reaction, for the same reasons as an increase in enzyme concentration. Again, adding further enzymes when no more substrate is available and all the active sites are full means that the enzyme concentration is the limiting factor for the reaction.

Cofactors and Coenzymes

Some enzymes will work only if there is another non-protein substance attached to them and these are known as cofactors. Cofactors may be organic or inorganic molecules and work by helping the enzyme to bind to the substrate. An example of an inorganic cofactor is manganese ions, which are cofactors for hydrolase enzymes which catalyse the hydrolysis of chemical bonds. Organic cofactors are also called coenzymes and these participate in the chemical reaction and are changed during the reaction, before being recycled for further use.

Enzyme Inhibitors

Enzyme activity may also be affected by enzyme inhibitors. Competitive inhibitors compete with the substrate molecules for attachment to the active site but do not result in a reaction. The higher the concentration of inhibitors, the more the reactions will be reduced.

Non-competitive inhibitors will bind to the enzyme at another point, that is, away from the active site, causing a change in shape to the enzyme. The enzyme will no longer work, and increasing the substrate will therefore have no effect. Inhibition may be reversible or non-reversible.

Metabolic Poisons

Metabolic poisons, such as cyanide, arsenic and malonate, can interfere with metabolic reactions within cells. Cyanide, for example, is a non-competitive inhibitor of cytochrome c oxidase in cellular respiration reactions. If cells cannot respire they will die. Arsenic is also a non-competitive inhibitor of pyruvate dehydrogenase again in cellular respiration reactions.

Drugs

Some drugs such as antibiotics and various antivirals are also enzyme inhibitors. Antibiotics, such as penicillin, inhibit an enzyme called transpeptidase which catalyses the production of proteins in bacterial cell walls. This weakens the bacterial cell wall and the bacterium then bursts under the resulting increase in osmotic pressure.

Summary Points

1) The four main classes of organic molecules are proteins, carbohydrates, lipids and nucleic acids. In addition, a reactively small number of inorganic ions such as sodium and potassium are essential for life as components of larger molecules or extracellular fluids.

2) Horses must have a supply of energy to fuel energy-requiring processes, such as sustaining life and movement. This is obtained from cellular respiration – the oxidation of organic molecules such as glucose into simpler molecules, namely carbon dioxide and water.

3) Water has an important chemical structure which means it is liquid at room temperature and many substances dissolve in it due to its weak polar nature. Thus water molecules have a weak attraction for each other and other inorganic ions which form large numbers of weak hydrogen bonds. These unique properties include acting as a universal solvent and low viscosity. This means water molecules tend to stick together, allowing water to flow, and this is ideal for transport of substances around the horse's body.

4) A 21st amino acid has now been found, namely selenocysteine (SeC), and this amino acid is not coded for directly in the genetic code. Instead, it is encoded in a special way by a UGA codon, which is normally a stop codon.

5) Horses start life as a zygote (single fertilised cell) which has a complete set of genes. The cells then divide by mitosis, copying exactly the complete set of genes, but some of these cells differentiate into nervous tissue, whereas others may turn into skin cells or muscle. This is achieved by a process known as gene expression. Gene expression is how different genes are switched 'on' or 'off' in different cells.

6) Genes code for proteins. It was previously thought that genes were specific sections of DNA which encoded all proteins including enzymes. This theory is now revised to the one gene/one polypeptide hypothesis. Genes also encode for functional RNAs (i.e. areas of non-protein coding DNA) that have specific regulatory functions in the cell. This refers to the old theory of 'junk' DNA, which we now know has an important function.

7) In RNA, the DNA base thymine (T) is replaced by uracil (U), a fifth nucleotide which is almost chemically identical to thymine, but lacks its 5′ methyl group.

8) The genetic code used by all cells is called a triplet code, with every three nucleotides being 'read' from a specified starting point in the mRNA. Each triplet is called a codon and each codon codes for a specific amino acid.

9) There are special codons that are known as stop codons which effectively cause

a full stop at the end of the synthesised protein. Codons in a row between the stops are called genes.

10) Scientists have found that the enzyme/substrate complex changes shape slightly to complete a fit, locking the substrate more tightly into the enzyme. This is known as the 'induced fit' model, as opposed to the old lock and key model.

Q + A

Q Name the essential fatty acids in the horse's diet.

A Linolenic (omega 3) and linoleic (omega 6) fatty acids are essential, that is, they must be provided in the diet of horses.

Q Briefly describe the structure of collagen.

A Collagen is made up of three polypeptide chains that are tightly coiled into a triple helix formation.

Q Briefly describe the structure of haemoglobin.

A Haemoglobin is a globular protein composed of four polypeptide units joined together: two identical alpha chains and two identical beta chains.

Q How many amino acids could be coded for if a codon consisted of only two nucleotide bases?

A 16.

Q What is meant by the term 'degenerate' relating to the genetic code?

A For each amino acid there may be more than one codon.

2

Cells, Tissues and Organs

Cells – Building Blocks of Life

It is now thought that all animals, plants and fungi are related to each other from a long distant common ancestor. This can be seen from the structure of DNA in cells and the use of adenosine triphosphate (ATP) for energy production. In fact, mitochondria have their own loops of DNA that mark them out as ancient bacterial symbionts (see 'Mitochondria').

All living things are made up of microscopic building blocks or cells (Figure 2.1). In the horse, body functions involve the interaction of an estimated 400 trillion cells – the functional units of life. The horse is therefore a highly complex animal composed of trillions of eukaryotic cells grouped into various tissues and organs. Many of the cells of the tissues and organs will be actively dividing at any one time. Some tissues and organs will need constant cell replacements, such as the digestive system, skin and blood, whereas others undergo less division through the horse's lifetime. Cells cannot arise spontaneously so they must undergo cell division to make new cells. All cells within the body except for the germ or sex cells or undifferentiated stem cells are called somatic cells.

Different tissues are combined to form organs. Tasks are mostly carried out by several organs working together. The organs make up a system, for example the digestive system or the respiratory system. The horse's body is like a tower block housing a complex organisation. In order to function efficiently

it requires a great deal of specialisation and communication between cells. Cells are self-contained units with a great variety of structure and function.

There are basically two types of organisms: prokaryotic and eukaryotic. Prokaryotic organisms are extremely small (<2-μm-diameter) single-celled organisms, that is, they consist of one prokaryotic cell. Eukaryotic organisms or eukaryotes are made up of many eukaryotic cells. These are larger (10–100 μm diameter) and more complex and include all animal and plant cells.

Prokaryotic Cells

The first living organisms on planet earth were thought to be prokaryotes. Prokaryote means 'before the nucleus', and therefore these organisms do not have a separate nucleus divided from the rest of the cell by a membrane. They do have genetic material (i.e. DNA), but this is circular, compared to linear DNA in eukaryotic cells. There are also no membrane-bound organelles such as mitochondria. Mitosis and meiosis are absent. The ribosomes are also smaller, at 20 nm or less.

The prokaryotes are divided into the domains bacteria and archaea. Bacteria are mostly rod- or spherical-shaped cells with a rigid cell wall made of peptidoglycan unique to bacteria. The cell wall sits upon the plasma membrane, which has a similar structure to eukaryotic cell membranes. Bacteria often have further modifications to the cell wall, such as a capsule (to prevent them from

Equine Science, Third Edition. Zoe Davies and Sarah Pilliner.
© 2018 Zoe Davies and Sarah Pilliner. Published 2018 by John Wiley & Sons Ltd.

Sectional view

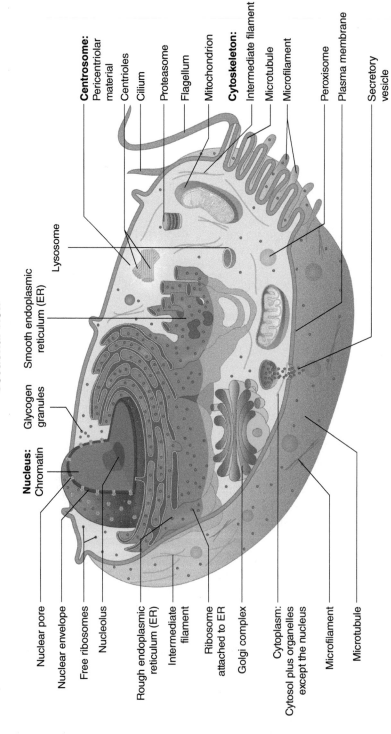

Nucleus:
Chromatin

Nuclear pore

Nuclear envelope

Free ribosomes

Nucleolus

Rough endoplasmic reticulum (ER)

Intermediate filament

Ribosome attached to ER

Golgi complex

Cytoplasm:
Cytosol plus organelles except the nucleus

Microfilament

Microtubule

Glycogen granules

Smooth endoplasmic reticulum (ER)

Lysosome

Centrosome:
Pericentriolar material

Centrioles

Cilium

Proteasome

Flagellum

Mitochondrion

Cytoskeleton:
Intermediate filament

Microtubule

Microfilament

Peroxisome

Plasma membrane

Secretory vesicle

Figure 2.1 Structure of a cell. *Source:* Tortora 2009. Reproduced with permission of John Wiley & Sons.

drying out) or flagella (for locomotion) or pili (for conjugation).

Archaea were shown to be a separate domain in 1977. Many archaea thrive under the extreme conditions of hot sulphur pools or in minerals and rock deep inside the Earth; however, they have since been found in numerous more common habitats. Archaea include Sulpholobales, Thermoplasmatales and Halobacteriales. Prokaryotes have higher metabolic and growth rates and shorter reproduction times compared to eukaryotes.

Eukaryotic Cells

Eukaryotic cells include all plants, fungi, protoctists and animal cells. Protoctists are unicellular or simple multicellular organisms belonging to the kingdom Protoctista and include protozoans, algae and slime moulds. There is no cell wall in animal cells, but plants have a cell wall made from cellulose and fungi have a cell wall made from chitin.

Eukaryotic cells have a 'true' nucleus and a highly organised cytoplasm containing cell organelles with various functions. Eukaryotes also have a cytoskeleton comprising microtubules, microfilaments and intermediate filaments which help shape and organise

the cell. The DNA in the nucleus is linear and divided into bundles known as chromosomes. Ribosomes are larger than prokaryotic cells. Eukaryotes are larger than prokaryotes. Mitosis and meiosis take place in eukaryotic cells. Table 2.1 summarises the similarities and differences between eukaryotic and prokaryotic cells.

The two most common units used to describe the size of cell organelles are micrometre (μm) (one thousandth of a millimetre) and nanometer (nm) (one-thousandth of a micrometre). The cellular structure described below is that of a eukaryotic animal cell.

Cell Function

The individual cells of the horse's body act, interact and react with each other – they are not independent. In order to function normally, there must be a continuous exchange of information, which is normally chemically or electrochemically controlled. These chemical compounds may be hormones or enzymes found in the fluid surrounding the cells (interstitial fluid) or directly transferred between adjacent cells (see 'Cell Signalling').

Table 2.1 Summary of the similarities and differences between eukaryotic and prokaryotic cells.

Eukaryotic cells	Prokaryotic cells
Large cells (10–100 μm)	Small cells (<2 μm)
Nucleus present	No nucleus, free DNA in cytoplasm
Linear DNA formed into chromosomes	Circular DNA known as plasmids
Organelles are membrane bound	No membrane-bound organelles (no mitochondria, for example)
Have a cell surface membrane	Have a cell surface membrane
Large ribosomes	Small ribosomes (<20 nm)
No cell wall – animals	Cell wall made from peptidoglycans
Cell wall made from cellulose – plants	
Cell wall made from chitin – fungi	
Yeast, amoeba, mammalian heart and liver cells	Bacteria – *Salmonella* and *E. coli*
Can be single-celled or multicellular organisms	Always single-celled organisms

Cytoplasm

Cytoplasm is the fluid contained within the cell that holds and surrounds the cell's organelles (apart from the nucleus which contains nucleoplasm) in a liquid environment which is necessary for many of the cell's vital functions to occur. The materials that are found within the cytoplasm are also typically found within the cell membrane. Typically, the cytoplasm contains materials that are known as cytoplasmic inclusions. These inclusions include starch granules, mineral crystals or lipid droplets that are floating around within the cytoplasm.

Cytosol

Cytosol is part of the cytoplasm. Cytosol is a gel-like translucent fluid which is not enclosed within cell organelles. Cytosol is responsible for suspending the cell organelles and inclusions within the cytoplasm. It makes up around 75% of the cell's total volume and includes protein complexes, salts and organic compounds. Cytosol consists mostly of water.

Movement of Substances in and around Cells

The transfer or transport of substances inside and around cells takes place via a number of different ways:

- diffusion
- osmosis
- facilitated diffusion
- active transport
- endocytosis
- exocytosis.

Diffusion is a passive process which does not require energy and is the net movement of particles from an area of high concentration to an area of lower concentration.

Osmosis is the movement of water molecules from an area of higher water potential to an area of lower water potential through a partially or semi-permeable membrane.

Facilitated diffusion is the net movement of particles from an area of higher concentration to an area of lower concentration using carrier or channel proteins. Carrier proteins aid diffusion of large molecules including large polar molecules and ions, whereas channel proteins aid diffusion of smaller ions and polar molecules. This is a passive process and does not require energy.

Active transport as the name suggests requires energy (ATP) and carrier proteins to transport molecules against a concentration gradient.

Endocytosis is the movement of large molecules such as proteins, dead cells and bacteria into a cell. The plasma membrane of the cell surrounds the large molecule and then pinches off to form a self-contained vesicle within the cell. This is an active process requiring energy.

Exocytosis is the movement of molecules out of a cell. The self-contained vesicles within the cell move to the outer boundary plasma membrane and fuse with it before releasing the contents of the vesicle. This is an active process requiring energy.

Cell Organelles

Within eukaryotic cells the cell membranes divide the cytoplasm into multiple compartments or organelles, each with different functions in the cell. For example, in the mitochondria the outer double membrane separates out those reactions that occur in mitochondria from those in the general cytoplasm. This allows the enzymic reactions of the Krebs cycle to be kept separate from the electron transfer chain. This is essential since both sets of reactions have different enzymes which function better under different pHs.

Cytoskeleton

The cytoplasm is not simply space filled with fluid in which the organelles are suspended. It contains a complex network of fibres known as the cytoskeleton (Figure 2.2) which provides structural support and helps the cell to maintain and change its shape when required. The cytoskeleton also helps the cell to move and moves materials within the cell. The cytoskeleton is made

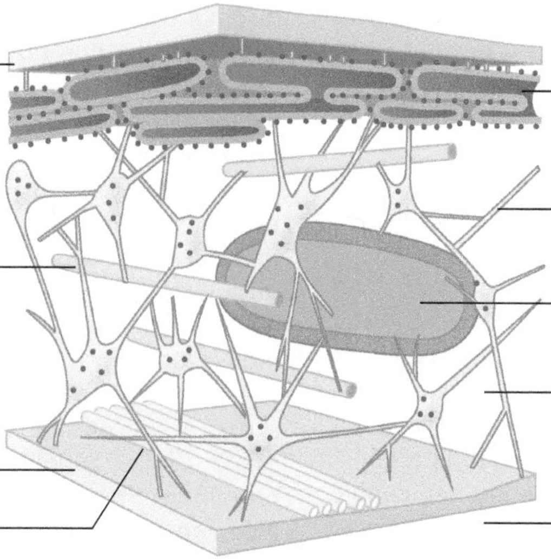
Plasma membrane
(phospholipid bilayer)
Rough endoplasmic
reticulum
Intermediate
filaments
Microtubules
Nucleus
Inside cell
Plasma membrane
Microfilaments
Outside cell

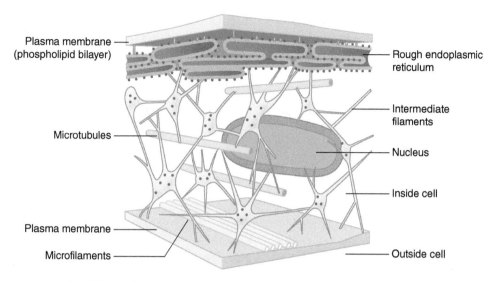

Figure 2.2 Cytoskeleton of the cell.

up of three protein-containing elements, namely microtubules, microfilaments and intermediate filaments.

Microtubules are the largest components of the cytoskeleton. They are slender hollow tubes approximately 24 nm in diameter, made from protein subunits, namely alpha and beta tubulin dimers. They can be longer or shorter, as tubulin subunits are added or removed from one end. They aid cell division by forming the spindle, and are a major constituent of cilia and flagella, that is, they are important for cell motility. This is why cilia and flagella are thought to be part of the cytoskeleton. They also help maintain cell shape and move organelles.

Microfilaments are long polymers of the protein actin (and sometimes myosin) and consist of two very fine intertwined strands approximately 6 nm in diameter. They can grow or shrink, as actin subunits are added or removed from either end. Microfilaments help to maintain cell structure by forming a network and aid in movement within cells. Actin microfilaments help with muscle contraction in muscle cells and cell division (during cytokinesis). They also aid the movement of pseudopodia in certain cells.

Intermediate filaments contain fibrous proteins such as keratin (found in hair). The fibres are wound into thicker rope- or cable-like structures around 10 nm wide. Intermediate filaments help to anchor the nucleus and organelles in place within the cell.

Cell or Plasma Membrane

The word membrane means 'very thin layer', an accurate description of the term. The cell membrane forms the outermost limits of the cell and separates it from other cells. Cell membranes also surround cell organelles, but the structure remains basically the same. Cells are very small and each one is a highly dynamic system with the ability to exchange a relatively large volume of fluid relative to its size. Cell membranes provide a boundary between the cell and its environment and they are vital for regulating what goes in and out of the cell.

Because cell membranes undertake these extremely important roles within cells it is important to understand their structure and function. The roles of cell membranes include cell transport, cell recognition and cell signalling. Scientists have been able to freeze cells and then cleave them, a process known as 'freeze fracture'. This has enabled them to see the structures of the inner membrane surfaces, providing far more information about their structure and function.

The Fluid Mosaic Model of Cell Membrane Structure

All cell membranes are basically the same. They are composed of lipids, proteins and carbohydrates (usually attached to lipids or proteins). The fluid mosaic model (Figure 2.3) describes the arrangement of these molecules within the membrane. Phospholipid molecules form a continuous double layer or bilayer. The bilayer is fluid because the phospholipids are continually moving. Protein molecules are interspersed throughout the bilayer like tiles in a mosaic, hence the name. Some proteins have a polysaccharide chain attached and are known as glycoproteins, whereas some lipids also have a polysaccharide chain attached and are known as glycolipids. Cholesterol molecules are contained within the bilayer. Fat- or lipid-soluble molecules, for example gases and steroids, can move through the cell membrane by diffusion, down their concentration gradient. The cell membrane is thus composed of five different components:

- phospholipids
- proteins
- glycolipids
- glycoproteins
- cholesterol.

Phospholipids form a barrier to dissolved water-soluble substances (Figure 2.4) and have a head and a tail. The head is water 'loving' (i.e. hydrophilic) and the tail is water 'hating' (i.e. hydrophobic). The molecules arrange themselves into a bilayer so that the water-loving heads face outwards towards water on either side of the membrane, whereas the water-hating components face inwards, that is, at the centre of the bilayer. This is very important as it prevents water-soluble substances such as ions and polar molecules diffusing (moving) through the membrane. At the same time it allows smaller non-polar substances such as carbon dioxide and water to diffuse through the membrane.

Proteins control movement in and out of the cell. Some proteins form channels within the membrane, allowing small charged (polar) water-soluble particles to pass through, such as calcium ions. Other proteins transport larger molecules and charged molecules across the membrane by active transport and facilitated diffusion, that is, across a concentration gradient. These are called carrier proteins. Most importantly, proteins act as receptors for certain molecules such as hormones involved in cell signalling. When a molecule binds to the protein a chemical reaction is triggered within the cell.

Glycolipids and glycoproteins provide stability to the membrane by forming hydrogen bonds with surrounding molecules of water. These act as receptors for messenger molecules in cell signalling. Glycolipids and glycoproteins provide the sites where hormones, antibodies and drugs bind to the cell. They play an important role in the immune response and cell-to-cell recognition. Glycoproteins also act as receptors for hormones and neurotransmitters.

Cholesterol is a lipid that is present in all cell membranes and acts as a packing molecule, giving stability to the membrane. It is not present in bacterial cell membranes. Cholesterol fits between the phospholipids (see Figure 2.4). It binds to the hydrophobic tails, causing them to pack more closely together. This makes the membrane less fluid and more stable. Cholesterol is a lipid and therefore also has hydrophobic regions, thus creating additional barriers to polar substances getting through the membrane.

The Role of Membranes in Cell Organelles

Many organelles in cells as well as all cells themselves are surrounded by membranes. These include the mitochondria, nucleus, Golgi apparatus, endoplasmic

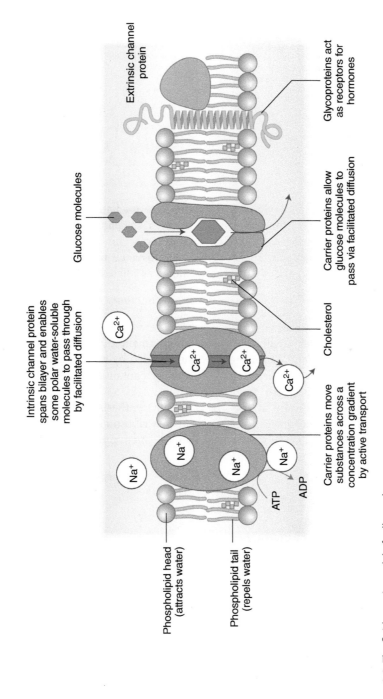

Figure 2.3 The fluid mosaic model of cell membranes.

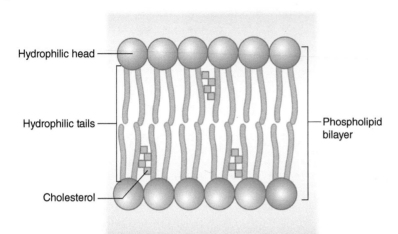

Figure 2.4 Phospholipid bilayer arrangement.

Hydrophilic head

Hydrophilic tails

Phospholipid bilayer

Cholesterol

reticulum (ER), lysosomes and vesicles. These membranes enable compartmentalisation of regions of the cell organelles and allow movement in and out of different substances.

There are three types of endocytosis (Figure 2.5):

- Pinocytosis or 'cell drinking' – pinocytosis occurs continuously in most cells, and the molecule engulfed is relatively small.
- Phagocytosis or 'cell eating' – during phagocytosis the cell ingests particles such as bacteria from the extracellular fluid. Phagocytosis occurs sporadically in specialised cells such as macrophages and neutrophils.

- Receptor-mediated endocytosis – this involves specific receptors that bind to large molecules in the extracellular fluid. The substance bound to the receptor is known as a ligand.

Some functions of membranes are given below.

- Containment of DNA – the nucleus is surrounded by an envelope of two membranes containing the DNA material within.
- Protein synthesis – some of this occurs on free ribosomes and some takes place on the membrane-bound ribosomes on

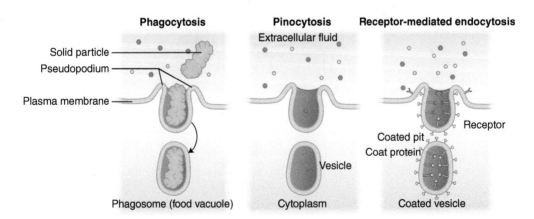

Phagocytosis

Solid particle

Pseudopodium

Plasma membrane

Phagosome (food vacuole)

Pinocytosis

Extracellular fluid

Vesicle

Cytoplasm

Receptor-mediated endocytosis

Receptor

Coated pit

Coat protein

Coated vesicle

Figure 2.5 Three types of endocytosis. *Source*: Peate 2011. Reproduced with permission of John Wiley & Sons.

the rough ER. The protein is made directly inside the space within the membranes of the ER.

- Energy production and transfer – the reactions of cellular respiration take place in the membrane-bound energy production systems in the mitochondria.
- Cell communication and recognition – glycoproteins and glycolipids act as cell identity markers, helping cells to arrange themselves in tissues and allowing foreign cells to be recognised so that the immune system can respond.
- Packaging and secretion – the Golgi apparatus produces lysosomes and packs and secretes substances such as proteins and hormones.
- Transport – carrier and channel proteins are involved in selectively transporting substances across the cell membrane. Cholesterol acts as a plug to prevent movement of polar molecules through the membrane.

- Entry and export of substances – the cell membrane can take up fluid or even solid material and form a membrane round it called a vesicle. These membrane-bound transport vesicles can move substances to the surface of the cell so they can be 'pinched off' by exocytosis (Figure 2.6).

Nucleus

The nucleus is the largest organelle in the cell, lying centrally and surrounded by cytoplasm. The nucleus is the 'brain' of the cell, containing genetic material responsible for the transmission of hereditary characteristics from cell to cell and from parent to offspring. The nucleus contains deoxyribonucleic acid (DNA). Nucleic acid contains all the necessary information to make a new copy of the cell and to control the cell's activities. In the dividing cell, DNA molecules condense into visible chromosomes. Each pair is known as a homologous pair and they both contain

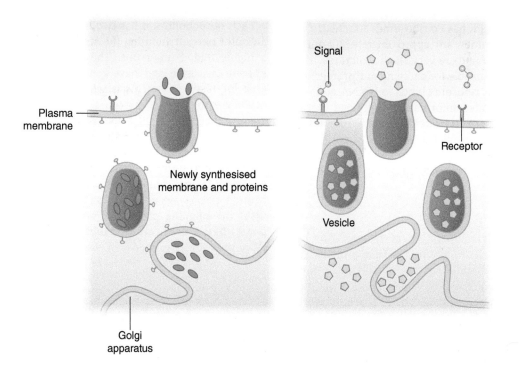

Figure 2.6 Exocytosis. *Source*: Peate 2011. Reproduced with permission of John Wiley & Sons.

genes at the same positions or loci. Alternative forms of genes are known as alleles.

At other times, the nucleus appears grainy as DNA material is dispersed within the nucleus as chromatin. Separate chromosomes are present, but the DNA is so spread out that it is impossible to distinguish individual chromosomes. The nucleus may have one or more nucleoli which produce ribonucleic acid (RNA), required for making ribosomes. The nucleus is bound by a nuclear membrane containing pores large enough for larger molecules to pass through, for example messenger RNA (mRNA).

Endoplasmic Reticulum and Ribosomes

Together with ribosomes, the ER is involved in the synthesis of protein within the cell. The ER is a series of complex channels where the narrow fluid-filled space between the membranes acts as a transport network, moving materials through the cell. The folded membrane creates a large surface area. Much of the outer surface of the ER is dotted with tiny ribosomes and this is known as rough ER. Smooth ER has no ribosomes attached.

Ribosomes are approximately 20 nm in diameter and are very small structures. They are responsible for carrying out protein synthesis. A ribosome binds to mRNA and uses the encoded information contained therein to assemble amino acids for protein synthesis. Ribosomes attached to the ER make proteins for export from the cell, whereas free ribosomes make proteins for use by the cell itself.

Golgi Body (Dictyosome)

The Golgi body consists of stacks of plate-like tubules. Its function is to take proteins and enzymes made by the ER and place them in membrane-bound packages or vesicles. Completed vesicles then 'pinch off'. The Golgi body is also involved in the secretion of protein from the cell, such as the release of digestive enzymes into the gut.

Mitochondria

Mitochondria are found in all living plant and animal cells. Mitochondria are thought to have originally existed as free-living Alphaproteobacteria and to have adapted to a symbiotic relationship within animal cells, approximately 1.5 billion years ago.

Mitochondria are semi-autonomous organelles, possessing their own unique genome separate to that of the equine cell's own genome (see Chapter 13) which is passed down the dam line. These cylindrical structures are responsible for the production of energy and are known as the 'powerhouses' of the cell. They are the sites of aerobic respiration, that is, oxidation of glucose to produce energy.

Mitochondria are responsible for producing approximately 95% of the eukaryotic cells' energy through the process of oxidative phosphorylation using the tricarboxylic acid (TCA) cycle. Mitochondria contain an ATP synthase, which is able to generate ATP from adenosine diphosphate. The great efficiency of mitochondria in ATP production is demonstrated by the ability to generate a net 36 molecules of ATP from the oxidation of one molecule of glucose.

Each mitochondrion has two membranes: an outer one surrounding the structure and a highly folded inner one. These folds are known as cristae and have a large surface area for respiration. This is where transfer of energy to form ATP occurs. ATP is the energy currency of all cells. The enzymes involved in cellular respiration are located in specific parts of the mitochondrion. This means that reactions can be localised and separated by membrane systems (Figure 2.7). Mitochondria have now been shown to regulate the ongoing process of apoptosis or programmed cell death of animal cells (see 'Apoptosis (Programmed Cell Death)').

Lysosomes

Although similar in shape to mitochondria, lysosomes have a quite different function. Lysosomes are vesicles containing digestive enzymes. They break down old or surplus cell organelles inside the cell. They may also break down substances brought into the cell by the process of endocytosis. The horse's body uses this 'destruction' process to break

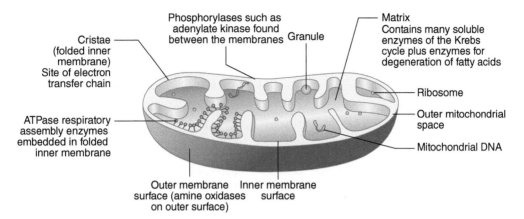

Figure 2.7 Mitochondrion showing location of different enzymes involved in cellular respiration.

down excess muscle in the uterus following birth and to reduce milk-producing tissue in the mare's udder following weaning.

Peroxisomes (Microbodies)

Peroxisomes are small, spherical bodies approximately 1 μm in diameter. They contain enzymes which oxidise certain molecules normally found in the cell, notably fatty acids and amino acids. Oxidation reactions produce hydrogen peroxide, which is the basis of the name peroxisome. This is a highly toxic by-product produced in the cell. Hydrogen peroxide is turned into oxygen and water, thereby rendering it harmless to the cell. Peroxisomes are found in greater numbers in the more active cells such as liver and muscle cells.

Centrosomes

Also known as centrioles, centrosomes are clearly visible during cell division, when they become the centre of the spindle apparatus that separates the chromosomes of the resulting cells.

Apoptosis (Programmed Cell Death)

Programmed cell death or apoptosis is a mechanism in multicellular organisms to help trigger the death of a cell. Apoptosis could also be referred to as cell suicide and is an entirely normal process. It has several functions within the horse's body:

- sculpting embryonic tissue;

- maintaining cell numbers in adults, replacing older cells;
- defence against damaged cells;
- defence against infected cells.

Apoptosis consists of a series of biochemical events that result in changes to the shape of the cell and ultimately end in the death of that cell. These changes include cell shrinkage, fragmentation of the nucleus, condensation of chromatin and chromosomal fragmentation of DNA. The remains of the cell are then safely disposed of by phagocytosis.

Excessive levels of apoptosis can lead to atrophy of tissues, whereas restricted apoptosis may result in cell proliferation or cancer. Apoptosis is not the same as necrosis, which involves traumatic damage which results in the cell spilling its contents. Apoptosis must be tightly regulated and is ultimately a balance between cell growth and cell death. Low rates of apoptosis may lead to overproliferation of cells, that is, cancer. Regulation of this important process occurs through a balance of positive and negative signals, namely:

- Positive signals
  - bcl-2 protein and growth factors;
  - interleukin-2, which binds to surface receptors to regulate metabolism.
- Negative signals
  - signalling proteins and peptides (e.g. lymphotoxin);
  - inducer signals from within the cell as a result of stress such as DNA damage or lack of nutrients or oxygen.

Cell Turnover

Foals grow because the cells divide by mitosis (see 'Cell Division (Mitosis and Meiosis)'), and cell production during growth out-numbers cell death. At adult size, the cell population stays reasonably constant. Different tissues have different cell turnover rates. Brain cells are not replaced, for example, and there is a steady decline in number from the adult stage. Other cells such as liver cells have a low turnover and, unlike the brain, can slowly regenerate if some cells are damaged or destroyed, such as following ragwort poisoning. Cells with the highest turnover are those in tissues with the most wear and tear, such as epithelium (e.g. skin and the gastrointestinal tract). The entire gut lining is replaced every couple of days. Much of the content of the gut cells is absorbed and recycled, but still these gut cells make up a significant proportion of the horse's droppings. Bone marrow cells also have a high division rate, as do the germ cells resulting in spermatozoa.

Cell Division (Mitosis and Meiosis)

An understanding of cell division is very important in equine biology. It is the process by which foals grow and develop. It is also vital for maintaining tissues and repair. There is a limit to the size of an individual cell and therefore to the size that tissues and organs can reach. For example, there is a limit to how long the limb of a horse will grow. Cells within the horse's limb can make different types of tissue, such as bone, muscle, tendon, nervous tissue and so on. Cells have specific instructions for cell division on what to do when and also when to stop.

Cell division is fundamental to all life in that cells can only arise from division of other cells. Mitosis and meiosis are processes that have very different purposes: mitosis is the simpler process and is responsible for cell growth and repair, whereas meiosis is concerned with producing sex cells or gametes for sexual reproduction in multicellular organisms such as the horse.

The majority of the horse's body cells are known as somatic cells. The only other cells are the reproductive or sex cells or gametes. This is important as they undergo two different processes for cell division, namely:

- Somatic (body cells) – nuclear division by **mitosis** results in two identical daughter cells with the same genes as the parent cell and containing two sets of chromosomes, that is, 64 (diploid), symbol '2n'.
- Reproductive – nuclear division by **meiosis** results in four new sex cells or gametes, be it sperm or ovum, with a single set of chromosomes, that is, 32 (haploid), symbol 'n'.

Diploid is derived from the Greek language meaning 'double number'. The requirement for gametes to have a haploid number of chromosomes, that is, 32, is due to the process of fertilization, when the genetic material of the ovum (n) and a single sperm (n) combine. The resultant zygote will have 2n, that is, $32 + 32 = 64$ chromosomes (the diploid number). The zygote then undergoes rapid cell division by mitosis, producing identical cells with the correct diploid number of chromosomes during growth as an embryo, foetus and then foal and adult.

The Cell Cycle

The cell cycle is the name for the sequence of changes from formation to division into two cells. In somatic cells (i.e. body cells except the gametes) this process is divided into two periods:

- interphase (cell not dividing);
- mitotic phase (cell dividing).

The stages of the cell cycle are shown in Figure 2.8.

The cell cycle can be thought of as one complete life of an individual diploid cell, beginning and ending with cell division. This consists of mitosis stages and interphase. Interphase is simply the period between cell division when the cell carries out its normal functions. Some cells do not divide in the

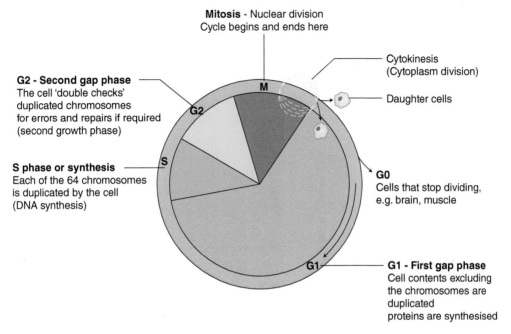

Figure 2.8 Four stages of the cell cycle. *Source*: Peate 2011. Reproduced with permission of John Wiley & Sons.

adult horse, such as muscle and nerve cells, and these are always in interphase. During interphase the chromosomes are unwound in the nucleus and therefore more available to code for proteins as per the normal function of that particular cell.

When a cell is about to divide, chromosomes condense and separate into homologous pairs. They appear like small pairs of rods under a light microscope. They both contain the genes at the same positions otherwise known as loci. One of these chromosomes came from the dam and one from the sire in each pair. So although homologous chromosomes carry the same genes, they are not necessarily the same version of that gene. This is very important for variation within a species. See also 'Chromosomes' in Chapter 13.

The appearance, number and arrangement of chromosomes in the nucleus are referred to as the karyotype. The equine karyotype is shown in Figure 2.9. Note the two XX chromosomes, denoting a female.

Mitosis

Mitosis is the division of the nucleus only and not the entire cell. Cytokinesis is the term for the entire cell splitting into two daughter cells. Interphase is not part of mitosis but prepares the cell for mitosis, and there are three stages of interphase, namely G1, S and G2 (see Figure 2.8). Interphase is a state of high metabolic activity as the cell grows and prepares to divide (Figure 2.10).

Key Events

Interphase (stages G1, S and G2)

→ Prophase → Metaphase → Anaphase

→ Telophase → Cytokinesis.

- Prophase – chromosomes condense, centrosome duplicates, microtubules for spindle fibres elongate and nuclear membrane breaks up.
- Metaphase – chromosomes line up in the middle of the cell at what is called the metaphase plate and all spindle fibres

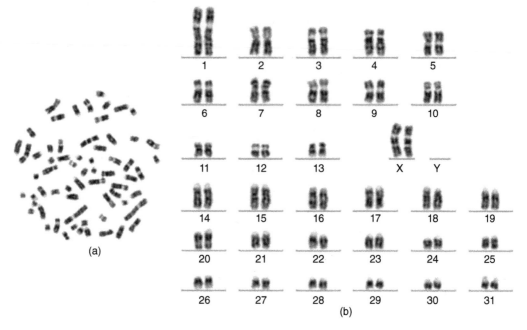

(a)

(b)

Figure 2.9 (a) A G-banded metaphase and (b) karyotype of a normal female horse (2n = 64XX). *Source*: Chowdhary 2013. Reproduced with permission of John Wiley & Sons.

should be connected to the kinetochores of the chromatids.

- Anaphase – sister chromatids are pulled apart and move to opposite poles by shortening of the microtubules.
- Telophase – nuclear membranes develop for **two** nuclei.
- Cytokinesis – the cell divides in two.

Interphase

Interphase is the period between cell division. Most of the time the nucleus appears grainy as DNA material is dispersed within the nucleus as chromatin. At the beginning of mitosis the chromosomes replicate themselves, forming a carbon copy within the nucleus of each chromosome. DNA replication takes place during interphase. Cells form new cell organelles to supply the daughter cells and build up a store of energy to support the process of cell division.

Prophase

Following replication, chromosomes contract and become visible as double strands under a light microscope. These chromosome strands (the parent cell strand and its carbon copy, the daughter cell strand) are known as chromatids and are joined together at their centre by a centromere. Later in prophase the mitotic spindle begins to form. This is a ball-shaped group of microtubules. Lengthening of the microtubules pushes the centrosomes to opposite or pole ends of the cell. The nuclear membrane breaks down.

Metaphase

The spindle spans the width of the cell. The centromeres with the chromatid pairs then attach to the centre of the spindle (see Figure 2.10). The midpoint region is now known as the metaphase plate.

Anaphase

The centromere splits in two, each taking one chromatid along the spindle fibres to the opposite ends of the cell. This takes place by the spindle fibres contracting and requires energy. As the 'chromosomes' are pulled by

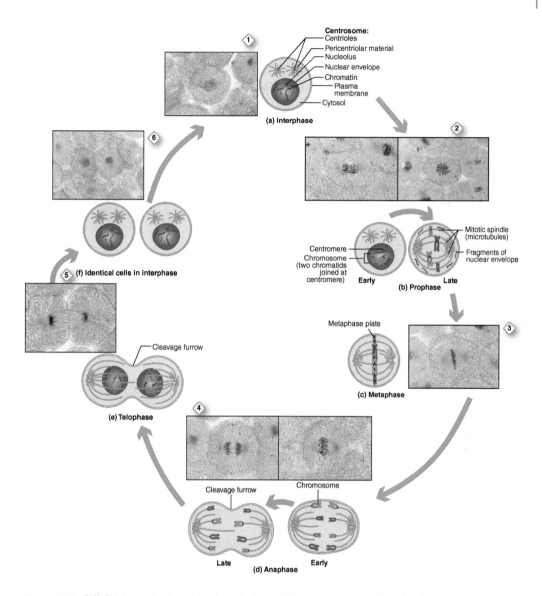

Figure 2.10 Cell division: mitosis and cytokinesis. *Source*: Tortora 2009. Reproduced with permission of John Wiley & Sons.

the microtubules of the mitotic spindle, they look V-shaped as the centromeres lead the way, pulling the trailing 'arms' behind them. Once separated the chromatids are now known as chromosomes.

Telophase

The final stage of mitosis begins when chromosome movement stops. The identical sets of chromosomes now have been separated from each other and lie at separate poles of the cell. The chromosomes uncoil and revert to their thread-like chromatin form.

Cytokinesis or Cytoplasmic Division

Cytokinesis is the division of the cytoplasm and organelles of the cell. The cell membrane begins to grow down between the two by invagination, and usually this starts in late anaphase. Two daughter cells are formed, beginning with a cleavage furrow, and the spindle fibres break down and disappear. The nuclear membrane reforms around each of the two nuclei and chromosomes regain their grainy appearance.

After cytokinesis the result is two new separate identical daughter cells with equal amounts of cytoplasm and organelles and identical sets of chromosomes. Interphase begins when cytokinesis is complete. Figure 2.11 is a diagram following one pair of homologous chromosomes through one mitotic division. Compare this with Figure 2.12 showing meiosis.

Meiosis

Meiosis is the division of only the nucleus in gametes or sex cells. It is the process of cytokinesis after meiosis that splits the

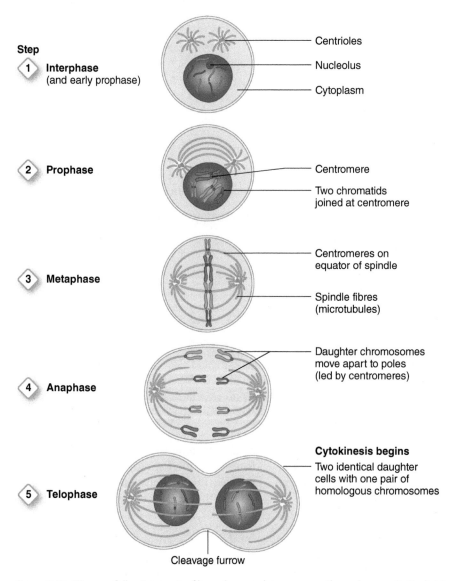

Figure 2.11 Diagram following a pair of homologous chromosomes through one mitotic division.

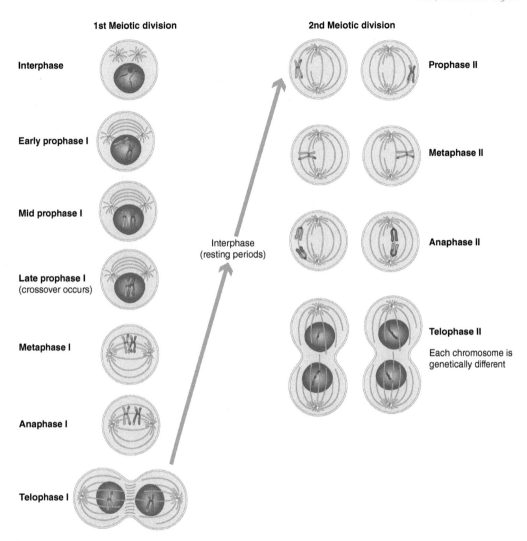

1st Meiotic division

Interphase

Early prophase I

Mid prophase I

Late prophase I
(crossover occurs)

Metaphase I

Anaphase I

Telophase I

Interphase
(resting periods)

2nd Meiotic division

Prophase II

Metaphase II

Anaphase II

Telophase II

Each chromosome is
genetically different

Figure 2.12 Meiosis.

entire cell. The result is four different haploid cells. Prophase I, the main event, is a cross-shuffling of sections of chromatids. This is the basis of genetic variation in offspring. The cell then divides and divides again. The main difference between meiosis and mitosis is the cross-shuffling or crossover (occurring at the chiasmata) of sections of chromatids that produces non-identical cells.

Meiosis involves two nuclear divisions and is a reduction division occurring during oogenesis in the ovary and spermatogenesis in the testes (see Figure 2.12).

Key Events

- DNA is replicated in the same way as during mitosis, resulting in chromosomes that consist of two identical chromatids.
- This is followed by the first meiotic division, during which crossing over occurs in prophase I. The sister chromatids from one chromosome are no longer identical to one another.
- Independent assortment then occurs in metaphase I.
- One chromosome from each homologous pair moves into each daughter cell. Which

individual chromosome of the homologous pairs moves to which daughter cell is completely random. This mixing among homologous pairs provides for genetic variation among the resultant offspring.

- After this first meiotic division, each daughter cell has a haploid number of chromosomes, but each chromosome consists of two chromatids.
- During the second meiotic division of the two daughter cells, each of the resulting four cells receives one of the chromatids.
- The overall result of meiosis is the production of four daughter cells, each of which has a haploid number of chromosomes.

Interphase DNA replicates, so cells that had two copies of each chromosome now have four.

First Meiotic Division

- Prophase I – chromosomes become visible, and centrioles move to opposite ends of the cell. Each homologous pair then comes together to form a bivalent and each chromosome in the bivalent forms two chromatids. Genetic mixing occurs at the chiasmata which are the points of crossover and are visible.
- Metaphase I – the bivalents arrange themselves on the equator of the spindle.
- Anaphase I – chromatid pairs from each homologous chromosome spilt apart and move to opposite poles of the cell.
- Telophase I – cytokinesis begins, forming two new daughter cells, but each of these is genetically different from the parent cell. This is the major difference between mitosis and meiosis.
- Interphase – resting state, which varies depending upon the type of cell.

Second Meiotic Division

- Prophase II – new spindle forms at right angles to the first one.
- Metaphase II – chromosomes align themselves near the equator of this spindle. Each chromosome is a pair of chromatids.

- Anaphase II – chromatids are pulled apart to form two chromosomes which then move to opposite ends of the cell.
- Telophase II – cytokinesis begins, forming four haploid cells knowns as a tetrad, each with a single chromosome (i.e. half of a pair), each of which is genetically different.

Cell Signalling

Cells must communicate with each other and therefore they use chemical messengers to gather information about and respond to changes in their environment. The membrane of the cell receives a chemical signal, for example from a sex hormone or from an endocrine gland, and this is followed by a signal transduction pathway. The pathway involves a series of enzymes and molecules within the cell which sets off a signal cascade, resulting in a large response from the cell. Cell signalling pathways may be short or long and are categorised accordingly (Figure 2.13):

- Endocrine pathway – transports hormones over long distances via the circulation to the target cells.
- Paracrine pathway – signal acts locally upon cells next to or very close to the target cell. This is important in embryonic development.

Cells can also make and respond to their own signals and this is known as autocrine signalling.

Cell Differentiation and Stem Cells

The horse's body also contains undifferentiated or unspecialised cells known as stem cells. Stem cells are found in all multicellular organisms. They have two special abilities:

- Self-renewal – an ability to undergo numerous cell divisions in this unspecialised state.
- Potency – an ability to differentiate into specialised cells.

Totipotent cells are the first cells produced in the few cell divisions following

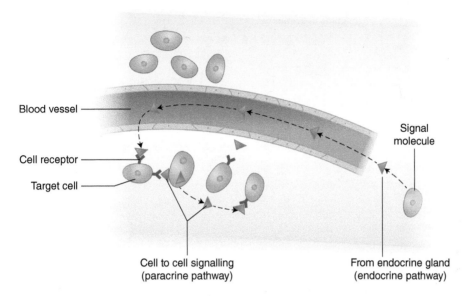

Figure 2.13 Cell signalling pathways.

conception and can develop into any cell type (embryonic in particular). Pluripotent cells are derived from totipotent cells and give rise to any of the cells produced by the three germ layers (endoderm, mesoderm and ectoderm) in early embryonic development. Embryonic and foetal stem cells are therefore pluripotent.

Adult somatic stem cells are multipotent; that is, they are undifferentiated cells found within tissues containing already differentiated cells. These adult stem cells can produce only a limited number of cell types as they are required to repair and replace worn tissues and cells. Adult stem cells are therefore limited to producing blood, heart, nerve and muscle cells, whereas embryonic/foetal stem cells can be used to produce many more different types of cells.

Stem cell therapy is now widely used in the repair of certain equine injuries such as tendon injuries.

Blood Cell Production from Stem Cells

In the equine foetus new blood cells are produced in the liver. After birth, the neonatal foal then makes new blood cells in the red bone marrow. All the different blood cell types are derived from a single stem cell known as a haemocytoblast which is a multipotent stem cell (Figure 2.14). Haemocytoblasts undergo cell division by mitosis and then differentiate into precursors of each of the different types of blood cell in the horse. When stem cells divide, one of the two daughter cells remains a stem cell, while the other is a precursor cell (see discussion on haematopoiesis under 'Blood' in Chapter 7).

Tissues and Organs

Most equine cells are microscopic, but the egg cell or ovum is just about visible with the naked eye. It is larger because it needs more room to house food reserves. The horse is multicellular, with body systems comprising complex tissues and organs that interact, working together to maintain the horse's internal environment. A tissue is a collection of cells that work together to achieve a particular function. Different tissues combine to form organs which are

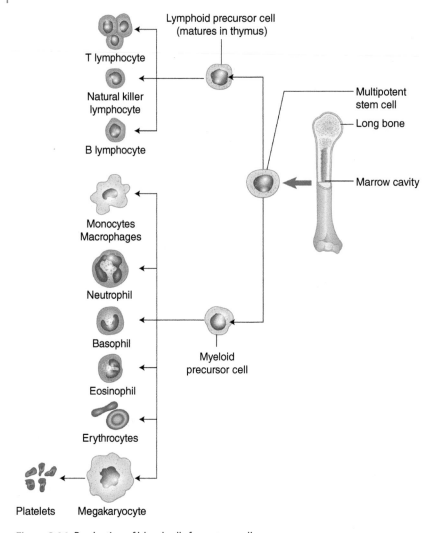

Figure 2.14 Production of blood cells from stem cells.

more complex in structure. Organs usually have a specific job in the horse, for example to hear sounds, to absorb food or to pump blood around the body. The study of tissues is much more interesting if the structure is related to its function in the equine body. Understanding whether tissues are behaving normally or abnormally is a vital part of equine management.

Each organ of the horse's body is made up of a combination of four basic tissue types:

- Epithelial tissue – lines body cavities, hollow organs and tubes, forms glands, includes skin.

- Connective tissue – protects and supports body organs, stores fat for energy, has an immune function, includes bone, cartilage and blood.
- Muscular tissue – generates physical force of movement (see Chapter 3).
- Nervous tissue – coordinates body activities and helps in homeostasis (see Chapter 8).

Epithelium/Epithelial Tissue

Epithelial tissues form continuous sheets that line and cover body structures and cavities such as the equine digestive system. Different

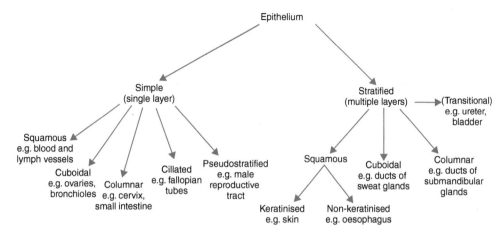

Figure 2.15 Classification of epithelium.

types of epithelial tissue are classified according to the **size** and **shape** of cells and the number of cell layers they contain (Figure 2.15). For example, simple squamous epithelium contains only a single layer of 'flat' cells and is therefore very thin and ideally suited to be a membrane where substances can pass in and out, such as is found in the alveoli of the lungs or Bowman's capsule within the kidney. On the other hand, stratified squamous epithelium is several cells thick and can be replaced continuously, making it ideal as a protective covering for the skin or the lining of the small intestine and oesophagus. Cells of the lower layers of stratified epithelium are more columnar in structure. Those near the top are often flattened and frequently dead. These may have been impregnated with the protein keratin, such as skin, mane/tail and hoof. Other epithelial tissue containing keratin includes parts of the digestive, respiratory and reproductive tracts, larynx and vocal cords, cornea, gums, hard palate and top of the horse's tongue. Epithelial tissues have little mechanical strength and therefore they are supported and attached to underlying connective tissue via a basement membrane. This is a continuous sheet made from collagen and other proteins. Epithelium, due to its lining function, tends to be subject to more wear and tear and therefore has a good capacity for cell renewal.

Epithelium mainly consists of closely packed cells with little extracellular material between them and is arranged in continuous sheets. Epithelial tissues vary in how much they allow passage of substances and so on between cells. Some epithelial cells are tightly joined together, that is, cell membranes are in tight contact with the neighbouring cells without any gaps. These are known as cell junctions. Some cell junctions are deliberately tightly held together, such as those in the lining of the digestive tract and bladder. This prevents leakage of the contents of these organs through the lining, such as in the gut wall, which could have devastating consequences. Some cell junctions are lightly held together, whereas others allow channels to run between them for the passage of molecules. This is very important as it allows communication between epithelial cells and allows passage of nerve impulses, for example.

Some epithelial cells are ciliated with tiny hairs on their apical surface which form a carpet to 'waft' particles and so on along. An example is the lining of the respiratory tract trapping inhaled dust and other particles, sweeping it up to the throat where it can be coughed up or swallowed. Also the fallopian tubes are ciliated to help move the ovum along from the ovaries. Epithelium lacks blood vessels and is therefore known as avascular. Nutrients are supplied to and waste products removed from epithelial cells via adjacent connective tissues. Epithelium also has a nerve supply. Because epithelial tissues tend to be subject to higher levels of wear and tear, they tend to also have a higher capacity for tissue renewal, that is, cell division. Epithelial tissue is the first tissue to be formed in the embryo.

Epithelium may be covering/lining or glandular.

- Lining epithelium – this covers and lines the skin, and some internal organs such as the heart and kidneys. It also lines blood vessel ducts or tubes and the inside of the digestive, respiratory, reproductive and urinary systems. Examples of lining epithelia are shown in Table 2.2.
- Glandular epithelium – this makes up the secretory portion of glands, such as the sweat glands of the horse. Glandular epithelium is secretory, and secretes substances onto its surface, into the blood or into ducts.

Epithelial Cell Shapes

- Squamous – flat and thin, allowing substances to easily diffuse through via osmosis, diffusion or secretion.
- Cuboidal – cube-shaped cells, may have microvilli, such as in intestinal wall, often involved in absorption and secretion.
- Columnar – taller and narrower cells, may have cilia or microvilli on the upper free surface, often involved in absorption and secretion (Figure 2.16). For example, ciliated epithelium is found in the lining of the respiratory tract.

Epithelial cells may also change shape over time, such as when stretched, as in the lining of the bladder, for example. Also cells may change in shape with wear; for example, skin cells start off taller on the basement membrane and as they move towards the skin surface the cells become flatter, that is, become squamous, before being sloughed off the top. Classification of epithelium is therefore based upon the shape of cells on the basement membrane, the number of cells and the number of layers.

Epithelial Arrangement of Cells

- Simple – single layer of cells, allowing movement of some molecules, ions and so on to pass through.
- Pseudostratified – single layered, therefore simple epithelium, but appears to be in

Table 2.2 Classification of lining epithelia.

Simple epithelium	Stratified epithelium
• Simple squamous	• Stratified squamous
E.g. endothelium lining heart and blood vessels, lungs and kidneys	May be keratinised, such as skin, or non-keratinised, such as mouth lining
• Simple cuboidal	• Stratified cuboidal
E.g. thyroid gland and kidneys	Mainly protective; relatively rare tissue
• Simple columnar	• Stratified columnar
Non-ciliated (may have villi) or ciliated	Protection and absorption; relatively rare tissue
E.g. goblet cells which secret mucus as lubricant in respiratory and digestive tracts	
• Pseudostratified columnar	• Transitional epithelium
Absorption and protection but without goblet cells or cilia	Tends to be elastic, such as within lining of bladder; no basement membrane

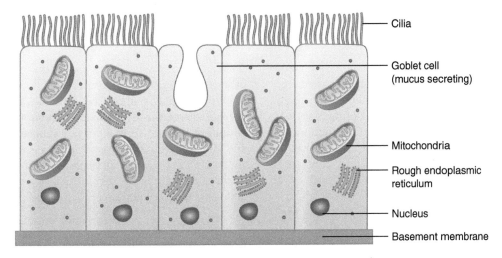

Figure 2.16 Columnar epithelium.

multiple layers because nuclei are found at different levels within the cells.

- Stratified – more than one layer, tends to be protective in function.

Glands may be endocrine or exocrine.

- Endocrine – diffuse into blood, no ducts, for example hormones.
- Exocrine – secrete into ducts that empty at a surface or lumen, for example skin (sweat glands), mucus within gut, digestive

enzymes and saliva from the salivary glands.

Connective Tissue

Connective tissue contains a variety of different types of cells entrenched in an intercellular substance known as the matrix. Connective tissue includes tissues such as bone and cartilage, lymph and blood (Figure 2.17). It is one of the most abundant

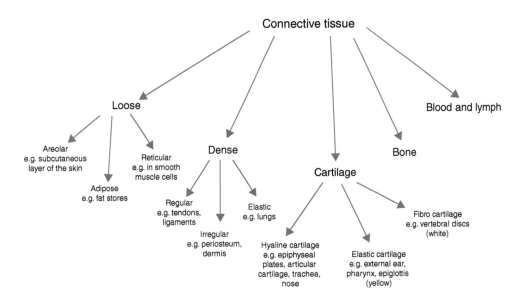

Figure 2.17 Types of connective tissue.

tissues in the horse's body. As the name suggests, it connects and binds tissues together, filling space. It also stores energy in the form of adipose tissue, which adds insulation. It supports, strengthens and compartmentalises tissues and allows movement, such as the skeletal muscle. Connective tissue also has an important immune function.

Connective tissue contains cells that are not packed closely together, in contrast to epithelial tissue, and are separated by an extracellular matrix or mesh which they secrete. This matrix varies depending upon the type of the tissue, but generally contains a ground substance which fills space between the cells and through which protein fibres run. The extracellular matrix gives connective tissue its specific properties; it may be fluid, gel-like or solid with fibres running through it.

For example, in cartilage tissue, the extracellular matrix is pliable but still firm, whereas bone is much harder and less malleable. Fibrous cartilage is an excellent shock absorber because it can be compressed, taking the considerable weight of the horse's body when the limbs are moving, without being damaged. It can also absorb significant impacts, such as when the horse is galloping or jumping. Tendons are made from fibrous connective tissue with a small amount of elasticity and contain closely packed collagen fibres. The tendons are structured in such a way as to withstand enormous forces when the horse is jumping and galloping for example.

Connective tissue tends to be found within the body and not within lumens or on surfaces and, unlike epithelia, has a good blood supply. It also has a good nerve supply, the exception being cartilage.

Ground Substance

Ground substance is an important component of connective tissue as it provides the important environment surrounding connective tissue cells, exchanging important nutrients and other substances with the blood supply. It also plays an active role in the development, migration and proliferation of connective tissue cells and, most importantly, how they function.

Ground substance contains water and other larger organic molecules, the nature of which depends upon the function and type or the connective tissue. For example, chondroitin sulphate is a ground substance and is a polysaccharide found in connective tissue such as bone and cartilage. Hyaluronic acid is a polysaccharide that lubricates joints and also helps to maintain eyeball shape.

Connective Tissue Cells

Connective tissue cells vary depending on the type of connective tissue, but include the following:

- Fibroblasts – move through connective tissue, laying down fibres and the ground substance of extracellular matrix.
- Macrophages – a type of leucocyte (white blood cell) which develops from monocytes, responsible for 'clearing up'; they surround and engulf bacteria and debris by phagocytosis, hence their name.
- Plasma cells – develop from B lymphocytes, secrete antibodies and are important for immune function.
- Mast cells – found alongside blood vessels that support connective tissue, secrete histamine and can destroy bacteria.
- Adipocytes – fat cells that store triglycerides.

Functions of connective tissue are shown in Table 2.3.

Connective Tissue Fibres

Fibres are very important in connective tissue as they provide support and structure. There are three different types of fibre found in the extracellular matrix between the cells of connective tissue:

- collagen fibres
- elastic fibres
- reticular fibres.

Collagen fibres are very strong and somewhat flexible. The fibres are often bundled

Table 2.3 Functions of connective tissue.

Connective tissue	Function
Bone	Skeleton supports and protects major organs of the body, provides support for movement and anchoring of muscles, etc.
Ligament	Supports joints such as suspensory ligament and attaches bone to bone
Tendon	Attaches muscle to bone and is a conduit for movement of limbs
Areolar tissue	Protects organs, blood vessels and nerves. More like a packing tissue
Cartilage	Found on ends of bones in joints to provide a smooth surface for movement; also found in trachea and bronchi to prevent collapse
Blood (liquid connective tissue)	Transports nutrients, oxygen, carbon dioxide and other important substances round the body
Adipose tissue	Provides insulation and stores excess energy as fat

together and positioned parallel to each other, such as found in tendons, ligaments and skin, to give increased strength. Collagen fibres consist of the protein collagen and this is produced by fibroblasts in the form of elongated fibrils. Collagen is the most abundant protein in the horse's body (approximately 25–35% of total body protein). Collagen fibres are found in most connective tissues, especially bone tendons, ligaments and cartilage.

Elastic fibres are smaller than collagen fibres and are made from elastin, a protein that is surrounded by a glycoprotein called fibrillin. Elastic fibres are quite strong and have the ability to return to their pre-stretched or relaxed shape after stretching. This property is known as elasticity. These fibres are commonly found in the horse's skin, lungs and blood vessel walls.

Reticular fibres are produced by fibroblast cells and consist of type III collagen and a coating of glycoprotein. They provide support to the walls of blood vessels. They also form a cross-linked fine mesh called reticulin, providing the support framework for many soft organs such as the liver, spleen and lymph nodes.

Tissue Repair

Tissue repair is vital to keep the adult horse's body working smoothly, replacing worn-out tissues and dead cells. New cells are produced by the parenchyma cells which support connective tissue. Each of the four main tissues, muscular, nervous, connective and epithelial, have different capacity for repair and renewal. Muscle regenerates poorly and any discontinuity is bridged by newly formed fibrous connective tissue which does not have the same contractile properties. Skeletal muscle fibres cannot replace themselves fast enough to replace extensively damaged muscle fibres, such as those damaged by rhabdomyolysis.

On the other hand, blood vessels and lymphatics, red and white blood cells, the epidermis of the skin and epithelia lining internal surfaces are constantly dying and being replaced. Their life expectancy can be measured in days or weeks rather than years. The cells of the epidermis live for about 27 days and these tissues never grow old.

Epithelial cells have a continuous renewal process, as there is a large amount of wear and tear where this tissue is found (see 'Cell Differentiation and Stem Cells') Bone can replace and repair itself well, whereas cartilage tissue is limited, as is muscle tissue. Parenchymal cells can regenerate injured tissue to a similar structure to the original, whereas fibroblasts produce new connective tissues that club together to produce scar tissue, causing fibrosis. This is not a specialised functional tissue but a 'healing' tissue, which does not perform the same as the original

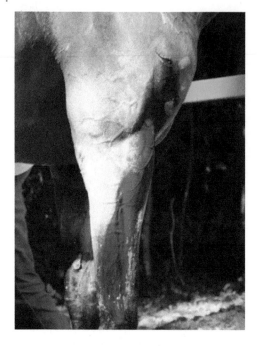

Figure 2.18 A fresh equine wound. *Source*: Dee.lite, https://commons.wikimedia.org/wiki/File:Polo_Schnittverletzung_Pferd.JPG. CC BY-SA 3.0.

tissue. Thus scar tissue can impair the original function, for example of the tendon or ligament. Scar tissue may also form adhesions which stick together and again impair the functionality of the damaged tissue.

Horses are very prone to accidental wounds due to their athletic nature and fight or flight response to perceived danger. Figure 2.18 shows a fresh equine wound.

The Four Stages of Wound Healing

Stage 1 – Traumatic Inflammatory Phase

The traumatic inflammatory phase (Figure 2.19) is also known as the defensive stage. Inflammation is initiated immediately there is any damage to tissues. Chemical messengers flow from the damaged cells to the adjacent areas where they stimulate undamaged cells into activity. Certain chemicals, namely bradykinin and histamine, cause the walls of small blood capillaries to become leaky, and some plasma and white cells and platelets are able to leak into the damaged

area and onto the wound surface, producing an exudate. If there has been extensive tissue damage, the blood capillaries may be overstimulated, causing excessive exudate, swelling (oedema) and pain.

The ends of severed blood capillaries are sealed by blood clotting which, through a series of chemical reactions, brings about the formation of a mesh of fibrin fibres with trapped red blood cells stuck to them. Any blood that clots within the tissue spaces and lies between the wound surface and the tissue spaces must be broken down and removed at a later date as it will obstruct healing.

Within 1 hour, circulation of specialised white blood cells known as polymorphonuclear leucocytes (PMNs) occurs. These cells originate from the bone marrow and they are attracted by chemicals released by bacteria. The PMNs begin to stick to the inner surface of the capillary walls in the vicinity of the wound. They then squeeze their way through the leaky blood vessels by changing their shape to become flat, and move into the surrounding tissues.

Bacteria are always present in wounds. They live on the skin and in the atmosphere and even pre-surgical asepsis techniques cannot get rid of them all. So all wounds, be they surgical or accidental, will contain significant numbers of bacteria. In serious injuries it is sometimes preferable to control the amount of inflammation to prevent permanent swelling. This is often the case with tendon injuries, where too much swelling can impair the healing process.

Stage 2 – Destructive Phase (0–3 Days)

The second or destructive phase begins after about 8 hours. The macrophages and mononuclear cells are carried by the blood to the affected area. The macrophages, which are part of the reticulo-endothelial system, scavenge for dead cells and bacteria and clear away any blood and damaged tissue fibres. These then try to remove any unwanted foreign material that has found its way into the wound and leave a clean pathway for the formation of new tissue which must follow.

Figure 2.19 Inflammatory response to injury.

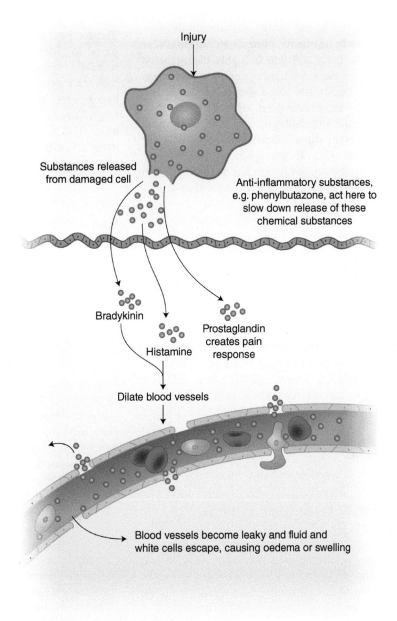

Injury

Substances released from damaged cell

Anti-inflammatory substances, e.g. phenylbutazone, act here to slow down release of these chemical substances

Bradykinin

Histamine

Prostaglandin creates pain response

Dilate blood vessels

Blood vessels become leaky and fluid and white cells escape, causing oedema or swelling

Macrophages also stimulate the production of fibroblasts, the cells that make the body's principal structural protein, namely collagen. Collagen can be found in fresh wounds within 48 hours, new blood capillaries also start to grow into the wound from the edges and fibroblasts start to multiply. The fibroblasts make collagen in the form of cross-linked fibrils which form a network of fibrous bundles. Then remodelling begins at the start of the third phase known as the proliferative stage.

Stage 3 – Proliferative Phase (3–24 Days)

Also known as the reconstructive phase, this is when the fibroblasts start to make a collagen network behind the macrophages. Collagen is the main constituent of skin, tendons, ligaments, bones, cartilage and scar tissue. Early collagen is highly disorganised and its early formation depends to a large extent upon the blood supply to the injured area. Fibroblasts need stimulating to produce the vital collagen, and one of the most important stimulators is vitamin C. Without vitamin C, collagen synthesis is inhibited. Since the horse's body cannot store vitamin C, the importance of good nutrition at this stage is apparent.

The considerable activity that occurs during this phase results in the formation of granulation tissue. This consists of newly formed and fragile capillary loops supported in a scaffold of collagen fibres. The amount of granulation tissue produced depends upon the amount of inflammation. As this proliferative phase continues there is a rapid increase in the strength of the wound. Any excessive movement at this stage will result in impaired healing, as the edges between the wound surface must be kept still. Usually, by about the fourteenth day, the wound has about one-quarter of the strength of the surrounding tissue. Factors that may impair healing at this stage are age, the amount of oxygen available and zinc deficiency.

Stage 4 – Maturation Phase (24 Days to 2 Years)

During the maturation phase there is a progressive decrease in the vascularity of the scar, shrinkage of the fibroblasts, enlargement and reorientation of the collagen fibres, and improved tissue strength. The dusky red colour of new vascular granulation tissue changes to the pale, white, avascular (no blood capillaries) scar tissue. After the first 6 weeks only half of the normal strength of the wounded skin is achieved. Strength of the pre-injured tissue is rarely achieved in practice. The scar then slowly reduces, causing flattening and softening of the scar. This may take up to a year.

Ageing Tissue

Tissues heal better in young horses, compared to older horses. Younger horses tend to have a higher metabolic rate which means cells can repair faster. Also, older tissues become less elastic and stiffer and the collagen fibres change in quality as horses get older. This means that older horses are more likely to suffer from injury/damage and do not repair as well as younger horses.

Stem Cell Therapy

Stem cell therapy may help many equine injuries and conditions but is most commonly used to assist the healing of tendon, ligament, bone and joint injuries/arthritis. Stem cell therapy involves removing stem cells from a source (bone marrow or fat) from the horse, processing it to concentrate the stem cells and then injecting it into the site of injury.

Stem cells from fat may be used by taking adipose cells from the fat pad over the tail of the horse; this may be more difficult with leaner fit horses. Mesenchymal stem cells are primitive cells with the ability to become any type of specialty connective tissue cell (bone, tendon, muscle, etc.). In horses, bone marrow is typically harvested from the sternum. This is a veterinary procedure and is done with the horse standing under local anaesthesia. The marrow is aspirated with a special needle and can be either injected directly into the tendon or processed to isolate the stem cells. Figure 2.20 shows a colony of embryonic stem cells, from the H9 cell line.

Stem cell therapy is most effective when carried out around a month or so post injury and before scar tissue has become established. Overall healing time is not necessarily faster with stem cell therapy, as tendons take a long time, usually 12 months or so, to heal to full strength. If returned to work too soon, the risk of re-injury increases. Stem cell therapy is now also helpful in fracture repair and intra-articular joint therapy, arthritis

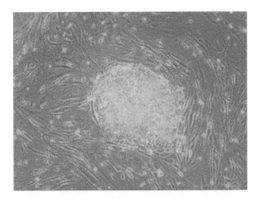

Figure 2.20 A colony of embryonic stem cells, from the H9 cell line (NIH code: WA09). Viewed at 10× magnification with a Carl Zeiss Axiovert scope. (The cells in the background are mouse fibroblast cells. Only the colony in the centre is human embryonic stem cells.) *Source*: Ryddragyn, https://en.wikipedia.org/wiki/File:Humanstemcell.JPG. CC BY-SA 3.0.

and osteochondritis dissecans (OCD), as the cells appear to be drawn to inflamed areas. Within a joint, stem cells will move to the areas of both cartilage and bone injury.

Stem cell injections to treat joint damage and therefore pain have improved and in many cases have resulted in a dramatic reduction in pain and improved mobility and repair of both cartilage and bone injury within the joint. This improvement has resulted from the use of autologous stem cells from the horse's own body rather than foetal bovine serum, which was originally used in the treatment.

Stem cell therapy may be combined with hyaluronic acid (HA), as HA increases the time stem cells stay in the joint. Injecting HA prophylactically into joints that are not inflamed is not useful, as the injected stem cells stimulate the production of growth factors similar to plasma-rich protein (PRP) and interleukin-1 receptor antagonist protein (IRAP), which blocks the inflammatory proteins that produce inflammation, breakdown of cartilage, pain and lameness. Future treatments may allow horse owners to have stem cells preserved long before their horse needs them. The cells could be frozen and stored in liquid nitrogen, similar to embryo and semen storage.

Another new treatment for tendon injuries that does not involve stem cells is a substance known as urinary bladder matrix (UBM) which is derived from the wall of a pig's bladder. It contains a mixture of proteins, including collagen. It does not contain cells, however, and so reduces any possible immune response. The absence of cells should eliminate the body's autoimmune (allergic) reaction to the substance. UBM is supplied in sheets which are ground to a fine powder and suspended in sterile saline. The mixture is then injected into the injured tendon or ligament. The proteins form a 3D scaffold onto which the cells that create tendon and ligament tissue can adhere.

Summary Points

1) All animals, plants and fungi are related to each other as they share a common ancestor. Mitochondria have their own loops of DNA known as mitochondrial DNA passed down via the dam.

2) The horse's cells act and interact with each other (they are interdependent) and this involves a continuous exchange of chemical and electrochemical messages.

3) The fluid mosaic model of the cell membrane structure is very important, as it regulates different substances passing in and out.

4) Mitochondria pose their own unique genome, separate from and smaller than that of the cells' own genome from DNA within the nucleus. This is passed from generation to generation via the dam's ova.

5) The horse's body also contains stem cells. These are undifferentiated or unspecialised. They have the ability to undergo numerous cell divisions in this unspecialised state and are also able to differentiate into specialised cells.

Q + A

Q Name the different ways substances are transported in and around cells.

A Diffusion, osmosis, facilitated diffusion, active transport, endocytosis, exocytosis.

Q Briefly describe the structure of a cell membrane using the fluid mosaic model.

A Cells are composed of lipids, proteins and carbohydrates (usually attached to lipids or proteins). The fluid mosaic model describes the arrangement of these molecules within the membrane. Phospholipid molecules form a continuous double layer or bilayer. The bilayer is fluid because the phospholipids are continually moving. Protein molecules are interspersed throughout the bilayer like tiles in a mosaic, hence the name. Some proteins have a polysaccharide chain attached and are known as glycoproteins, whereas some lipids also have a polysaccharide chain attached and are known as glycolipids. Cholesterol molecules are contained within the bilayer.

Q What is apoptosis and why is it important?

A Apoptosis is programmed cell death. It has several functions within the horse's body – sculpting embryonic tissue, maintaining cell numbers in the adult, replacing older cells, defence against damaged cells and defence against infected cells.

Q Cell signalling pathways may be short or long. How are they categorised?

A Endocrine pathway – this transports hormones over long distances via the circulation to the target cells. Paracrine pathway – signal acts locally upon cells next to or very close to the target cell. Cells can also make and respond to their own signals and this is known as autocrine signalling.

Q Why do tissues heal better in young horses?

A Younger horses have a higher metabolic rate, which means cells can repair faster.

Q When is the best time to undertake stem cell therapy?

A Around 1 month following the injury.

3

Equine Support and Movement

Points of the Horse

Being familiar with the surface anatomy of the horse will help to identify the underlying structures (Figure 3.1).

The Skeletal System

The skeletal system consists of all the bones and joints within the horse's body. It provides a framework for the attachment of muscles and protects important organs and structures within. Bone is a highly dynamic and complex tissue, being continuously remodelled throughout the life of the horse. Each bone is an organ, with several different tissues working together including cartilage, dense irregular connective tissue, epithelium, nervous and adipose tissue and bone marrow which forms new blood cells.

Functions of the skeletal system include:

- Giving support and rigidity for movement – provides points of attachment for muscles, ligaments and tendons and acts as levers for the muscles to work against. Most skeletal muscles attach to bones, resulting in movement when muscles contract and/or relax.
- Protecting the internal organs – for example, the brain which is housed in the skull for protection, the rib cage provides protection for the heart and lungs.
- Providing homeostasis of minerals – particularly calcium, phosphorus and magnesium. When required, bone is able to

release minerals into the blood to support plasma levels and other tissues.
- Involvement in haematopoiesis (sometimes termed haemopoiesis) – production of blood cells from red bone marrow. Red bone marrow is found within certain adult bones such as the pelvis, ribs, sternum, skull and vertebrae and the end of the forelimb bones and femur. In the foetus red bone marrow is present in all bones during development. It contains developing blood cells, macrophages, adipocytes and fibroblasts. In newborn foals all bone marrow is red and this slowly changes to mainly yellow in colour in the adult horse.
- Storing triglycerides – adipose (fat) cells in the form of yellow bone marrow.
- Providing autologous mesenchymal stem cells (MSCs) from bone marrow – which are now often used as a primary stem cell source for regenerative tissue repair of tendon by veterinary surgeons.

Bone

Bone makes up the largest component of the skeleton. There are 205 bones in the equine skeleton, 34 of which are found in the skull. There are 20 bones in each of the limbs and 37 bones in the horse's rib cage. There are approximately 54 vertebrae in the vertebral column helping protect the spinal cord. The number of vertebrae in the tail may vary slightly with different horse breeds.

Bone is one of the hardest tissues in the horse's body and bone tissue needs to be

Equine Science, Third Edition. Zoe Davies and Sarah Pilliner.
© 2018 Zoe Davies and Sarah Pilliner. Published 2018 by John Wiley & Sons Ltd.

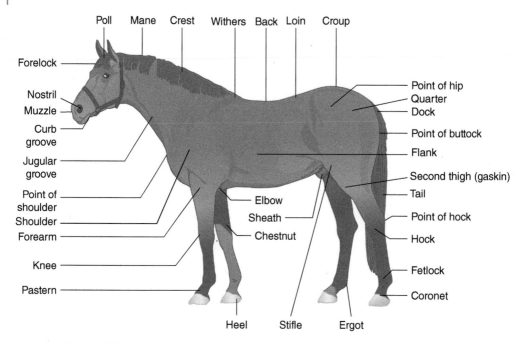

Figure 3.1 Points of the horse.

tough and resilient. Thus bone has two important properties: it is both rigid, giving strength, and elastic, allowing some flexibility, without which bone would be brittle and easily broken. About 30% of an adult horse's bone consists of living, organic fibrous tissue or collagen. This provides flexibility to bone. The remaining 70% consists of inorganic bone salts of which the most important is hydroxy-apatite $(Ca_{10}(PO_4)_6(OH)_2)$. Calcium and phosphorus are thus essential in the diet to maintain bone structure, but sodium, magnesium, potassium, chloride, fluoride, bicarbonate and citrate ions are all present in variable amounts. Essentially bone consists of a matrix of collagen and polysaccharides (glycosaminoglycans (GAGs) – containing chondroitin sulphate) encrusted with mineral salts which impart strength. Approximately 80% of the mineral salts are calcium phosphate, with the rest being mainly calcium carbonate and magnesium phosphate. Calcium phosphate is found mainly in hydroxyapatite crystals which give hardness to bone. The proportion of organic and inorganic material in bone varies with

age. Thus young horses have 'soft' bones containing up to 60% fibrous tissue, while old horses develop 'brittle' bones with a low fibrous content. While bone may look inelastic and almost lifeless it is a highly dynamic structure – the entire calcium content of the skeleton is replaced every 200 days. This ability to mobilise minerals allows the skeleton to act as a mineral reservoir in times of need. A lactating mare, for example, can make up the required calcium for milk from her body reserves should her diet lack calcium. No other tissue in the body is capable of as much growth and absorption as bone.

Bone can therefore be damaged or diseased and will try to repair any damage that is not catastrophic. Bone will also adapt to environmental stress which includes exercise.

Classification of Bone Tissue

There are two types of bone tissue: dense or compact, and spongy or cancellous.

Dense or Compact Bone

Compact bone is solid except for microscopic spaces. Its structure consists of

Figure 3.2 Haversian system or osteon structure.

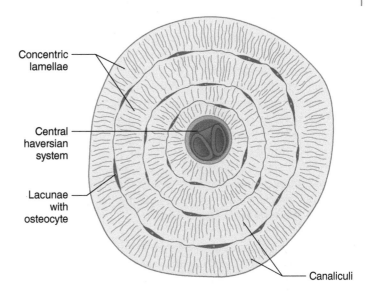

Concentric lamellae

Central haversian system

Lacunae with osteocyte

Canaliculi

repeating structural units called haversian systems or osteons (Figure 3.2). Each osteon consists of a central haversian canal and its concentrically arranged lamellae.

Compact bone is deposited in sheets called lamellae which are arranged as cylinders within cylinders, that is, they are highly structured, and these are similar in appearance to the growth rings round a tree. Nerves, lymph and blood vessels run inside a central canal, and this compacted structure gives immense strength. The tube-like osteons form a series of cylinders which run parallel to each other in long bones along the same axis as the bone. Between the lamellae are small spaces called lacunae (meaning little lakes) housing osteocytes. Radiating in all directions from the lacunae are the canaliculi which are filled with extracellular fluid, providing oxygen and nutrients to the bone and removing waste materials. The canaliculi therefore connect between each other and the central canals, providing a system for movement of important substances within bone. Larger blood and lymph vessels and nerves transverse through the periosteum and enter the bone via Volkmann's canals which penetrate into the bone, connecting eventually with the central haversian canals.

Spongy or Cancellous Bone

Spongy bone is much lighter than compact bone and so it is easier for muscles to move the bone if required. Spongy bone is found in the ribs, sternum, vertebrae, pelvis and ends of the long bones. These locations contain red bone marrow for haematopoiesis. Spongy bone is not made up of osteons but consists of slender, irregular 'finger like' trabeculae or bars which branch and unite to form a latticework of thin columns of bone. There are much larger spaces between the trabeculae which are filled with red bone marrow. Each trabeculae contains concentric lamellae, lacunae housing osteocytes and canaliculae radiating outwards.

Types of Bones

Each bone has a characteristic shape which is determined by its function within the skeleton. Bones are classified into four main types based upon their shape, namely:

- long bones
- flat bones
- short or cuboidal bones
- irregular bones.

Long bones act as supporting columns and levers, for example the cannon bone. They have greater strength and width. They consist of a shaft (diaphysis) and mostly two ends (epiphyses). Long bones include the femur, tibia and fibula, humerus, radius and ulna, cannon bones and phalanges. Compact bone makes up the shaft of a long bone and is organised in a tube-like form surrounding red or yellow bone marrow (the medullary cavity). Each end of the long bone is spongy bone covered by a thin shell of compact bone. Long bones are characteristic of limbs and have terminal enlargements which are associated with joints, for example the end of the femur and tibia. There are two reasons for this:

- to spread the pressure over a larger articular surface and thus reduce the wear and tear on the joint surfaces;
- the joint is more stable and less likely to move out of alignment, that is, to become dislocated.

Flat bones consist of two plates of compact bone enclosing a middle layer of spongy bone. They are generally thin and provide extensive points for muscle attachments. Flat bones include the skull, sternum, scapulae and ribs.

Short or cuboidal bones, for example the carpal bones of the knee and the tarsal bones of the hock, act as shock absorbers.

Irregular bones generally have a specialist function, such as the vertebrae and some facial bones in the skull. Most irregular bones consist of spongy bone covered by a thin shell of compact bone.

Regardless of their shape, the composition of these bones is similar. The gross structure of a long bone is shown in Figure 3.3. A cross-section of a long bone shows an outer layer of compact bone for strength and then an inner layer of spongy bone (Figure 3.4).

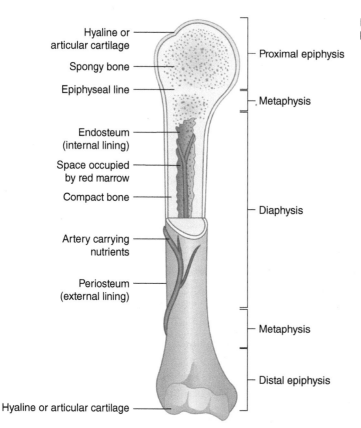

Hyaline or articular cartilage

Spongy bone

Epiphyseal line

Endosteum (internal lining)

Space occupied by red marrow

Compact bone

Artery carrying nutrients

Periosteum (external lining)

Hyaline or articular cartilage

Proximal epiphysis

Metaphysis

Diaphysis

Metaphysis

Distal epiphysis

Figure 3.3 Gross structure of a long bone.

Figure 3.4 Cross-section through a long bone.

Periosteal outer covering

Dense compact bone

Bone marrow cavity

Spongy bone

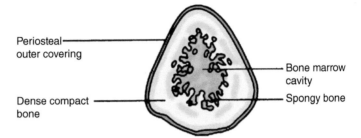

The diaphysis is the shaft, the epiphyses are the ends (singular epiphysis) and the metaphysis is the area where the shaft of the bone in a mature horse joins the epiphysis. In a growing horse such as a foal or yearling, the metaphysis contains the growth plate (epiphyseal plate), a layer of hyaline cartilage enabling growth and lengthening of the long bone. Once the bone stops growing the cartilage in the epiphyseal plate turns to bone and is known as the epiphyseal line.

Compact bone is thickest where stress is the greatest. Surrounding the compact bone is a dense connective tissue membrane called the periosteum which acts as an attachment point for tendons and ligaments. The periosteum helps nourish and protect bone and is a tough sheet of connective tissue which lines the bone surface except for where articular cartilage is situated. It also helps repair damage to the bone surface, particularly micro fractures such as sore shins and splints (Figure 3.5).

The periosteum has associated blood vessels within and is lined with cells called osteoblasts (see below), which secrete new bone matrix that makes the bone thicker in diameter but not in length, as lengthening occurs at the epiphyseal plates. The articular cartilage covers the part of the epiphysis that forms a joint with another bone. Cartilage reduces friction and wear and tear on the ends of the bones within a joint and also acts as a shock absorber. Articular cartilage lacks a perichondrium and therefore has limited ability to repair itself when damaged. The perichondrium is a layer of dense irregular

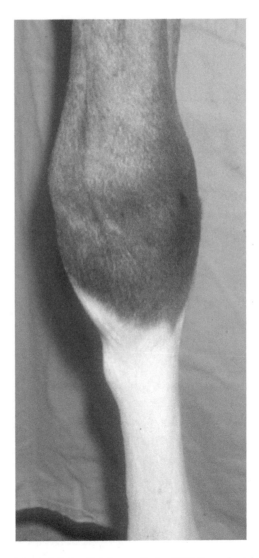

Figure 3.5 A splint. *Source*: Baxter 2011. Reproduced with permission of John Wiley & Sons.

connective tissue that surrounds the cartilage of developing bone.

The amount of space within bone determines if it is spongy or compact. Approximately 80% of the equine skeleton contains compact bone and 20% spongy bone.

Microscopic Bone Structure

There are four main cell types in bone (Figure 3.6):

- Osteogenic cells – unspecialised stem cells from mesenchyme tissue, the only bone cells able to divide.
- Osteoblasts – bone-building cells that become trapped in the extracellular bone matrix and eventually turn into osteocytes.
- Osteocytes – mature bone cells, which nourish bone and do not divide.
- Osteoclasts – large cells derived from the fusion of many monocytes, found in the endosteum (a thin membrane lining the medullary cavity) and responsible for resorption of bone.

Bone Formation and Growth

In the unborn foal there are two main types of bone formation or ossification:

- intramembranous bone formation;
- endochondral ossification.

Intramembranous bone formation gives rise to flat bones such as the skull, jaws and pectoral girdle, and involves ossification of the dermis. Mesenchyma cells become differentiated into rows of osteoblasts which begin to lay down bony plates. The osteoblasts also increase in number and lay down bone salts onto the plates, resulting in an increase in size.

The best example of endochondral ossification takes place in the long bones (Figure 3.7a and b). In the embryo, bone

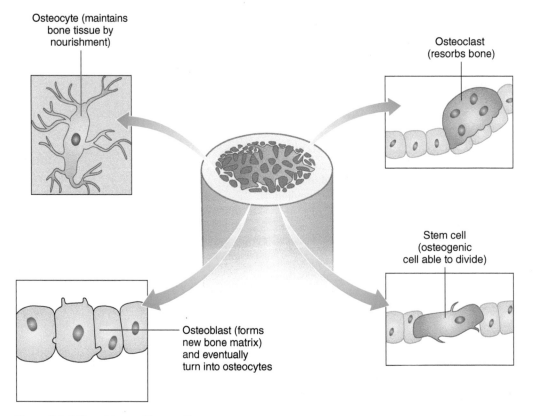

Figure 3.6 Different types of bone cell.

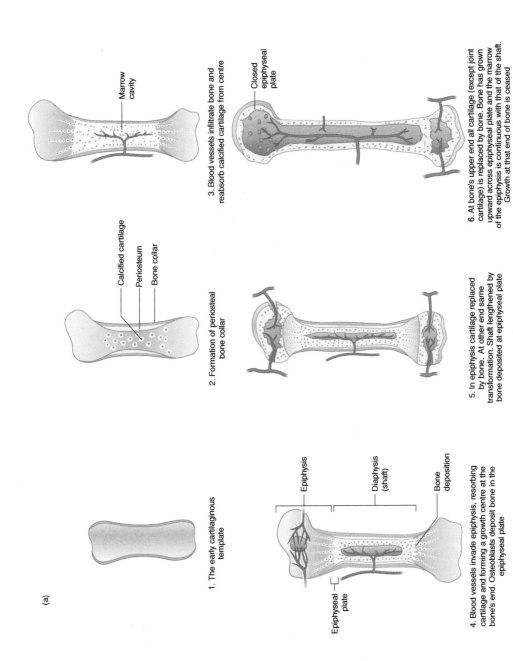

(a)

1. The early cartilaginous template

2. Formation of periosteal bone collar

Calcified cartilage
Periosteum
Bone collar

3. Blood vessels infiltrate bone and reabsorb calcified cartilage from centre

Marrow cavity

4. Blood vessels invade epiphysis, resorbing cartilage and forming a growth centre at the bone's end. Osteoblasts deposit bone in the epiphyseal plate

Epiphysis
Diaphysis (shaft)
Bone deposition
Epiphyseal plate

5. In epiphysis cartilage replaced by bone. At other end same transformation. Shaft lengthened by bone deposited at epiphyseal plate

6. At bone's upper end all cartilage (except joint cartilage) is replaced by bone. Bone has grown upward across epiphyseal plate and the marrow of the epiphysis is continuous with that of the shaft. Growth at that end of bone is ceased

Closed epiphyseal plate

Figure 3.7 Growth and development of a long bone. (a) How cartilage is turned into bone. (b) How the bone enlarges in length and width as the young horse grows.

(b)

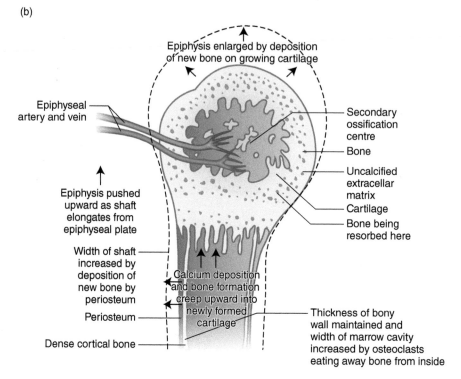

Figure 3.7 (*Continued*)

begins as cartilage; then osteoblasts invade the cartilage and lay down bone matrix. Mineral salts are deposited in the matrix, a process called calcification, resulting in bone. By the time the foal is born, calcification is complete in most bones.

Once the bone is formed it grows; growth involves an increase in diameter (from the periosteum) as well as in length (epiphyseal plates). The increase in length takes place at two narrow bands of cartilage called the epiphyseal growth plates. Cartilage grows continuously on the side of the growth plate nearest the end of the bone; meanwhile the cartilage on the shaft side of the growth plate is invaded by osteoblasts and converted to bone. Gradually the osteoblasts 'catch up' on the cartilage, so that when the bone is the correct length the growth plate 'closes'. The growth plates close at different times in horses:

- Lower end of radius, bottom of radius/ ulna, that is, just above the knee: 2 years

- Top of radius: 2.5–3 years
- Humerus: 3–3.5 years
- Knee bones: 1.5–2.5 years
- Vertebrae: 5.5–6 years
- Scapula: 3.5–4 years
- Pelvis: 3–4 years
- Femur: 3–3.5 years
- Hock: 4 years
- Coffin bone: fused at birth
- Short pastern: birth to 4 months
- Long pastern: 6 months to 1 year
- Lower end of cannon bone: 9–18 months
- Fetlock: 8–9 months

Growth in length of the cannon bone stops with fusion of both growth plates at around 1.5 years, and growth of circumference or girth of the cannon bone does not finish until around 5 years. This is mostly true for other bones too. The closure of the plates is affected by the sex hormones. Colts and fillies grow at a similar rate until they reach puberty, when testosterone, the male sex hormone, stops the closure of the plates, so that colts continue to grow. Oestrogen promotes the closure of the plates and the growth rate of fillies slows down. Anabolic steroids tend to hasten the closure of the plates, and if given to the young horse will stunt the growth of the skeleton while enhancing muscle development.

The increase in diameter is brought about by osteoblasts which line the periosteum. In simple terms, the osteoblasts lay down new layers of bone over the old in a similar way to the growth of a tree which gives rise to rings that can be seen when the tree is felled. Simultaneously the old bone lining the marrow cavity is eaten away by osteoclasts, cells that reabsorb bone. This means that the bone marrow cavity will enlarge but the wall of the shaft does not become too thick and heavy.

Developmental Orthopaedic Disease

The causes of growth-related problems or developmental orthopaedic diseases (DOD) are multifactorial and include genetics, nutrition, particularly poor or imbalanced mineral supply, and trauma. The term was coined in 1986 to encompass all orthopaedic problems seen in the growing foal and has become the generally accepted term. DOD encompasses all general growth disturbances of horses and is therefore quite non-specific. When first used, the term included the following:

- osteochondritis dissecans (OCD)
- subchondral cystic lesions
- angular limb deformities (ALD)
- physitis (Figure 3.8)
- flexural limb deformities (FLD) (may be secondary to osteochondrosis or physitis)
- cuboidal bone abnormalities
- juvenile osteoarthritis.

In a study of Thoroughbreds (TBs) in Ireland the peak incidence of DOD problems occurred between weaning at approximately 6 months and the end of December. This study also showed that approximately 70% of the horses showed some evidence of

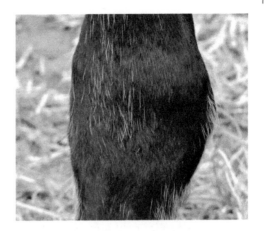

Figure 3.8 Weanling with physitis of the forelimb fetlock. *Source*: Courtesy of Zoe Davies.

DOD, but only 11% required treatment. DOD appears to commonly involve ALD and physitis problems that spontaneously self-correct. It is the ones that do not self-correct, such as OCD and subchondral bone cysts, that often need further investigation/ treatment.

Fast-growing foals and yearlings with higher potential adult bodyweights will have faster growth rates and therefore be more susceptible to mineral imbalances. Nutrigenomics may also play an important role. Using horses before the closure of the plates may lead to growth-related long-term skeletal problems which in future may compromise the ability of the horse to undertake a successful athletic career. The distal radial plates do not close until well into the racing career of a flat racehorse. The cartilage of the open epiphysis is very sensitive to jarring which can give rise to large lumpy swellings immediately above the knee.

DOD should not be used synonymously with osteochondrosis. It is considered an inappropriate term for all subchondral cystic lesions, physitis, ALD, FLD and cervical vertebral malformations (wobbler).

ALD refers to deformity in the limbs:

- carpal or fetlock valgus abnormal angulation away from the midline (if the fetlock or knee 'turns out');

- carpal or fetlock varus abnormal angulation toward the midline (if the fetlock or knee 'turns in' – known as 'pigeon toed').

The most common ALD is carpal valgus, the second most common is fetlock varus and tarsal valgus is the least common.

FLD is divided into two broad categories:

- Flexor laxity – in which the joints are hyperextended due to loose supporting structures.
- Flexor contracture – normal extension of joints is limited and the joints are permanently flexed due to tight supporting structures.

Flexor laxity and contracture include:

- the distal interphalangeal (DIP) joint – contracture of the deep digital flexor tendon and club foot;
- the metacarpophalangeal joint – flexural deformity;
- flexural deformity of the carpus;
- congenital hyperextension deformities.

Bone Remodelling

Throughout the horse's life bone undergoes a remodelling process, which is a balance between the breakdown of old bone and the formation of new bone. Remodelling occurs to allow the bone to act as a mineral store and also to let the bone adapt to stress such as exercise. Bone is a plastic tissue, capable of growth and repair and adaptation to the stresses placed upon it.

Remodelling starts when the foal is about 3 months old, when the newly formed bone begins to rearrange itself into haversian systems. These systems consist of a series of vertically aligned tubules through which the blood vessels travel. If the haversian systems are formed too quickly with too little mineral content, the bone becomes porous and not as strong as dense bone. It is essential that there are adequate and balanced amounts of calcium and phosphorus and other important trace minerals in the diet to allow effective remodelling to take place.

Bone acts as an important store of calcium and phosphorus and other minerals which can be readily called upon, for example, during pregnancy and lactation. The soft red bone marrow found in the ribs, sternum and long bones of young foals produces red blood cells. As the animal matures the red bone marrow in the long bones is replaced by yellow bone marrow and the red cell production is taken over mainly by the spleen.

Bone is similar to skin in that it continues to replace old tissue with new, mostly due to wear and tear. Remodelling therefore involves breaking down old bone tissue and removing minerals and collagen fibres by specialised cells known as osteoclasts (see 'Microscopic Bone Structure'). This is replaced by osteoblasts that build up bone by deposition of minerals and collagen fibres. Remodelling takes place continuously in the horse's skeleton, but at different rates in different areas of the body. It takes place in the adult horse, not just those horses that are growing. There is a balance between osteoclast and osteoblast activity.

Hormones and their Effect on Bone Growth

Several hormones affect bone growth, particularly long bones. These include growth hormones and sex hormones (androgens and oestrogens). Growth hormone promotes elongation of the long bones. The sex hormones promote growth and epiphyseal closure. Growth hormone does not directly affect chondrocytes but instead stimulates production of peptides know as insulin-like growth factors (IGFs) in the liver. These act on chondrocytes to produce more cartilage, in which bone can then form to increase the length of the bone.

The sex hormones can cause growth spurts, with androgens having a greater effect than oestrogen, particularly around puberty. Androgens increase the secretion of growth hormone and colts are therefore generally bigger than fillies. Sex hormones are also responsible for closure of the epiphyseal plates.

Effect of Exercise on Bone Tissue

Bone is a smart issue and can change to a certain extent in response to the mechanical stresses placed upon it over time. Increased mechanical stress results in the laying down of more collagen fibres and minerals in the bone to increase strength. In the absence of mechanical stress, bone will become weaker as resorption rates exceed bone formation and demineralisation occurs. This may happen to horses on box rest. Bones of equine athletes with regular training which subjects the bones to increasing stresses become thicker than those not working. It is important to take this into account in the post-injury training process.

Calcium Homeostasis

Ninety-nine percent of total body calcium of the horse is found within bone in the adult horse. The main calcium source is the diet, but if calcium levels are low or there are other mineral interactions, then plasma calcium levels must be maintained through homeostasis. This involves the use of bone as a calcium reservoir, which may happen when calcium plasma levels start to fall. Small changes in plasma calcium levels can have devastating effects on the horse, and so it is vital the level is kept within relatively narrow margins. Calcium is required for heart, muscle and nerve function, is a cofactor for several enzymes and is important in blood clotting.

Calcium homeostasis involves the release of calcium ions from bone via the osteoclasts when plasma levels fall, and deposition of calcium ions back into bone via the osteoblasts when plasma levels increase. Plasma calcium levels are regulated by parathyroid hormone (PTH), which is secreted by the parathyroid glands which are embedded in the posterior surface of the thyroid gland and works via negative feedback. If plasma calcium levels begin to fall, receptors within the parathyroid glands increase production of cyclic adenosine monophosphate (AMP) in response. The gene for PTH within the nucleus of parathyroid gland cells detects this increase in cyclic AMP and PTH production is increased and released into the plasma. PTH also conserves calcium, thereby reducing losses in urine, and increases absorption of calcium from the gut via calcitrol (the active form of vitamin D). Calcitrol is released from the kidneys in response to PTH. PTH increases the activity of osteocytes, which increases bone resorption and thereby increases calcium levels in the plasma. The rising calcium levels past normal levels will trigger parafollicular cells of the parathyroid gland to release the hormone calcitonin which inhibits osteoclast activity, thereby reducing calcium levels.

Bone Fracture and Repair

Horses are athletic animals and are used for equestrian sports, some of which put the risk of bone fractures at a high level, such as flat and jump racing, show jumping and eventing. Fractures of the limbs in particular are common. Some fractures are repairable and others less so due to the site and extent of the injury. Other factors include age, presence of infection, degree of repair required, future athletic potential and damage to surrounding tissues. Repair is faster in young horses.

A bone that has been broken goes through a number of stages of repair. Although bone has a rich blood supply, healing can sometimes take many months. The nervous supply also means that bone fractures are very painful to the horse. A break in the bone may interfere with the blood supply to the bone temporarily and this will result in a delay in healing. Severe fractures will completely disrupt blood supply and these are often catastrophic injuries that cannot be repaired and the horse will need to be euthanised.

The stages a broken bone goes through during repair are as follows:

- Fracture of bone followed by an inflammatory response.
- Phagocytes remove dead tissue from the damaged area.

- Chondroblasts form fibrocartilage at the site of fracture.
- Fibrocartilage is converted to spongy bone by osteoblasts.
- Bone remodelling occurs.
- Dead bone is absorbed by osteoclasts.
- Spongy bone is converted to compact bone.

The Skeleton

The skeleton (Figure 3.9) comprises bones, cartilage and joints and can be divided into two parts:

- the axial skeleton consisting of the skull, vertebral column (or spine), ribs and sternum;
- the appendicular skeleton consisting of the forelimbs and hindlimbs.

The Axial Skeleton

The Skull
The horse's skull consists of 34 bones and its main function is to protect the brain and house important sense organs such as the eyes and ears. The skull has four cavities:

- Cranial cavity – encloses and protects the brain.
- Orbital cavity – protects the eye.
- Oral cavity – provides a passageway to the digestive system.
- Nasal cavity – provides a passageway to the respiratory system.

These cavities are important for making the skull lighter in weight or it would be too heavy for the horse to carry. The nasal cavity is framed by the conchae or turbinate bones which are highly folded and scroll-like and light in weight. They arise from the lateral walls of the nasal chambers and are lined with mucous membranes to help warm inspired air when the horse is breathing in.

The cranium houses the brain, that is, within the upper part of the skull, and is formed by the occipital, parietal, interparietal, temporal, sphenoid, ethmoid and frontal bones. The frontal bones create the horse's forehead. The orbit is a bony socket which protects the eye and is framed by the zygomatic arch. The maxilla and zygomatic

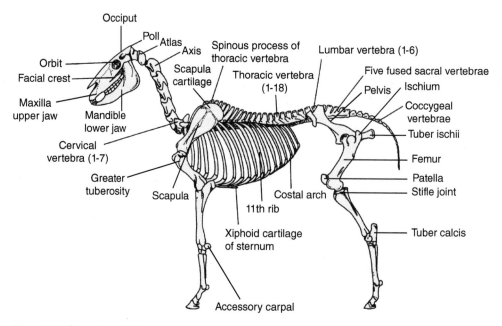

Figure 3.9 The equine skeleton.

bone create a sharp ridge known as the facial crest, and this can be seen and felt externally. Diverticula or paranasal sinuses are found within the frontal, nasal, maxillary, sphenoid and palatine bones. The oral cavity or mouth cavity contains the teeth, the roof of the mouth being formed by the maxillary bone, whereas the lowest part of the jaw is the mandible, which is the largest bone in the horse's skull.

The Vertebral Column or Spine

The spine provides longitudinal support for the body and the necessary strength for suspending the enormous weight of the horse's gut. It is relatively rigid and incompressible, compared with the flexible spine of cats, for example. The vertebrae themselves are wholly incompressible; bending is allowed by the joints between the vertebrae, while the cartilaginous discs between each vertebra allow slight compression. The spine (apart from the neck) can only move slightly in three planes dorsoventral flexion, lateral bending and axial rotation. Researchers found, using kinematics (skin markers placed along the dorsal midline), dorsiflexion (extension of the back) during the first half of a diagonal stance and ventroflexion during the second part, with a very small range of motion of less than 4°. Studies have also found that the most movement in the equine spine (apart from head, neck and tail) occurs at the lumbosacral joint.

The spine can be divided into five regions:

- Neck: 7 cervical vertebrae.
- Upper back: 18 thoracic vertebrae.
- Loins: 6 lumbar vertebrae.
- Croup: 5 fused sacral vertebrae.
- Tail: 15–21 coccygeal vertebrae.

The vertebrae make up a long bony chain housing and protecting the spinal cord (Figure 3.10). At each vertebra a pair of spinal nerves branch off from the spinal cord to penetrate every part of the body.

Each vertebra has the same basic shape:

- the vertebral body or centrum;

- an arch surmounted by the dorsal spine;
- a pair of transverse processes of very variable size and shape;
- two pairs of articular surfaces.

The spinal, lateral and articular processes allow for the attachment of muscles and ligaments, and the body and arch protect the spinal cord.

Intervertebral Discs The vertebral column, also known as the backbone or spinal column, is a strong semi-flexible rod through which passes the spinal cord. The cervical, thoracic and lumbar vertebrae can move to varying degrees, but the sacrum is fixed. The coccygeal vertebrae of the tail can move, for example in swishing the tail. Between each vertebra from the second cervical to the sacrum are intervertebral discs. There are no discs between the atlas and axis. The discs form strong joints and help protect the spinal cord and absorb shock, such as when the horse lands after jumping. Each disc has an outer ring of fibrocartilage but no soft elastic pulpous part in the middle, unlike humans and dogs.

In horses, it has been suggested that degenerative disc disease does not occur because of the absence or poor development of this gelatinous nucleus pulposus in the disc and the fact that the discs are very thin in horses. It is thought that degeneration of the lumbosacral intervertebral disc (intervertebral disc disease (IVDD)) is a routine finding in older horses and that this may be found in up to 50% of veterans. Most bone spurs on the vertebrae are a result of damage from wear and tear and occur between the 10th and 17th thoracic vertebrae. This is the region of the thoracic spine where the greatest amount (although limited) of lateral bending and axial rotation occurs. IVDD has only recently been recognised in horses. Once damaged, the normally soft and cushioned disc can become hardened and calcified. Not all calcified discs will cause pain or disability. Many horses are predisposed to injury or damage due to weakened ligaments that hold the vertebrae and discs in place.

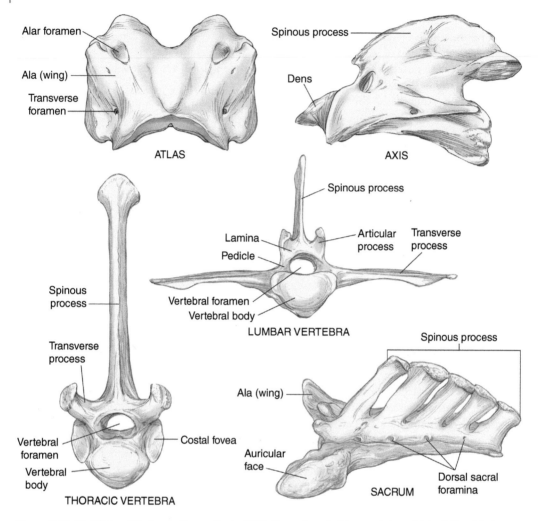

Figure 3.10 Vertebrae of the horse. *Source*: Baxter 2011. Reproduced with permission of John Wiley & Sons.

Cervical Vertebrae The horse's neck is a complex S-shaped structure and consists of seven cervical vertebrae (see Figure 3.8). The first is the atlas, which consists of a short tube with large wings; it articulates with the skull at the occiput, allowing the horse's head to nod. The horse's neck is able to stretch longer than most other herbivores. The wings of the atlas can be felt on either side of the neck below the poll and behind the jawbone. The second is the axis united to the atlas by a tooth-like projection, the odontoid process, which allows the head to move from side to side. The atlas and axis are different from the rest, that is, the five remaining cervical vertebrae (see Figure 3.9) which are some of the longest vertebrae in the horse's spine.

There are no intervertebral discs between the atlas and axis.

Over one-hundred muscles help support and move the seven bones of the horse's neck. These house the highly sensitive and important spinal cord and the peripheral nerves which intersect the vertebrae, before tracking down the forelegs. The long, strong ligament of the neck, the nuchal ligament, attaches to the axis; it helps hold up the horse's very heavy head and neck, and allows the head and neck to be raised and lowered. In fact, the horse carries its head higher than most other herbivores and this requires considerable muscular effort, hence the amount of muscle found in the neck. The neck constitutes 6% of the horse's bodyweight. The joints between the other cervical vertebrae enable the horse to bend its neck sideways and to arch its neck. The curves formed by the vertebrae are deep in the neck and do not follow the crest.

There is also a system of short stabilising muscles known as axial muscles which encase the vertebrae, keeping them in position. The long muscles work with the axial muscles to keep the horse's neck stable. The neck also houses the trachea, oesophagus, jugular vein and many tendons, ligaments and cartilage.

Spinal cord and peripheral nerve compression can occur due to congenital (present at birth) spine malformations, injuries that break or reshape the bone, degenerative joint disease or a combination of the above. A common symptom is ataxia, or a lack of coordination in the gaits. Other neurologic signs affect muscle strength, skin sensation and body awareness and usually accompany ataxia.

Peripheral nerve signs or 'referred pain' and paresthesia (pins and needles and numbness) are more difficult to diagnose in horses. A compressed or irritated nerve root in the neck can refer signs to the forelimb with or without local neck pain and it is therefore difficult to determine the presence and severity of referred pain from the neck into the forelimbs. In other words, some horses might display signs of poor performance or even lameness as a result of neuromuscular dysfunction originating in the neck.

Traumatic neck injuries do happen and are more often seen in jumping horses hitting fences head-on. Rotational falls, where the horse flips over its head, usually over a cross-country obstacle, can also cause serious trauma. Such falls can cause fractures, accelerate arthritic degeneration or compound the effects of developmental disease, such as vertebral malformations, with long-lasting, often fatal consequences.

A fractured vertebra may cause damage to the spinal cord, leading to ataxia and other neurologic disorders such as incontinence and tail weakness.

Overriding Dorsal Spinous Processes Overriding dorsal spinous processes (ORDSP) or 'kissing spines' is becoming increasingly discussed as a cause of poor performance or lameness in athletic horses. As a result, X-rays of the lateral spine are often requested for pre-purchase examinations. Many equine veterinarians are now being asked questions by owners concerning saddle fitting, fitness and so on. Treatment of this condition ranges from analgesia either by injection or oral and shockwave therapy. Recently, new surgical techniques have been devised to treat it.

ORDSP is only one potential cause of lameness and poor performance and does not always result in poor performance or gait alterations in horses that have the condition.

Thoracic Vertebrae The back consists of 18 thoracic vertebrae, five or six lumbar vertebrae, the sacrum and the coccygeal vertebrae. The thoracic vertebrae are typical vertebrae linked by cartilaginous pads called discs; the spinous processes are very large, giving the horse its pronounced withers and allowing extensive muscle and ligament attachment (see Figure 3.10). The withers are the highest point of the thoracic spine and are formed by the spinous processes of the third to tenth thoracic vertebrae. The withers are held firmly in place by ligaments between the spines and other muscles and ligaments attached to the spines, including the funicular portion of the nuchal ligament. The way the spinous processes are directed is of great importance to the athletic horse; there are two articulations, one between the discs and the bodies of the vertebrae, and the lateral articulations on each side of the vertebrae. The movement between the horse's thoracic vertebrae is strictly defined and limited in comparison to many other animals.

Lumbar Vertebrae The lumbar vertebrae make up the loin region and, as with the thoracic vertebrae, have a strictly defined and very limited degree of movement. In fact, apart from the neck and tail, the horse's back shows very little movement; some movement only is seen between the last thoracic and first lumbar vertebrae and between the first three lumbar vertebrae as previously discussed. The degree of movement depends on the thickness of the intervertebral discs, which are firmly attached to the vertebrae, almost like part of the bone that has not yet become calcified or bony. Indeed, as the horse ages it is common to find that the discs do become calcified, thus joining the vertebrae together. There may even be further outgrowths of bone acting as bridges across neighbouring vertebrae; two adjacent lumbar vertebrae may be joined by the transverse process on one side and not the other, and this will cause pain until both sides become fused.

Sacrum The sacrum (see Figure 3.10) is a composite bone made up of five vertebrae, situated beneath the loins in the croup region. The pelvic bones are attached to either side of it by the sacro-iliac joint.

Coccygeal Vertebrae There are usually 18 coccygeal or tail vertebrae, but the number can vary from 15 to 21 in number according to breed, and they decrease in size and complexity from first to last.

The total length of the spine is a series of curves, so that it is slightly arched at the upper end of the neck and concave above in the lower third of the neck (Figure 3.11). At the junction of the neck and the chest there is a marked change in direction, followed by a gentle curve, concave below, through the thoracic and lumbar region, which helps to support the horse's bodyweight. The dorsal spines of the thoracic vertebrae are held in position by strong ligaments. The design of the equine spine is similar to that of a suspension bridge and these curves give it the strength needed to carry the enormous weight of its gut (up to 200 kg in a 16.2-hh horse) and also in the mare, to enable carriage of the foetus and the associated fluid and membranes.

Sometimes large dips occur in the central area of the spine (Figure 3.12). This condition is known as lordosis or swayback (other terms include saddle-backed, hollow-backed, low in the back, 'soft' in the back or down in the back). It is a common back condition, particularly in older horses. Swayback is caused in part by a loss of muscle tone in both the back and the abdominal muscles, plus a weakening and stretching of the ligaments. It may be influenced by pregnancy and is sometimes seen in a broodmare that has had multiple foals.

Congenital lordosis is thought to be associated with incomplete development of thoracic vertebrae T5–T10 causing overextension of the vertebral joints. However, it is also common in older horses whose age leads to loss of muscle tone and stretched ligaments. A swayback is less able to support a rider. Short-backed horses may be more prone to kissing spines on dorsiflexion and long-backed horses more likely to suffer strain of soft tissues. These may be congenital or acquired. At walk the spine can be seen to move sideways, but at faster paces there is increased muscular resistance which minimises any movement. Above the spine the longissimus dorsi muscle and below the spine the psoas minor muscle contract to stop the horse flexing its back; when this synchronisation fails, for example if the horse falls, the back is vulnerable to damage.

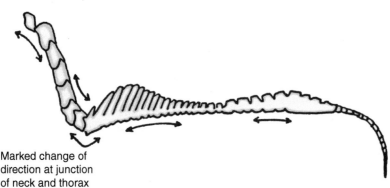

Figure 3.11 The spine is a series of curves.

Marked change of direction at junction of neck and thorax

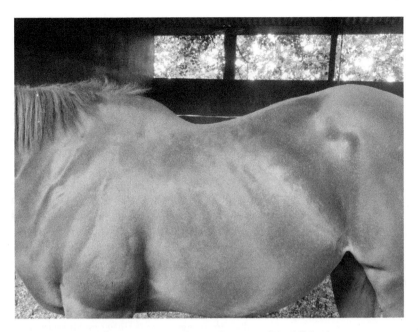

Figure 3.12 Dipped spine in a mare. *Source*: Courtesy of Harthill Stud.

The ligaments associated with the vertebrae include the supraspinous ligament, which runs along the top of the spines of the vertebrae and unites the summits of all lumbar and thoracic vertebrae. It divides to go up either side of the neck, becoming the nuchal ligament. The nuchal ligament consists of two parts:

- the funicular part is a rope-like ligament which supports the head and runs along the top of the neck;
- the lamellar part is a band attaching to the cervical vertebrae which restrains the movement of the dorsal spines and supports the weight of the head.

Joints of the Vertebral Column

The spine contains the smallest joints of the equine skeletal system, which are moved by some of the largest muscles of the horse's body, that is, those situated over the spine. There is a broad range of spinal movement, but it is nowhere near as flexible as the human spine.

In the horse's spine there are 48 small synovial joints and these joints are often overstressed, especially when the horse is moving very fast, such as racing, or over a wide range, such as dressage and show jumping. There is slightly more flexion in the thoracic part of the spine than the lumbar part in horses.

Ribs

Each thoracic vertebra carries a pair of ribs, and thus there are 18 pairs of ribs. Eight true ribs are attached to the sternum and ten pairs of false ribs are connected to the sternum indirectly via cartilage and form the costal arch. Indirect attachments give more freedom of movement. Ribs consist of a head, neck, tubercle, body and costochondral junction.

Sternum

The sternum or breastbone forms the floor of the chest and supports the true ribs. The rear of the sternum is drawn out into the xiphoid cartilage.

The Appendicular Skeleton

The appendicular skeleton is attached to the axial skeleton by the pelvic girdle and the pectoral girdle. However, the horse has no collar bone, so that the pectoral girdle is attached only by muscles and ligaments to the spine, ribs and sternum. This means that the forehand of the horse is designed to support the body and absorb concussion, not to propel the horse forwards.

Forelimb

The forelimb (Figure 3.13) consists of the following:

- scapula
- humerus
- radius and ulna
- carpus or knee
- three metacarpals (cannon and splint bones)
- three phalanges (long and pastern bones and the pedal bone)
- three sesamoid bones (the 'sesamoids' and the navicular bone).

Scapula

The scapula is a triangular, flattened bone which glides back and forth over the rib cage. There is no bony attachment between the scapula and the spine, so that the thorax is slung between the two scapulae, allowing the horse freedom of movement and compensating for the lack of flexibility of the spine. The length of the scapula will determine the slope of the shoulder and hence the length of stride of the horse. The scapula is divided lengthways by a prominent ridge called the scapular spine which can be felt through the skin. The supraspinatus muscle lies in front of the ridge and the infraspinatus muscle behind the ridge. The trapezius muscle and deltoid muscle are also attached to the scapular spine.

Humerus

The shoulder joint is formed between the scapula and the humerus. The humerus is one of the strongest bones in the body. The angulation of the humerus allows for shock absorption, and it is also the site of attachment for many muscles.

Radius and Ulna

Unlike the human, the radius and ulna of the horse (equivalent to our lower arm) are fused together to prevent any twisting of the horse's forearm. The ulna has become very small except for the olecranon process which forms the point of the elbow. The elbow joint itself is a hinge (ginglymus) joint which allows movement in one direction only.

Carpus (Knee)

The horse's knee is equivalent to the human wrist and consists of seven or eight small carpal bones; in the upper row are the radial, intermediate and ulnar carpals, with the pisiform bone or accessory carpal bone at the back of the knee (see Figure 3.13). The lower row consists of the first, second, third and fourth carpal bones. The knee is a hinge joint allowing movement in only one direction and the arrangement of the small carpal bones is designed to absorb shock.

Metacarpals

The three metacarpal bones are better known as the cannon bone and the two splint bones. The splint bones are a legacy from when the horse's ancestors had several toes, but while they do support the knee they are no longer weight-bearing. The cannon bone is capable of carrying substantial weight, having little spongy or cancellous bone surrounded by solid bone. The amount of 'bone' a horse has is determined by the circumference of the leg just below the knee and indicates the weight-carrying capacity of the horse.

Phalanges

The three phalanges are known as the long pastern, short pastern and pedal bone, and are equivalent to the human finger. The tendons from the muscles of the forearm attach to these bones, giving increased leverage and a powerful stride. The joint between the cannon bone and the long pastern bone is the fetlock joint, and is another hinge joint. It is

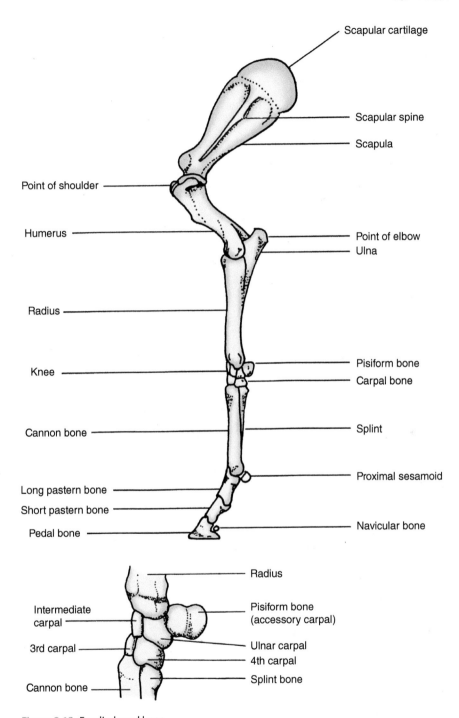

Scapular cartilage

Scapular spine

Scapula

Point of shoulder

Humerus

Point of elbow
Ulna

Radius

Knee

Pisiform bone

Carpal bone

Cannon bone

Splint

Proximal sesamoid

Long pastern bone

Short pastern bone

Navicular bone

Pedal bone

Radius

Intermediate
carpal

Pisiform bone
(accessory carpal)

3rd carpal

Ulnar carpal

4th carpal

Cannon bone

Splint bone

Figure 3.13 Forelimb and knee.

subjected to large amounts of stress and has a great deal of movement. The pastern joint is between the long and short pastern bones and has limited movement. The coffin joint is between the short pastern and the pedal bone and has a good range of movement.

Sesamoid Bones

The horse has three sesamoid bones; the proximal sesamoids, known as the 'sesamoids', are situated at the back of the fetlock joint, while the distal sesamoid or navicular bone is found inside the hoof at the

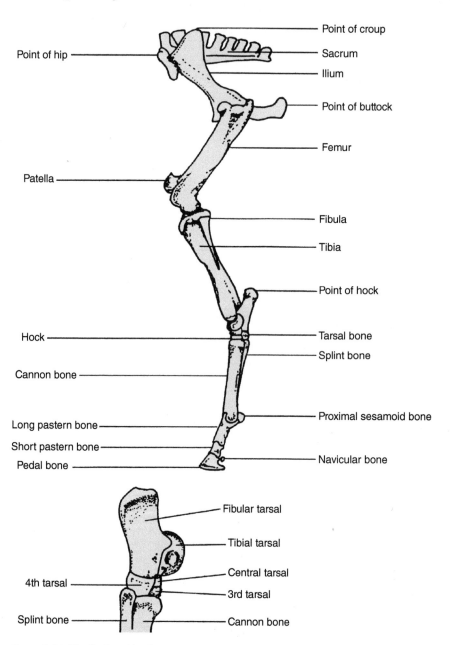

Figure 3.14 Hindlimb and hock.

back of the coffin joint. Their role is to act as pulleys, enabling the tendons that run over them to exert their pull on the phalanges.

Hindlimb

The hindlimb (Figure 3.14) has a bony attachment to the spine, allowing the propulsive forces to be transmitted to and along the spine to generate movement. The hindlimb consists of:

- pelvis
- femur
- tibia and fibula
- tarsus or hock
- three metacarpals (cannon and splint bones)
- three phalanges (long and short pastern bones and the pedal bone)
- three sesamoid bones (the 'sesamoids' and the navicular bone).

Pelvis

The pelvic girdle consists of the pelvic bones, the sacrum and the first three coccygeal vertebrae. Each half of the pelvis (Figure 3.15) is made up of three flat bones, the ilium, ischium and the pubis, which are fused into one. The upper portion of the pelvis, which is attached to the sacrum, is called the ilium. The front of the pelvic floor is the pubis and the rear portion is the ischium. All three bones meet at the acetabulum which articulates with the head of the femur to make the hip joint. The ilium is the largest bone and its outermost angle is seen as the tuber coxae – the point of the hip. Where the ilium attaches to the sacrum is the sacro-iliac joint which is characterised by strong muscle attachments. At the highest point of the hindquarters the two sides of the tuber sacrale form the croup. The points of

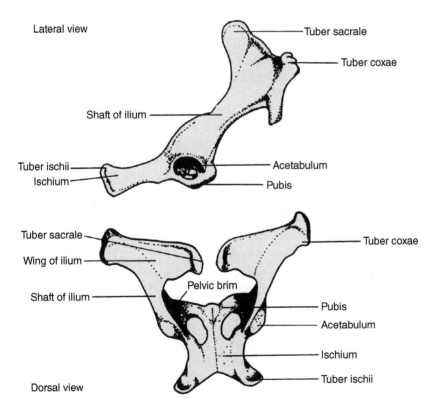

Figure 3.15 The pelvis.

the buttocks are the thickened ends of the ischium known as the tuber ischia.

The hip joint is deep in the hindquarter of the horse and is most easily seen when the hind leg is flexed. It is the joint between the pelvis and the femur and is capable of a wide range of movement. It acts to protect the internal organs, as a site for muscle attachment and to allow the efficient transfer of force to the spine.

Femur

The femur is a very strong bone designed to act as the medium between the hip joint and the stifle joint and is adapted for the attachment of the muscles of the hindquarter.

Tibia and Fibula

The tibia is a long bone running down and back between the stifle and the hock joints. The upper end provides attachment for the muscles acting on the hock and lower limb. The horse's fibula is so reduced in size as to be practically vestigial.

Tarsus (Hock)

The hock consists of six or seven short, flat tarsal bones arranged in three rows. In the upper row are the talus and the calcaneus, in the middle row is the central tarsus and below that the fused first and second tarsal and the third tarsal. The fourth tarsal occupies both the middle and lower row. A long bony process, the tuber calcis of the calcaneus, gives rise to the point of hock and guides the Achilles tendon of the gastrocnemius muscle over the hock, allowing tremendous leverage.

Below the hock the arrangement of bones is the same as in the forelimb. The patella is a sesamoid bone and the equivalent of the human kneecap. It is associated with the stifle – the joint between the femur and the tibia.

Stay Apparatus

See Chapter 16.

The Mechanics of Movement

Horses are able to perform exaggerated movements with training, such as seen in dressage horses. These are achieved through the action of muscles. Contractions where the length of muscle shortens and movement occurs are known as isotonic contractions. When muscle contracts against something immovable and does not shorten this is called isometric. Skeletal muscles are attached to bones by tendons. Muscles have two attachments, namely the origin and insertion, creating movement across joints when they contract. The amount and type of movement depends upon the individual joint and where the muscle is in relation to that joint. Muscles can only pull; they cannot push and therefore movement occurs through the action of opposing sets of muscles.

The skeleton acts as a system of leavers. The joints act as a fulcrum or pivot, the muscles exert the force and the weight of bone being moved represents the load. The flexion (bending) and extension (unbending) of the horse's limbs is caused by the action of antagonistic muscles. These work in pairs and their actions oppose each other. Every movement is coordinated and requires the use of force by the muscle. This is achieved by the actions of agonists, antagonists and synergists. The opposing action of agonists and antagonists working at a low level results in muscle tone. Either muscle in the pair may act as the agonist or prime mover, depending upon the movement required, that is, flexion or extension.

Joints

All vertebrates have a jointed skeleton, including horses. Joints in the skeleton arise where two bones meet, giving the skeleton flexibility and allowing movement. Most joints are moveable, but some such as those in the skull, sacrum and pelvis are immovable as they are fused. Ligaments bind bones together, while tough elastic, slightly stretchy tendons attach muscle to bone.

The function of joints is to allow movement and also to absorb the force of impact and transfer the force via cartilage to bone. Joints are the result of a complex process of development where several different tissues of the body interact. However, the basic structure of all joints is similar (Figure 3.16). The joint capsule is composed of two layers:

- an outer fibrous layer which is attached to the periosteum of the bone
- an inner synovial membrane which secretes joint oil or synovial fluid that supplies nutrition to the articular cartilage. The fluid also acts as a lubricant to the joint. The synovial membrane of a joint occasionally produces abnormal amounts of synovial fluid in response to low-grade trauma, resulting in conditions such as bog spavin and articular windgalls.

Joint or articular cartilage covers the ends of the bone to give protection. This cartilage does not have a blood or nerve supply, and thus damage to the cartilage does not result in pain. Any pain experienced by the horse is caused by inflammation of the synovial membrane and the joint capsule. Articular cartilage has limited ability to repair itself; thus damage to the cartilage is not completely repaired.

The joint capsule and its ligaments provide the joint with stability. Both are attached to the periosteum, the fine membrane covering the bone, and stretching of the ligaments can result in tearing of the periosteum, leading to pain and new bone formation.

The joints of the limbs below the knee and hock are essentially hinge joints which allow movement in only one direction. The capsular ligaments which support the joint are very strong strap-like ligaments that have very little stretch. A ligament that is forced to stretch by, for example, holding a joint open beyond normal limits, will become sprained, showing inflammation, pain and swelling.

Types of Joints

Functional classification of joints is based on the amount of movement:

- Synarthroses – no joint movement, relatively rigid (syndesmosis, synchondrosis).
- Amphiarthroses – a small amount of movement (symphysis).
- Diarthroses – a wide range of movement, monaxial, biaxial and triaxial (hinge, sliding, ball and socket, pivot and ellipsoid, all of which are synovial joints).

Structural classification of joints is as follows:

- fibrous – fixed
- cartilaginous
- synovial.

Fibrous Joints

Fixed or fibrous joints have no movement. They are made up of fibrous tissue between the ends of bones. They are key in equine

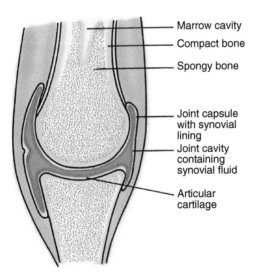

Marrow cavity

Compact bone

Spongy bone

Joint capsule with synovial lining

Joint cavity containing synovial fluid

Articular cartilage

Figure 3.16 Basic structure of a joint.

development as they allow the extension of individual bones during growth. Types of fibrous joints are described below.

- Suture – these fibrous joints consist of a thin layer of dense irregular connective tissue. They are gradually eliminated and once fixed following growth, they are classified as synarthrosis (immovable).
- Syndesmoses – facing areas of two bones, joined by connective tissue ligaments. They allow very limited movement, for example joints of the metacarpus. A gomphosis is the attachment of the tooth to the bone within its socket in the jaw (dentoalveolar joint) and is an example of a syndesmosis.
- Interosseous membrane – a substantial sheet of dense irregular connective tissue binding neighbouring long bones and permitting slight movement (amphiarthrosis).

Cartilaginous Joints

Cartilaginous joints are only slightly moveable. They consist of a pad of fibrocartilage between bones, such as that found between the vertebrae of the spine, and move by compression of the cartilage. There is no synovial cavity as the bones are held together by cartilage. Types of cartilaginous joints are described below.

- Synchondroses – the connecting material is hyaline cartilage, for example joints between epiphyses and diaphyses of juvenile long bones which disappear on maturity (see closure of growth or physeal plates). Permanent synchondroses – include the joint between the skull and the hyoid bone. Functionally they are immovable joints (synarthroses).
- Symphysis – a cartilaginous joint where the ends of the articulating bones are covered with hyaline cartilage and bones are connected by a broad flat disc of fibrocartilage. This type of joint is found in the pelvis and in the intervertebral joints. Functionally it is a slightly movable joint, that is, amphiarthrosis.

Synovial Joints

Synovial joints are articulated joints which are freely moveable. They are separated by a fluid-filled joint capsule, which is bound by a synovial membrane. The synovial membrane is a pink connective tissue sheet that is vascular and has a nervous supply. It may be unsupported (i.e. in the form of a pouch), or resting on an outer fibrous capsule, or separated from the capsule by pads of fat. There is not a continuous covering of cells. Cells that do exist produce the lubricant (aminoglycans) found in synovial fluid. Synovial fluid is produced by the synovial membrane and from blood plasma. Its function is to nourish and lubricate the articular cartilage. Joints of horses may contain as much as 20–40 ml of synovial fluid, which appears pale to light yellow in colour and is usually quite thick and viscous, due to containing hyaluronic acid.

Frequently, the synovial membrane is also reinforced by a fibrous capsule and strap-like ligaments. This restricts joint movement, providing stability to the joint. It also encloses bone and muscle insertions within the joint capsule and is supplied by blood vessels and a nerve supply.

Articular cartilage covers the articular surfaces and is made up of hyaline, although fibrocartilage or fibrous tissue may substitute. Articular cartilage does not have a blood or nerve supply and nutrients enter via diffusion from the synovial fluid and nearby blood vessels.

Some joints possess intracapsular discs or menisci, allowing complicated movements, for example the temperomandibular joint and the paired menisci of the stifle joint. There is limited response to injury and little repair capacity to articular cartilage. There are seven different types of synovial joint in horses:

- ball and socket (spheroidal joint)
- hinge
- gliding
- pivot
- ellipsoid
- condylar
- saddle.

Ball and socket joints are the most moveable, allowing all of the following movements: extension, flexion, adduction, abduction, rotation and circumduction. Examples are the shoulder and hip joints.

Hinge joints allow movement in one plane only, giving flexion and extension inhibited by collateral ligaments and/or bony protuberances. Examples are the elbow joint, joints between the phalanges, pedal bone, short pastern and long pastern bones.

In gliding joints the bones glide over each other and this is the least movable type of synovial joint. Examples are found in the carpals and tarsals.

Pivot joints allow movement round one axis and a rotational movement like a peg fitted into a ring. Examples are the atlas and axis, and the first two cervical vertebrae, which allow the horse's head to rotate to a certain extent.

Ellipsoid joints allow movement in two planes at right angles with limited rotation (e.g. the radiocarpal joint).

Condylar joints are knuckle-shaped condyles (a rounded projection on a bone, usually for articulation with another bone) which vary in distance from one another, allowing uniaxial movement with limited rotation (e.g. the femorotibial joint).

A saddle joint is a synovial joint where one of the bones forming the joint is shaped like a saddle with the other bone resting on it like a rider on a horse. Saddle joints provide stability to the bones while providing more flexibility than a hinge or gliding joint.

Movement of Joints

- Sliding joint – flat surfaces slide against each other, producing no change in orientation of their bodies.
- Rotation – a moving bone revolves around its own longitudinal axis.
- Flexion (palmar flexion) – the angle between two parts of a limb is reduced.
- Extension – the angle between two parts of a limb is increased.

- Overextension (aka dorsal flexion) – for example posture of equine fetlock standing at rest.
- Adduction – movement of bone toward the midline.
- Abduction – movement of bone away from the midline.
- Circumduction – a combination of flexion abduction, extension and adduction that allows a limb to move in a circular motion.

Ageing of Joints

Horses are athletic animals and for those involved in hunting, polo, eventing, show jumping and/or racing at speed or exaggerated athletic movements as seen in dressage the forces applied to joints can be excessive, particularly over time. Joints, particularly those in the limbs, can therefore be prone to injury and premature ageing. With age there is reduced production of synovial fluid and the cartilage becomes thinner, leading to degenerative changes. Many older horses have evidence of osteoarthritic changes in their joints, but some younger athletic horses also have these changes. Hyaluronic acid is sometimes used by veterinary surgeons as an injection into the joints to help improve lubrication.

It is not currently possible to cure osteoarthritis, but treatment may halt or slow the cycle of inflammation that brings further damage, ease pain and stiffness and/or support the regeneration of cartilage as much as is possible to keep the horse working and pain free.

Muscles

The horse's skeleton is incapable of movement on its own; all movements, from a simple flick of the tail to the most difficult dressage manoeuvre, are brought about by a complicated system of movements by skeletal muscles. Depending on how much subcutaneous fat a horse has, it is often possible to picture many of these muscles and to feel the faint grooves that represent the divisions between them. Entire males such as colts and stallions have more skeletal muscle than mares and fillies. All horses, regardless of breed, fitness and age, have the same arrangement of skeletal muscles, but some muscles may be better developed in particular horses due to their genetic muscle fibre type composition or specialist training. There are, however, three types of muscle found in the body, each of which has its own characteristics and functions:

- cardiac muscle
- smooth muscle
- skeletal muscle.

Cardiac Muscle

Cardiac muscle (Figure 3.17) is highly specialised and is found only in the heart, forming the majority of the heart wall. Under the microscope it appears striped or striated and has branching fibres that interconnect via intercalated discs that allow the heart to act as a unit. Cardiac muscle is involuntary, that is, not under conscious control of the horse.

The heart is composed of three major types of cardiac muscle – atrial muscle, ventricular muscle and neuromuscular muscle fibres – which provide a transmission system for rapid conduction of the cardiac excitatory signal throughout the heart. This means that these specialised cardiac muscle fibres must keep all of the heart muscles working together in rhythm. Of the three, ventricular muscle is by far the thickest and most powerful. This is because the ventricles are responsible for providing the most powerful thrust to propel blood out of the heart and around the whole body.

Cardiac muscle contractions are rapid and powerful, and the fibres do not tire. Cardiac muscle:

- is only found in the heart
- is striated with branching fibres
- enables the heart to work as a unit
- has rapid powerful contractions and does not tire
- is not under conscious control.

Smooth Muscle

Under the microscope, smooth muscle does not appear striated and cells are spindle-shaped with a central nucleus (Figure 3.18). Smooth muscle is not under conscious control. The stimuli for contraction

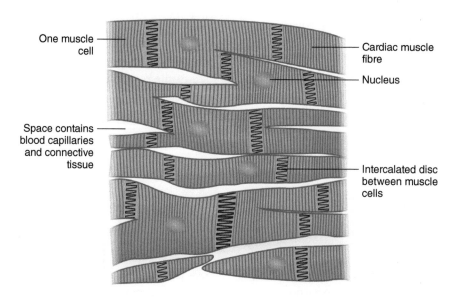

One muscle cell

Cardiac muscle fibre

Nucleus

Space contains blood capillaries and connective tissue

Intercalated disc between muscle cells

Figure 3.17 Cardiac muscle.

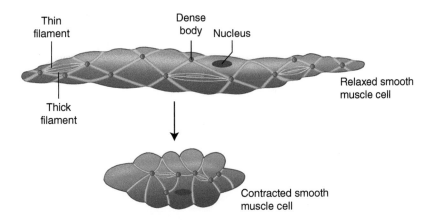

Figure 3.18 Smooth muscle.

vary and include both nervous stimuli and chemical stimuli such as hormones. Smooth muscle is spread throughout the body organs, especially those of the gut. Contraction of a smooth muscle fibre is much slower and lasts much longer than that of skeletal muscle fibres.

There are two functional categories of smooth muscle:

- multi-unit (consisting of individual fibres with their own motor nerve ending)
- single-unit (visceral) types.

Multi-unit smooth muscle occurs in the walls of some of the largest arteries and large pulmonary air passages, in the pilo-erector muscles of the hair follicles in the skin and in the internal muscles of the horse's eye. Each motor unit contracts independently of the others, hence the name of this muscle type. Multi-unit smooth muscle fibres have few if any gap junctions. The cells rely on individual nervous stimulation and respond to the individual stimulation on an independent basis. This is very similar to skeletal muscle cells.

Single-unit smooth muscle is more widespread. It occurs in most blood vessels and in the digestive, respiratory, urinary and reproductive tracts – thus it is also called visceral muscle. Single-unit smooth muscles are held together via electric adjacent cells. The electrical synapse of these muscles

creates numerous gap junctions. This means the muscle fibres act as a single unit.

Smooth muscle can sustain rhythmic contractions for quite long periods, which allows for movement such as the peristaltic waves of the gut that propel the digesta along its length. Smooth muscle:

- is non-striated
- consists of spindle-shaped cells with a central nucleus
- is not under conscious control
- lines body cavities and blood vessels.

Skeletal Muscle (Voluntary or Striated Muscle)

Skeletal muscle (Figure 3.19) can be seen grossly as muscles under the skin that are influenced through horses working. Horses have unusually large muscle masses compared to many other mammals, especially TB sprinters. Approximately 53% of the total body mass is taken up by muscle in horses. Under the microscope, skeletal muscle, also known as striated or voluntary muscle, appears striped and it is under conscious control. Each skeletal muscle is a separate organ organised into bundles of muscle cells or fibres. Each fibre is a single muscle cell with many nuclei and each fibre is also a bundle of smaller myofibrils that are very specifically arranged in a lengthways manner.

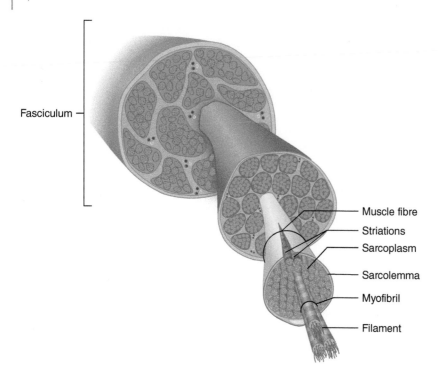

Fasciculum

Muscle fibre
Striations
Sarcoplasm
Sarcolemma
Myofibril
Filament

Figure 3.19   A skeletal muscle fibre. *Source*: Peate 2011. Reproduced with permission of John Wiley & Sons.

Each myofibril is further arranged into two kinds of microfilaments, namely thick and thin, which overlap, forming light and dark bands, giving the skeletal muscle its striated appearance. Each sarcomere is bound by the dark z lines (which form the borders of the sarcomere) and a sarcomere is one complete contractile unit.

All muscle fibres are supplied by branches of motor neurons which terminate in a motor end plate (also known as the neuromuscular junction). The motor neurons and all the fibres it innervates are known as a motor unit and each one may contain several hundred fibres. The response of the muscle is not always the same – there are grades of response – and this is achieved by varying the number of motor units that are active at any one time. Individual muscles are also surrounded by connective tissue which helps protect them and keep them separate from other tissues such as skin and bone. Skeletal muscle is either striated or under conscious control.

When muscles contract they do so by shortening their length; when they relax there is an increase in length. Total relaxation, however, never occurs, a slight contraction in one muscle being counter-balanced by slight contraction in another, leading to tension known as muscle tone. Muscle tone means that muscles are always ready for action – this is important in an animal such as the horse, whose main means of survival is fight or flight.

Each myofibril is composed of sarcomeres which are crossed by regular bands that give rise to the striations seen under the microscope. The lighter coloured areas are the 'I' bands which alternate with darker 'A' bands. The bands are made up of proteins called actin (A band) and myosin (I band). Electrical impulses from the nerves supplying the muscle cause the thin filaments of actin to slide over the thick filaments of myosin to shorten the whole muscle (Figure 3.20).

Within a myofibril the thin filaments are held in place by Z-lines (see Figure 3.20). An action potential arriving at the motor end plate sets off a series of events, causing the thin and thick filaments to slide past each other, causing contraction or shortening of the muscle fibre. The sarcomere and the I-band shorten and the H-band is seen to shorten or even disappear (under the microscope).

A single muscle fibre may contract fully or not at all in response to an action potential. This is known as the all-or-none law of muscle contraction. If the stimulus is too weak to produce an action potential then the muscle fibre does not respond. However, as mentioned previously, skeletal muscles as a whole can produce varying levels of contraction within a muscle by varying the number of motor units that are active at any one time. These graded responses are achieved by changing the frequency of nervous stimulation and the number and size of motor units recruited. Muscles contract maximally when action potentials arrive at a rapid rate and a large number of motor units are recruited at the same time. This sliding motion is known as the sliding filament model.

The Sliding Filament Model

The sliding of thick and thin filaments over each other during contraction is possible due to their structure and arrangement. Cross-bridges or heads are studded into the ends of the thick myosin filaments, linking the thin actin filaments next to them. The thin filaments also contain a regulatory protein complex, so when the cross-bridges of the thick filaments connect to the thin filaments this results in a change of shape which moves one filament over the other. The cross-bridge formation is essential and this requires:

- ATP – on the myosin;

- calcium ions released from the sarcoplasmic reticulum following an action potential.

As these cross-bridges with sarcomeres attach and detach, they shorten the muscle cell as follows:

- Binding sites on actin molecules (to which myosin heads will relocate) are blocked by a complex of two proteins – tropomyosin and troponin.
- Before the muscle contracts, ATP binds to the heads of the myosin molecules, putting them in a high energy state.
- An arriving action potential causes the sarcoplasmic reticulum to release calcium ions, which bind to troponin, causing the movement of the blocking complex and thereby exposing the myosin binding sites on the actin filament.
- The heads of the cross-bridging myosin molecules now attach to these binding sites on the actin filament. This requires the use of ATP. Energy release from ATP creates a change in the actin–myosin cross-bridge, resulting in a bending action or the power stroke. This makes the actin filaments slide past the myosin filaments towards the centre of the sarcomere.
- New ATP attaches to the myosin molecules, releasing them from the binding sites on the actin molecules and therefore preparing for a repeat movement.

Muscle Anatomy

The musculature of horses consists of deep postural muscles or stabilising muscles. Deep postural muscles keep the axial skeleton in place, whereas stabilising muscles produce movement via the appendicular skeleton. Postural muscles such as those holding the spinal vertebrae in place appear to have mainly slow twitch type 1 muscle fibres (see 'Muscle Fibre Types'). These postural muscles are those required to hold the horse in an outline, which riders aim to improve by schooling.

Skeletal muscles enable the horse to adjust to the surrounding environment and make

(a)

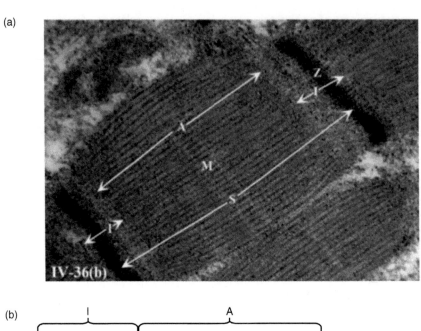

(b)

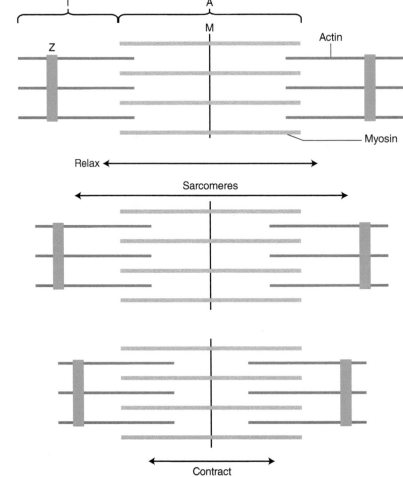

Figure 3.20 (a) Contractile units in a myofibril in human muscle. *Source*: Hossler 2014. Reproduced with permission of John Wiley & Sons.

necessary movements such as grazing and running. They are attached to, and hence move, various parts of the skeleton and body. There are approximately 700 separate skeletal muscles in the horse's body, making up about one-third of its total weight (Figures 3.21 and 3.22).

Muscles create movement by acting across joints. There are two sets of muscles: flexors, which are placed behind the bone and pull it backwards, bending the joint, and extensors, which are placed in front of the bone and pull it forwards, straightening out the joint from its bent position. Remember that muscles not only produce movement, but also control and limit normal movement and prevent undesirable movements.

Each end of the muscle tapers from a larger muscle belly into a tendon – fibrous tissue which is continuous with the connective tissue of the muscle at one end and blends with the thin membrane covering the bone (periosteum) at the other. When a muscle contracts, the fibres within it shorten and exert, via the tendon, a pull on the skeleton. Muscles are often large and bulky, so tendons help concentrate their pull onto a small area of the bone. The horse is unusual in that it has no muscle below the knee and hock; in order to move the hoof, the muscles have to act from a distance and their power is transmitted by cord-like tendons which allow the limbs to remain streamlined and lightweight. The movement of the knee (carpal joint), fetlock and pastern joints is produced by the muscles of the forearm. Muscles that move the limb away from the body are called abductors, while those that carry the limb towards the body are adductors.

Muscle bellies vary in size and shape; some are large, flat sheets, such as the latissimus dorsi muscle, others are long and strap-like,

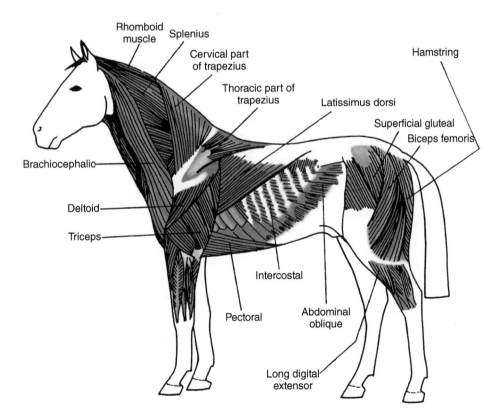

Figure 3.21 Superficial muscles.

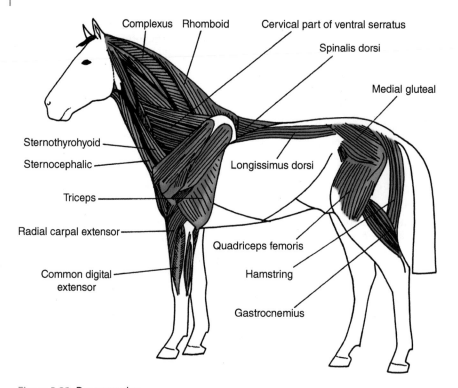

Figure 3.22 Deep muscles.

for example the brachiocephalic muscle. In both of these cases the fibres that make up the muscle belly run parallel to the long axis of the muscle. In other muscles, for example the common digital extensor muscle of the forearm, the individual fibres run obliquely to the long axis, with the muscle belly attached to either side of the tendon. These are called pennate muscles because they resemble a feather with the barbs radiating out from the quill. The length of the muscle fibres within the muscle belly determines the range of movement possible, while the power of contraction is due to the number of fibres present. Thus the long thin muscles allow substantial extension and retraction but cannot exert much force. The shorter pennate muscles do not allow as great a range of movement, but because there are a large number of fibres these muscles have greater strength.

In order for muscles to produce movement they must be attached at both their ends.

These ends are sometimes classified as the 'origin' and the 'insertion', the origin being the least movable of the two ends, so that when the muscle contracts the insertion end is brought closer to the origin. However, in the brachiocephalic muscle either end can be the origin or the insertion; if the forearm is kept still and the head dipped, the insertion is at the back of the head and the origin at the base of the neck. If the head is kept still and the forearm moved, then the attachment at the head becomes the origin and that at the forearm becomes the insertion.

Muscles are always arranged in opposing groups which perform opposite actions; this results in smooth and even movements. Muscles use energy to contract but do not have a way of stretching themselves again; instead the contraction of the opposing muscle is used to relax the tensed muscle. Thus as one group contracts, the other relaxes to a corresponding degree; if the splenius at the top of the neck contracts, the head is lifted but the sternocephalic on the underside of the neck acts in opposition so that the degree of head-lifting is controlled.

The name often describes the main action of the muscle; for example, the digital extensor extends the toe. Some muscles are named after their places of attachment; the brachiocephalic, for example, extends from the arm (brachium) to the head (cephalic).

Muscles of the Neck and Shoulder

Table 3.1 shows all the muscles of the neck and shoulder and the main muscles are discussed below. In the absence of a bony attachment, the muscles of the shoulder help to tie the limb to the body. Bearing in mind that two-thirds of the horse's bodyweight is taken on the forehand, these muscles act as weight supporters and shock absorbers.

Brachiocephalic

Behind the lower jaw or mandible lies the parotid gland, the largest of the salivary glands. Below and behind the ear the parotid gland meets the brachiocephalic muscle. The brachiocephalic muscle is a long, flattened muscle arising from the mastoid process of the temporal bone behind the ear, the wing of the atlas and the transverse processes of the second, third and fourth cervical vertebrae. The muscle runs down the length of the neck and inserts onto the humerus, forming the upper boundary of the jugular groove. When the muscle contracts it pulls the forearm forwards, and the position of the horse's head will affect its efficiency. Horses move more freely in front when the head and neck are extended, unlike the position demanded of the dressage horse. It is a powerful muscle with a two-way action: when the head is extended and the neck held firmly by its own muscles, contraction of the brachiocephalic carries the arm and knee forward; when the horse is standing still, contraction helps turn the head.

- Origin – wing of atlas.
- Insertion – humerus.

- Acts on the cervical vertebrae, extends the shoulder joint and produces sideways movement of the head and neck.

Sternocephalic

The sternocephalic muscle or sternomandibularis is a long, narrow muscle which extends from the sternum to the jaw, forming the lower boundary of the jugular groove. Underneath the neck the trachea can be felt through the thin sternothyroid muscles. The oesophagus lies on the left side along the upper surface of the trachea and can be seen dilating when the horse swallows food or water.

- Origin – sternum.
- Insertion – back of jaw.
- Flexes the head and neck forward and down.

Splenius
- Origin – thoracic vertebrae.
- Insertion – wing of atlas and cervical vertebrae.
- Flexes the cervical vertebrae to lift the head and to turn the head and neck from side to side.

Trapezius

The trapezius is a flattened triangular sheet of superficial muscle, the base of which arises in the area of the neck, withers and thorax from the funicular part of the ligamentum nuchae and the supraspinous ligament back to the tenth thoracic vertebra. The point of the muscle inserts into the spine of the scapula.

Trapezius – Cervical Part
- Origin – cervical vertebrae.
- Insertion – scapular.
- Draws the scapula up and back to lift the shoulder.

Trapezius Muscle – Thoracic Part
- Origin – thoracic vertebrae.
- Insertion – scapula.
- Draws the scapula up and back to lift the shoulder.

Table 3.1 Muscles of the neck and shoulder.

	Brachiocephalic	Sternocephalic	Splenius
Location			
Joint action	Cervical vertebrae; flexor laterally extends shoulder joint	Flexor of cervical vertebrae and inclines to one side	Lateral flexor of cervical vertebrae
Body action	Sideward movement of head and neck, when acts singly	Flexes head and neck forwards and downwards	Elevates head and turns head and neck to one side
Origin	Wing of atlas and mastoid process, temporal bone, nuchal crest	Manubrium of sternum and cariniform cartilage	Spines of 4th to 6th thoracic vertebrae
Insertion	Humerus – deltoid tuberosity and fascia shoulder and arm	Mandible to caudal border of ramus	Nuchal crest, transverse vertebral processes of 3rd to 5th cervical mastoid process and wing atlas
Nerve supply	Spinal accessory nerve, cervical nerve, axillary nerve	Spinal accessory nerve, 11th cranial nerve, ventral branch	Last six cervical nerves, dorsal branches
Blood supply	Inferior cervical artery, carotid artery, vertebral artery	Carotid artery	Deep cervical artery, dorsal artery
Development problems	Gait not level in front: worse on turns and circles; not going forwards, choppy strides	Overdeveloped: horse takes a pull; no control of athletic performance	Stiff neck in lateral flexion; tight neck

	Trapezius	Rhomboideus	Multifidus cervicus	Longissimus capitis
Location				
Joint action	Draws scapula upwards and backwards	Draws scapula upwards and forwards	Rotates head to opposite side of flexion	Rotate atlas
Body action	Lifts shoulder	Elevates shoulder	Extends neck and flexes to side of contraction	Extends head and neck, flexes head and neck laterally if acting singly
Origin	Dorsal midline and supraspinous ligament above 3rd cervical to 10th thoracic vertebrae	Occiput – dorsal midline of neck thoracic spine 2–7	Last five cervical vertebrae articular processes	Transverse processes of 1st two thoracic vertebrae
Insertion	Cervical part inserts along whole scapular spine, thoracic part only along proximal part of spine	Scapular cartilage – medial surface on dorsal border	Cervical vertebra – spinous and articular processes	Mastoid process wing of atlas, tendon in common with splenius and brachiocephalicus
Nerve supply	Spinal accessory nerve, dorsal branch	6th and 7th cervical nerves, ventral branches	Last six cervical nerves, dorsal branches	Last six cervical nerves, dorsal branches
Blood supply	Dorsal artery, deep cervical artery	Dorsal artery, deep cervical artery	Vertebral artery	Vertebral artery and deep cervical artery
Development problems	Underdeveloped: dip in neck, little lifting of shoulder or forehand, lack of coordination and forward movement	Loss of activity in shoulders/forehand. Affects coordination; stiff/tight muscles cannot stretch	Resistance in neck action, feels tight, poor contact with bit	Head unlevel; neck tight and stiff. One side difficult to flex and does not take contact. Head shaking, unsteady. Cannot extend head

(Continued)

Table 3.1 (Continued)

	Brachiocephalicus	Supraspinatus	Infraspinatus	Subscapularis
Joint action	Extensor	Extensor and support – acts as lateral ligament	Supports and stabilizes, acts as lateral ligament	Support; adducts humerus
Body action	Protracts forelimb, raises shoulder and pulls it forward	Advances forelimb	Abducts forearm and rotates outwards	Adductor of forelimb; prevents limb moving outwards
Origin	Wing of atlas and mastoid process, nuchal crest	Scapula – cartilage and spine; supraspinous fossa	Scapula – infra-spinous fossa and cartilage	Subscapular fossa, medial side
Insertion	Humerus – above deltoid tuberosity and distal crest, elongated line attachment	Humerus – lateral tuberosity	Humerus – caudal part of lateral tuberosity	Humerus – medial tuberosity
Nerve supply	Spinal accessory nerve and dorsal and ventral branches; axillary nerve, cervical nerve	Suprascapular nerve	Subscapular nerve	Subscapular nerve
Blood supply	Inferior cervical artery, carotid artery, vertebral artery	Suprascapular artery	Circumflex scapular artery	Subscapular artery
Development problems		Causes shoulder tightness or joint instability		
Location	Superficial pectoral	Deep pectoral	Coracobrachialis	Deltoideus
Joint action	Supporter	Pulls humerus back	Flexes shoulder joint; holds joint in apposition	Flexes shoulder joint
Body action	Adductors of forelimb	Retractor and adductor; helps raise thorax relative to limb	Adducts arm, supports forelimb	Abducts forelimb
Origin	Sternum – xiphoid and costal cartilage	Sternum – xiphoid cartilage, cartilages ribs 1–4	Scapula – cranial border of coracoid process	Scapula – lateral caudal edge
Insertion	Humerus – humeral crest and antebrachial fascia	Humerus – medial tuberosity	Humerus – cranio-medial part of shaft proximal end	Humerus – deltoid tuberosity
Nerve supply	Pectoral nerve	Pectoral nerve	Musculocutaneous nerve	Axillary nerve
Blood supply	Cranial circumflex humeral artery	Intercostal artery, internal and external thoracic, inferior cervical, anterior circumflex	Anterior circumflex artery	Subscapular artery
Development problems		Short stride and inability to spread over a fence. Sore on girthing up		

Rhomboideus

Underneath the trapezius is the rhomboideus which ties the scapula into the sides of the spinous processes of the thoracic vertebrae and the ligamentum nuchae. Like the trapezius, it has cervical and thoracic parts.

- Origin – occiput.
- Insertion – top of scapula.
- Lifts the shoulder up and forward.

Deltoideus

The deltoideus arises from the scapular spine; it can be felt on the outside of the shoulder joint as it runs down to meet the brachiocephalic muscle before inserting on the humerus.

- Origin – scapula.
- Insertion – humerus.
- Flexes the shoulder joint to abduct the forelimb.

Triceps

The triceps is made up of three muscles running from the scapula to the point of the elbow. They make up a rounded muscle mass lying alongside the ribs just above the elbow joint. The long head of the triceps originates on the scapula and flexes the shoulder as well as extending the elbow joint. The lateral and medial heads are shorter and originate on the humerus and extend the elbow joint.

- Origin – scapula/humerus.
- Insertion – olecranon process (point of elbow).
- Extends the elbow joint.

Muscles of the Trunk

The trunk consists of the back and loins, the chest and the barrel or abdomen. Table 3.2 shows the muscles of the trunk.

Latissimus Dorsi

The latissimus dorsi lies behind the shoulder, covering the side of the chest and extending up onto the back. It has a broad origin at the midline in the thoracic and lumbar regions which inserts on the humerus.

- Origin – thoracic/lumbar vertebrae.
- Insertion – humerus.
- Flexes the shoulder joint and draws the scapula down and back, retracting the forelimb.

Pectorals

The pectoral muscles pass down and out from the sternum to insert on the humerus to form a triangular sheet with the base on the sternum and the apex on the humerus. The superficial pectorals are easily seen on the front of the chest.

- Origin – sternum.
- Insertion – humerus.
- Supports and pulls the humerus back so that the forelimb is adducted.

Muscles of the Forearm

Digital Extensor

The muscle mass at the front of the forearm originates on the humerus and radius. These are known as the digital extensor muscles and their role is to carry the limb and foot forward. The extensor carpi radialis acts on the knee and the common digital extensor acts on the knee and digit (foot).

- Origin – upper ends of radius and ulna.
- Insertion – via digital extensor tendons to long pastern, short pastern and pedal bones.

Digital Flexor

The muscle mass at the back of the forearm originates on the humerus and point of the elbow. It includes the muscles that flex the knee, fetlock and foot. The tendons of the flexor muscles run down the lower limb to influence the bones of the limb and effect movement.

- Origin – upper ends of radius and ulna.
- Insertion – via superficial and deep digital flexor tendons to short pastern bone and pedal bone.

Table 3.2 Muscles of the trunk.

	Latissimus dorsi	Seratus ventralis	Levatores costarum	Longissimus costarum
Location				
Joint action	Draws scapula down and back, also draws humerus up and back; supports dorsal part of thorax; flexes shoulder joint	Cervical and thoracic part acts as 'sling' for trunk	Rotation and lateral flexion of spine	Extends spine; depresses and retracts ribs; expiration
Body action	Retracts forelimb and draws trunk forwards when limb fixed	Lifts body in relation to scapula; suspends trunk between scapulae	Draws ribs forwards for inspiration	Lateral flexion of trunk
Origin	Thoracic spines, withers and an aponeurosis continuous with thoracolumbar fascia over caudal thorax	Ribs – lateral surfaces of 1st to 9th	Transverse processes of thoracic vertebrae	Lumbar transverse processes last 15 ribs – anterior lateral surfaces lumbodorsal fascia
Insertion	Humerus – teres tuberosity	Scapula – serrated face on medial surface	Lateral surfaces and anterior borders of upper ends of ribs	Posterior borders of ribs; transverse process of last cervical vertebra
Nerve supply	Thoracodorsal nerve	Cervical nerves – 5th to 8th	Intercostal nerve	Thoracic nerve
Blood supply	Subscapular artery, intercostal artery, lumbar artery	Dorsal artery, vertebral artery, intercostal artery	Intercostal artery	Intercostal artery
Development problems	←Stiff in forehand; shows in turns and circles as stiffness→		←Causes sore, tight backs and a stiff wooden feel to the rider→	

Muscles of the Abdomen

The four layers of the abdominal muscles are strong, extensive muscles which form most of the abdominal wall. They support the digestive and reproductive organs. By compressing the abdomen they aid in defection, urination, expiration, coughing and parturition. They also flex the trunk laterally.

Intercostal Muscles

The intercostal muscles and other deeper muscles are responsible for the movements involved with breathing in and out. The external intercostals extend downward and backward from each rib to the next rib back. Their action increases the size of the thorax by rotating the ribs up and back. The internal intercostals lie beneath the external intercostal muscle and extend from each rib down and forward to the next rib in front. They rotate the ribs backwards, decreasing the size of the rib cage and thorax.

- Origin – thoracic vertebrae.
- Insertion – ribs.

Longissimus Dorsi

The longissimus dorsi is the largest and longest muscle in the body. Along with other muscles, it forms the contours of the horse's back. These muscles lie above the spine and between the processes of the vertebrae, extending longitudinally from the croup towards the withers.

- Origin – pelvis/sacrum.
- Insertion – thoracic vertebrae.
- This is the muscle on which the saddle, and hence the rider, sits. Its role is to transmit to the forehand the propulsion generated by the hindlimbs.

Muscles of the Hindlimb

The hindquarters extend out and back from the point of the croup and consist of a mass of muscle clothing the pelvis and femur and running down the thigh to the hock and lower leg. Table 3.3 shows the muscles of the hindlimb.

Gluteal

The gluteal muscles make up the bulk of the muscle mass that gives the quarters their rounded appearance. The gluteals arise from the shaft of the ilium and insert onto the femur.

- Origin – pelvis.
- Insertion – femur.
- Strong hip extensors involved in rearing, kicking and galloping.

Biceps Femoris

The hind part of the quarters is made up of a muscle mass called the biceps femoris extending from the sacral and coccygeal vertebrae to attach to the femur and stifle joint.

- Origin – sacral vertebrae.
- Insertion – femur.
- Extends and abducts the hindlimb; in other words, it is involved with propulsion, rearing and kicking.

Semitendinosus

The semitendinosus muscle is a long muscle extending along the rear of the biceps femoris down the back of the thigh. The division between these two muscles is known as the poverty line and is clearly seen in thin and fit horses.

- Origin – pelvis.
- Insertion – tibia.
- Extends the hip and hock and flexes the stifle so that the limb is rotated inwards and provides propulsion. These muscles make up the hamstring group and are important in locomotion.

Digital Extensor

Below the stifle the digital extensor and hock flexor muscles make up the gaskin or second thigh.

- Origin – femur.
- Insertion – lower limb.
- One of the muscles of the second thigh that attaches to the tendons of the lower leg, transmitting movement to the toe.

Table 3.3 Muscles of the upper hindlimb.

	Biceps femoris	Semitendinosus	Gastrocnemius	Gluteus medius
Location				
Joint action	Extends hip joint; flexes stifle joint; main belly flexes hock; anterior part extends stifle	Extends hip and hock and flexes stifle	Flexes hock	Extends hip joint
Body action	Extends and abducts hindlimb; propulsion; rearing; kicking	Propulsion of trunk; rotates limb inwards; rearing	Adducts hindlimb	Abducts limb; strong hip extensor; rearing; kicking; propulsion
Origin	Ischiatic spine; tuber ischium; sacral vertebrae; sacroiliac ligaments	Tuber ischium – mid-ventral area; illium – mid shaft	Femur	Illium – gluteal surface and crest; aponeurosis of longissimus lumborum
Insertion	Femur – 3rd trochanter, patella and lateral ligament; crest, crural fascia to hock	Tibial crest and fascia part joins tarsal tendon of biceps which attaches to tuber calcis	Hock via Achilles tendon	Femur – trochanter major
Nerve supply	Posterior gluteal nerve; sciatic nerve and branches; caudal, gluteal and peroneal nerves	Great sciatic nerve	Great sciatic nerve	Cranial and gluteal nerve
Blood supply	Gluteal artery and obturator branch; deep femoral artery; posterior femoral artery	Posterior gluteal artery; obturator artery; deep femoral artery; posterior femoral artery	Posterior gluteal artery; obturator artery; femoral artery	Gluteal artery; ileolumbar artery; iliacofemoral artery
Development problems	———	Shortening of forward stride; resists lateral movements; discomfort in hind joints		⟶

Gastrocnemius

The gastrocnemius runs down the back of the limb ending in a powerful tendon. It is associated with the tendon of the deeper lying superficial flexor muscle and the combined tendon is palpable above the hock as the Achilles' tendon. The tendon of the gastrocnemius attaches to the hock, while the superficial flexor tendon runs over the hock and down the back of the limb to the foot.

- Origin – femur.
- Insertion – hock.
- Attached to the Achilles tendon (one of the largest tendons in the body) and moves the hock.

Table 3.4 Slow twitch versus fast twitch muscle.

Characteristic	Slow twitch	Fast twitch
Colour	Red	White
Diameter	Small	Large
Rate of contraction	Slow	Fast
Rate of ATP production	Slow	Fast
Metabolism	Aerobic – high oxidative	Anaerobic – low oxidative
Power	Low	High
Fatigue rate	Slow	Fast
Reduce lactate	Yes	No

The Importance of Muscle Fibres in Equine Performance

Muscle Fibre Types

There are several different types of fibre within each muscle, but there are two basic fibre types, namely fast and slow twitch muscle fibres (Table 3.4). This is the same for horses and humans and has been studied using a technique called muscle biopsy, a safe and painless way of taking tiny samples of living muscle tissue for study under the microscope.

Initially, muscle fibre types are identified by colour; red muscle is associated with long-term or endurance work (chickens, for example, have dark leg meat and they use their legs for standing on all day). This dark red colour reflects the high myoglobin content and consequently the muscle's ability to store and use large amounts of oxygen; it is known as high oxidative muscle. The breast meat of chickens, on the other hand, is white. This muscle is used for power, for example getting a chicken off the ground and flying. This muscle has a lesser ability to use oxygen and is known as low oxidative muscle.

More scientifically, muscle fibres can be divided into two major groups depending on their contractile behaviour, that is, how fast they contract and relax. Identification is via muscle biopsy and uses the myosin ATPase staining process in the laboratory.

- Type I – slow twitch muscle has a slower contraction time and a greater ability to use oxygen (highly oxidative), which means that it has less power but can work steadily for long periods of time (i.e. endurance). Arabs have more type I fibres.
- Type II – fast twitch muscle has fast, powerful contractions. Fast twitch fibres differ in their ability to use oxygen.
- Type IIA fibres are both high and low oxidative. These can generate power and fibres are capable of utilising both aerobic and anaerobic metabolism to produce energy for work for a longer time. Type II A fibres are used to maintain speed.
- Type IIB fibres are low oxidative, meaning they are highly anaerobic. These fibres are used to give explosive power rapidly, for example for rapid acceleration and jumping. These tend to fatigue quickly.
- A further type IIC may be found in regenerating muscle and contains both fast and slow twitch myosin.

There is another classification system of muscle fibre types that is currently very expensive to use, namely myosin heavy chain (MHC) protein, where horse MHC protein is compared to rat MHC protein. The classifications in these cases are I, IIA and IIX.

Fast twitch, high oxidative fibres (type IIA) can generate power but also have a good ability to use oxygen and can therefore continue working for long periods of time. This makes these fibres very important to horses that need to sustain speed over long distances.

Muscle Fibre Recruitment

Most muscles consist of a mixture of these three fibre types. During muscle contraction it is unlikely that all the muscles need to exert maximum strength; in other words, not all the fibres in one muscle are stimulated at once. There is an orderly selection of muscle fibres depending on the amount of exertion; for walking and standing, only slow twitch fibres are used, but as the speed increases, fast twitch, high oxidative fibres are recruited, and when the horse is accelerating, galloping and jumping the fast twitch, low oxidative fibres are brought into play.

Muscle fibres are usually recruited in the following order: type I, type IIA, type IIB. To maintain posture or outline, mainly type I and type IIB are recruited at rest and at slow speeds. For speed and acceleration, then type IIB are recruited for sprinting and jumping. For endurance horses that would mainly use type I and type IIB, during a long event when glycogen is very much depleted then type IIA may be recruited later too.

Different muscles throughout the individual horse's body contain different muscle fibre types depending upon the function of that muscle. The muscles of the horse's hindquarters will have a higher number of type II fibres for propelling the horse forward. Muscles moving the forelimbs are more supportive and therefore have more type I muscles than the hindquarters. Even within a muscle the muscle fibres are not randomly placed, there are more type II on the outside than the inside of the muscle.

Table 3.5 Slow twitch fibres in different breeds.

Type of horse	Percentage of slow twitch fibres
Quarter-horse	7
Thoroughbred	13
Arab	14
Standardbred	18
Shetland	21
Pony	23
Donkey	28
Endurance horse	28
Heavy horse	31

Studies of human athletes have shown that the best marathon runners have a very high proportion of slow twitch fibres, while sprinters have more fast twitch fibres. This has a highly genetic basis and TBs can now be tested for this, which will help selection and training. This is discussed in Chapter 13.

A similar trend can be seen in different breeds and types of horses; even an unfit Quarter-horse, which is a sprinting specialist, has a greater proportion of fast twitch fibres than the Arab (Table 3.5). The physique of these two types of horses is also different; fast twitch fibres have a great diameter in order to generate power. In those horses better suited to endurance-type work the muscle fibres are thinner, allowing blood carrying oxygen and other nutrients to reach the fibres easily. Thus the Quarter-horse has a bulky, muscular physique, much like the powerful human sprinter, while the long-distance horse, the eventer and the hunter chaser, are more rangy and lean. The crossing of different breeds with different muscle fibre types such as warmblood (predominantly slow twitch) with a TB (predominantly fast twitch) results in offspring that may look more like a warmblood but that have higher levels of fast twitch fibres. These horses may be trained inappropriately for their muscle fibre types and this may lead to pain and discomfort.

Fatigue

The aim of getting a horse fit is to be able to work for longer before tiring, in other words to delay the onset of fatigue. A horse is said to be fatigued when it can no longer continue the exercise at that level – a horse cannot keep galloping at the same rate. If the horse is not allowed to slow down, exhaustion will set in eventually, exhaustion being the complete inability to continue work.

Causes of Fatigue

There are a number of different areas that may contribute to fatigue:

- fatigue of the energy-generating systems within muscle tissue
- accumulation of metabolic by-products, for example lactic acid, and failure of the muscle contraction
- disturbances to homeostasis, heat stress and dehydration
- lameness.

Lactic Acid Accumulation

As the speed increases, so does the energy demand from the muscle, and the blood is no longer able to supply oxygen quickly enough to satisfy these demands. At the same time, the fast twitch, low oxidative fibres are recruited, and these use the energy produced from glycogen in the absence of oxygen, a process called anaerobic respiration. This results in the by-product of anaerobic respiration being produced in muscles – namely lactic acid. At fast speeds there is so much lactic acid being produced that it builds up in muscle fibres. This lactic acid build-up

stops the muscle functioning correctly and eventually the horse has to slow down. Once the horse has slowed down sufficiently to return to aerobic work the blood can carry away the excess lactic acid. A successful training programme must aim to reduce the amount of lactic acid produced in the muscles. Lactic acid build-up is rarely an issue with endurance horses.

Summary Points

1) The skeletal system consists of all the bones and joints within the horse's body. It provides a framework for the attachment of muscles and protects important organs and structures within.
2) The term developmental orthopaedic disease (DOD) was coined in 1986 to encompass all orthopaedic problems seen in the growing foal and has become the generally accepted term. DOD encompasses all general growth disturbances of horses and is therefore quite non-specific.
3) The musculature of horses consists of deep postural muscles or stabilising muscles. Deep postural muscles keep the axial skeleton in place, whereas stabilising muscles produce movement via the appendicular skeleton.
4) There are two functional categories of smooth muscle, namely multi-unit (consisting of individual fibres with their own motor nerve endings) and single-unit (visceral) types.
5) Articular cartilage does not have a blood or nerve supply and nutrients enter via diffusion from the synovial fluid and nearby blood vessels.

Q + A

Q How many bones are there in the equine skeleton?

A There are 205 bones in the equine skeleton

Q Muscle fibres are recruited in what order?

A Muscle fibres are usually recruited in the following order: type I, type IIA, type IIB.

Q How do muscles create movement?

A Muscles create movement by acting across joints. There are two sets of muscles: flexors which are placed behind the bone and pull it backwards, bending the joint, and extensors which are placed in front of the bone and pull it forwards, straightening out the joint from its bent position.

Q Describe the functional classification of joints.

A This is based on the amount of movement as follows:

- Synarthroses – no joint movement, relatively rigid (syndesmosis, synchondrosis).
- Amphiarthroses – a small amount of movement (symphysis).
- Diarthroses – a wide range of movement, monaxial, biaxial and triaxial (hinge, sliding, ball and socket, pivot and ellipsoid, all of which are synovial joints).

Q Describe the difference in metabolism in slow twitch and fast twitch fibres.

A Slow twitch are aerobic and high oxidative; fast twitch are anaerobic and low oxidative.

4

The Lower Limb

As the horse evolved into a fleet-footed herbivore, the proportions of the limbs changed, so that the modern horse stands on the equivalent of the tip of the human middle finger (Figure 4.1). To achieve greater speed the lower limb was kept as light as possible, therefore the horse has evolved to have no muscles below the knee. The pull of muscles is transmitted to the bones of the lower leg and foot via long tendons, which can be easily felt running down the back of the horse's leg. The length of these tendons plus the fact that they lie close to the skin mean that they are susceptible to injury.

It is important to be able to identify the structures of the lower limb in the healthy horse so that signs of over-use or lameness can be located and acted upon before permanent damage is done. The cannon and two splint bones can also easily be felt under the skin. Each splint bone ends in an obvious small lump about three-quarters of the way down the inside of the cannon bone.

Tendons and Ligaments of the Lower Limb

The tendons and ligaments of the lower limb are shown in Figure 4.2.

Tendons

Tendons attach muscle to bone and are relatively inelastic. The function of tendons is to exert a pull on parts of the skeleton, initiated by muscle contraction. A tendon is not a separate entity; it is a strong extension of a muscle which attaches to bone. Muscle is elastic, but tendons are almost rigid compared to muscle. Tendons and muscles act together to allow movement, bear weight and accommodate stretch.

Tendons run from the forearm muscles downward in grooves of the bone across the knee and fetlock. They are held in position because the grooves are converted into canals by connective tissue called annular ligaments. Annular ligaments encircle tendons at the top and bottom to keep the tendons in the proper track. As tendons move in these canals they are subject to friction from all sides. To prevent damage, tendons are surrounded by tendon sheaths. These have an outer layer attached to the lining of the canal and an inner layer (epitenon) attached to the surface of the tendon (Figure 4.3). Oil-like synovial fluid is secreted between the two layers to allow the surfaces to run over each other smoothly.

The two layers form the mesotenon which carries blood vessels to the tendon. Inside this, the tendon consists of groups of fibres called fascicles, which run longitudinally, that is, in the same direction as the forces acting on the tendon. These are dense regular connective tissue fascicles encased in dense irregular connective tissue sheaths. Fascicles are bound by the endotendineum, which is a delicate loose connective tissue containing thin collagen fibrils and elastic fibres. Groups of fascicles are bounded by the epitenon. Filling the interstitial spaces within the fascia where the tendon is located is the paratenon

Equine Science, Third Edition. Zoe Davies and Sarah Pilliner.
© 2018 Zoe Davies and Sarah Pilliner. Published 2018 by John Wiley & Sons Ltd.

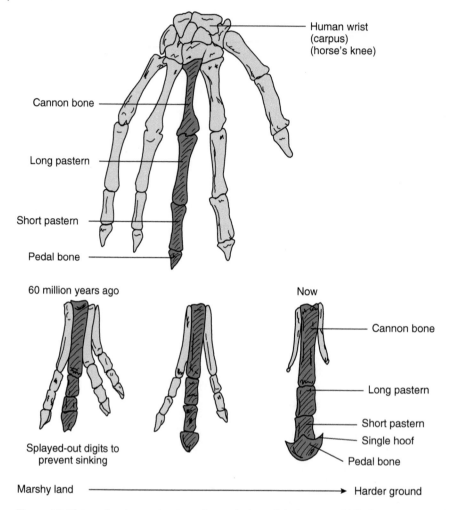

Figure 4.1 The modern horse stands on the equivalent of the human middle finger. *Source*: Adapted from Introduction to Horse Biology by Zoe Davies, Figure 1.2.

which is fatty tissue. The internal tendon bulk does not contain nerve fibres, but the epitenon and paratenon contain nerve endings. The collagen in tendons is held together with proteoglycan molecules including decorin and, in compressed regions of tendon, aggrecan, which are capable of binding to the collagen fibrils at specific locations.

Specialised cells called tenocytes produce the collagen molecules, which line themselves up end-to-end and side-to-side to produce collagen fibrils. Fibril bundles are organised to form fibres, with the elongated tenocytes closely packed between them. Tendon fibres as a whole show 'crimp'; rather than being straight they bend in a regular zig-zag pattern, giving the tendon a degree of elasticity, or rather a slight ability to lengthen. When the muscle contracts and puts pressure on the tendon, the crimp straightens before exerting its pull on the bone to which it is attached. Providing that the tendon is not overstretched, it returns to the crimp formation when the load is removed. Tendons have high tensile strength but restricted elasticity. At 3% extension the crimp disappears and at around 8% extension fibres rupture.

Tendon Repair

Collagen is produced by tendon fibroblasts, special cells arranged parallel to the fibrils.

Figure 4.2 Tendons and ligaments of the lower limb.

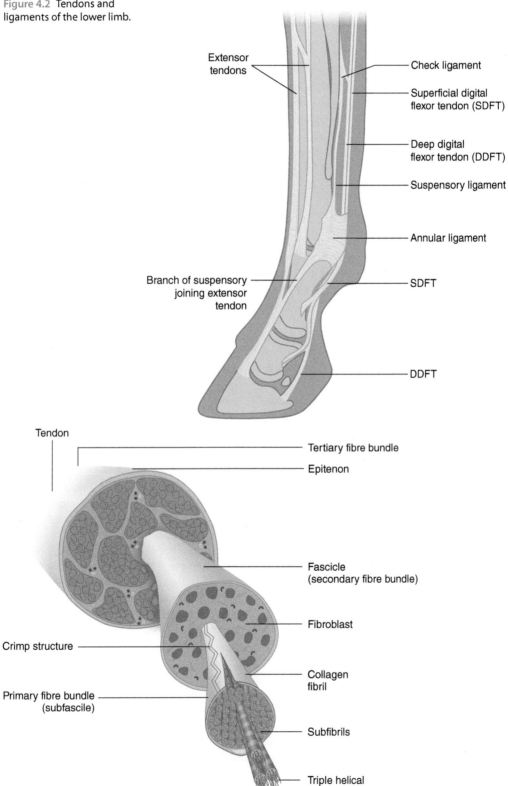

Extensor tendons

Check ligament

Superficial digital flexor tendon (SDFT)

Deep digital flexor tendon (DDFT)

Suspensory ligament

Annular ligament

Branch of suspensory joining extensor tendon

SDFT

DDFT

Tendon

Tertiary fibre bundle

Epitenon

Fascicle (secondary fibre bundle)

Fibroblast

Crimp structure

Collagen fibril

Primary fibre bundle (subfascile)

Subfibrils

Triple helical collagen molecule

Figure 4.3 Tendon structure.

All collagen tissue is replaced every 6 months. There are several types of collagen which are found in different parts of the body. Normal tendon is composed of type 1 collagen which is relatively elastic. However, if the tendon is damaged, the repair tissue is made of type 3 collagen, which is not as resilient, resulting in weakness so that the tendon is more susceptible to re-injury. In addition, the new collagen bundles are laid down randomly, not in parallel, which further weakens the tendon. Controlled exercise has a significant role in re-aligning the new collagen.

New therapies for tendon injuries include the following:

- Extracorporeal shock wave therapy (ESWT) – thought to increase blood flow, stimulate healing and possibly numb pain.
- Bone marrow transplant – bone marrow from the horse's sternum is extracted and then transplanted into the area of damage. Within the bone marrow are chemical and cell mediators that stimulate healing, including stem cells.
- Stem cell therapy – see Chapter 2. Stem cells are extracted from the horse's own fat and then placed in the damaged tendon. Stem cells are undifferentiated cells with the potential to become skin, bone, tendon or ligament cells.
- Interleukin-1 receptor antagonist protein (IRAP) – a chemical mediator in blood that prevents inflammatory chemical mediators in the blood from causing damage, allowing good chemical mediators to work more effectively. Blood from the horse is taken and incubated on special glass beads which grow IRAP. IRAP is then harvested and injected into the injury site.

Extensor Tendons

The common digital extensor tendon runs down the front of the cannon bone from the knee, attaching to the pedal bone within the hoof. The lateral digital extensor tendon runs from the side of the knee, outside the common digital flexor tendon, to insert onto the long pastern bone. Both the superficial and deep digital flexor tendons begin above the knee; the superficial tendon is joined by a strong fibrous band, the radial or superior check ligament, which fuses with it at the back of the knee.

Flexor Tendons

The deep and superficial digital flexor tendons pass down through the carpal canal in a synovial sheath to the cannon region. At the lower end of the cannon the superficial flexor tendon flattens and widens to form a ring which surrounds the deep flexor tendon. The deep flexor tendon runs through this ring behind the fetlock, surrounded by a synovial sheath. Below the fetlock the superficial flexor tendon divides into two parts, attaching to either side of the long and short pastern bones. The deep flexor tendon runs down through this fork, within the digital synovial sheath, to attach to the bottom of the pedal bone at the semi-lunar crest, crossing the underneath of the navicular bone (distal sesamoid). The navicular bursa lies between the deep flexor tendon and the navicular bone.

Ligaments and Suspensory Apparatus

A ligament originates from, and is attached to, bone. Ligaments are even less elastic than tendons. Thus a ligament has no muscular attachment as it connects bone to bone.

Check Ligament

In the upper part of the cannon the deep flexor tendon lies underneath the superficial flexor tendon and is attached to the back of the knee by the fibrous carpal check ligament. The check ligament can be palpated just below the knee if the horse's foot is picked up so that the tendons are relaxed.

Suspensory Ligament

The suspensory ligament differs from other ligaments in that it is a modified muscle and contains some muscle tissue, which gives it considerable elasticity compared to other ligaments. It lies between the deep flexor tendon and the cannon bone, and

The Lower Limb | 107

is sometimes mistaken for the splint bone, as it feels very rigid when the horse's leg is bearing weight. The suspensory ligament is a flat band originating from the back of the knee and passing down the back of the leg in a channel between the cannon bone and the two splint bones. At the level of the sesamoid bones it divides into two branches which pass forwards to join the extensor tendon on the front of the pastern. The rest of the suspensory ligament is attached to the sesamoid bones.

The suspensory ligament is part of the stay apparatus, which is discussed in Chapter 19. Its function is to suspend the fetlock, support the leg and prevent overextension of the fetlock joint. This support of the joint is helped by the superficial and deep flexor tendons along with the proximal sesamoid bones. Together, these structures carry much of the horse's weight during movement.

Blood Supply to the Lower Leg

The blood supply to the lower limb is shown in Figure 4.4. The median artery passes down behind the knees through the carpal canal with the deep digital flexor tendon and continues as the common artery on the inner side of the flexor tendons. It then passes between the back tendons and the suspensory ligament and divides above the fetlock into the lateral and medial digital flexor arteries passing across the fetlock to follow the borders of the deep digital flexor tendon into the foot. Within the foot the two digital arteries enter the underside of the pedal bone to form a terminal arch. Branches from this arch pass through the bone to nourish the sensitive structures within the hoof. Veins run alongside the arteries, draining from a coronary venous plexus which circles the upper part of the foot. On the outer side of the limb the lateral digital vein merges into the lateral palmar metacarpal vein, while on the inner aspect the medial digital vein joins the common digital vein before merging with the cephalic vein which continues above the knee.

Nerves accompany the arteries; the lateral palmar nerve runs alongside the lateral palmar metacarpal artery on the outer aspect of the leg (Figure 4.5). On the inner aspect the medial palmar digital nerve runs parallel to the common digital artery. The two nerves are connected by a communicating branch, which can be felt running diagonally across the superficial flexor tendon in thin-skinned horses. Both palmar nerves branch dorsally into the front of the pastern, the remainder of the nerves penetrating the foot and supplying the sensitive tissues within the hoof. The nerves can be 'blocked', that is, injected with local anaesthetic, either below or above the fetlock, during the location of the seat of lameness investigation, for example.

The Hoof

The old adage 'No foot, no horse' is still as true today as it has always been. The horse's hoof comprises a structure that surrounds the distal phalanx of the third digit of each of the four limbs of the horse. Different structures in the hoof contain different amounts of water.

- Hoof wall: 25% water
- Sole: 33% water
- Frog: 50% water.

These amounts vary slightly depending upon environmental conditions. The internal structures of the hoof are shown in Figure 4.6.

The Hoof as a Plastic Structure

Hooves are now considered to be plastic structures which can adapt their shape and strength depending upon the stresses and strains placed upon them. It is widely known that bone, cartilage, muscle, tendons and ligaments are able to do this. However, the plasticity of the hoof capsule is a relatively new area of veterinary science. The hoof and all the above tissues can change to a limited extent to improve strength and function as a result of the mechanical strains placed upon them by conformation and exercise. Foals

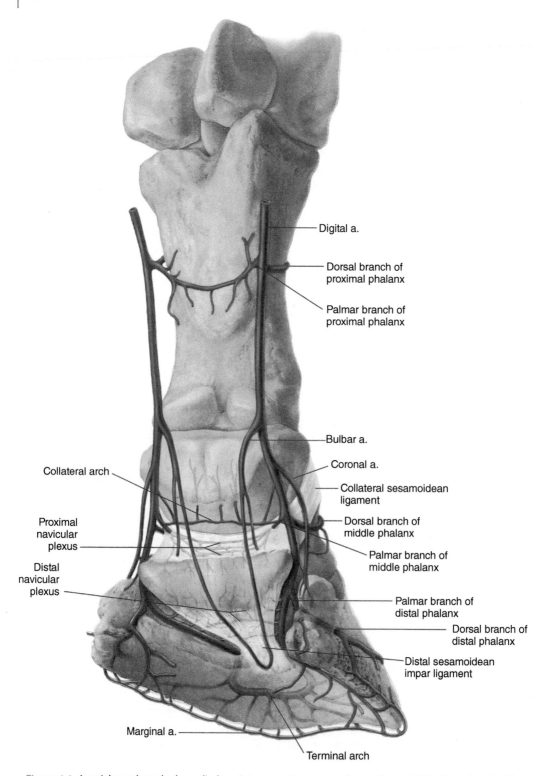

Digital a.

Dorsal branch of
proximal phalanx

Palmar branch of
proximal phalanx

Bulbar a.

Coronal a.

Collateral sesamoidean
ligament

Collateral arch

Dorsal branch of
middle phalanx

Proximal
navicular
plexus

Palmar branch of
middle phalanx

Distal
navicular
plexus

Palmar branch of
distal phalanx

Dorsal branch of
distal phalanx

Distal sesamoidean
impar ligament

Marginal a.

Terminal arch

Figure 4.4 Arterial supply to the lower limb. a, Artery; v, vein; n, nerve. *Source*: Baxter 2011. Reproduced with permission of John Wiley & Sons.

that exercise freely are known to have better chondrocytes, for example, than those that are confined.

Hooves are flexible and elastic under load. Loading of bone will cause the bone to remodel itself and become stronger, and vice versa – horses that are stabled for longer periods of time develop weaker bones due to bone turnover as loading is decreased. Horses that swim post injury do

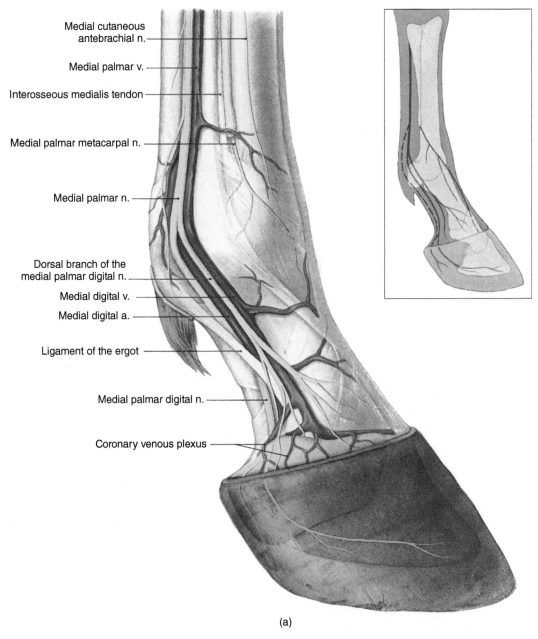

Medial cutaneous antebrachial n.

Medial palmar v.

Interosseous medialis tendon

Medial palmar metacarpal n.

Medial palmar n.

Dorsal branch of the medial palmar digital n.

Medial digital v.

Medial digital a.

Ligament of the ergot

Medial palmar digital n.

Coronary venous plexus

(a)

Figure 4.5 Medial (a) and lateral (b) aspects of the distal metacarpus, fetlock and digit, showing distribution of major nerves of the lower limb. a, Artery; v, vein; n, nerve. *Source*: Baxter 2011. Reproduced with permission of John Wiley & Sons.

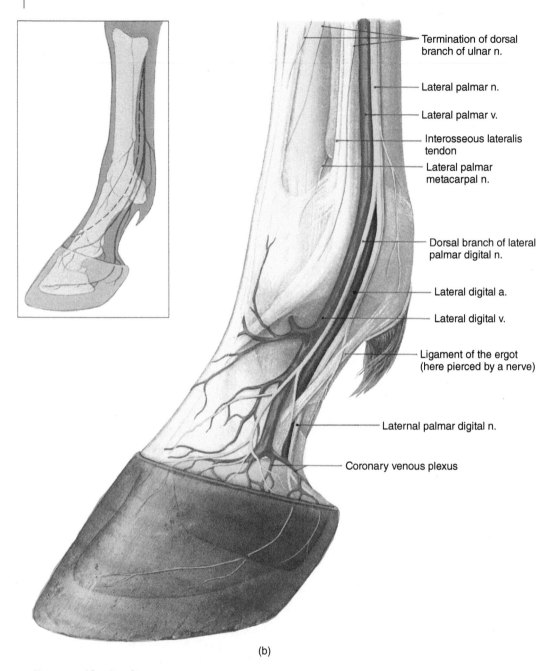

Termination of dorsal branch of ulnar n.

Lateral palmar n.

Lateral palmar v.

Interosseous lateralis tendon

Lateral palmar metacarpal n.

Dorsal branch of lateral palmar digital n.

Lateral digital a.

Lateral digital v.

Ligament of the ergot (here pierced by a nerve)

Laternal palmar digital n.

Coronary venous plexus

(b)

Figure 4.5 (*Continued*)

not build better bone as loading is reduced. Because of the hoof's adaptability it is often thought of as a smart tissue. Recovery under transient loading is central to the horse's movement and shock absorption. The hoof may be shod and/or trimmed frequently by farriers and foot trimmers and so is not 'normally' left to its own devices to grow and develop completely naturally. This in itself may lead to stress and strain on the hoof even from a simple foot trim and ultimately may change the shape and function of the hoof

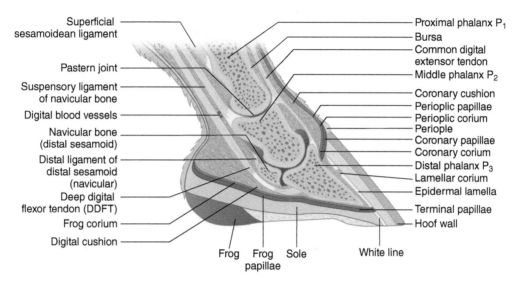

Figure 4.6 Internal hoof structures.

Superficial sesamoidean ligament

Pastern joint

Suspensory ligament of navicular bone

Digital blood vessels

Navicular bone (distal sesamoid)

Distal ligament of distal sesamoid (navicular)

Deep digital flexor tendon (DDFT)

Frog corium

Digital cushion

Frog

Frog papillae

Sole

White line

Proximal phalanx P$_1$

Bursa

Common digital extensor tendon

Middle phalanx P$_2$

Coronary cushion

Perioplic papillae

Perioplic corium

Periople

Coronary papillae

Coronary corium

Distal phalanx P$_3$

Lamellar corium

Epidermal lamella

Terminal papillae

Hoof wall

over time. This may be temporary or more permanent.

The front of the hoof is not designed as a major shock absorber, and so horses with pain in the heel will 'land' on the front part of the hoof and this could cause damage to the toe area. The back half of the hoof seems to play a major role in overall hoof health. Changes to this area may then affect the way the hoof copes with impact and may be beneficial or deleterious, affecting soundness. Impact of the hoof on the ground sends major shockwaves through the structure which are absorbed by the soft tissues of the hoof. These soft tissues therefore have to be adaptable. More studies are required to research the mechanical effects of different surfaces on the 'normal' hoof.

Repeated deformations to the hoof may be temporary; for example, each time the hoof impacts the ground the hoof internal structures expand slightly and then return to normal as the weight is lifted off. Other changes may be less reversible, such as changes to the soft tissues, contracted heels and ringbone. The long-term adaptive process of the hoof in response to deformations may result from stimuli (direct or indirect) which increase stress and strain and therefore elastic deformation of the hoof. The

sensory nerves detect this and this results in a response at cellular level to attempt to correct hoof tissue and return to normal.

The heel plays a major role in the mechanics of the hoof in cushioning impact. A large frog and prominent heels are likely to provide better cushioning of the hoof on impact with the ground. Horses with higher heel volumes tend to recover to soundness faster in some laminitic horses. Palpation of the heels can help assess the digital cushion underneath, and ideally this should barely deform on maximum pressure from the thumbs. The frog and heel tissues contain a high concentration of mechanoreceptors.

Effect of Movement on Hoof Structure

The hoof is structurally designed to be weight bearing and absorb concussion as the horse moves, with the limb acting as a spring from the shoulder down (forelimb). As the hoof hits the ground and the horse's movement and bodyweight (60% forelimb) exerts downward force, some energy is stored in structures such as ligaments and tendons as they stretch. Following stretch the next phase is recoil, using this stored energy as the hoof lifts off the ground and structures return to pre-stretch position. This uses little extra energy. In addition, as the frog hits the ground, the frog and digital cushion are compressed and flatten and physical pressure on the ungulate (lateral) cartilage, bars and hoof wall causes spreading of the heel. This helps squeeze blood out of the vascular bed. The blood also provides hydraulic assistance and further helps absorb some concussion. This flattening and stretching also helps push venous blood back up the lower limb. As the hoof lifts off the ground more blood refills the blood vessels.

Functions of the Hoof

The main functions of the hoof are:

- shock absorption
- storage of energy (see 'Effect of Movement on Hoof Structure' above)
- grip
- circulation
- as a lever for muscles of the upper limb to attach to phalanges (see 'Blood Supply to the Lower Leg').

Shock Absorption

The forelimb hooves carry 60% of the horse's bodyweight and therefore are subjected to greater load compared to the hindlimb. The front hooves are mainly shock absorbing, whereas the hind hooves are shock absorbing but also help propel the horse forward. These differences can be seen in the different shapes of fore compared to hind hooves.

The hoof is adapted to accommodate concussion when it hits the ground, with the wall bearing most of the impact. In the unshod horse, the frog strikes the ground first, then the heels, bars, quarters and finally the toe. As the frog comes under pressure the heels and bars expand; this expansion is limited by the toe which is immovable. Thus shoes are not nailed at the heel. Concussion is transmitted through the wall to the laminae and to the periosteum of the pedal bone and the rest of the bones of the limb. There is slight yielding of the pedal bone which is cushioned by the lateral cartilages. There is also some movement in the joint between the pedal bone and the short pastern. Concussion is also reduced by the cushioning effect of the frog and the digital cushion, but this is only applicable if the frog is in contact with the ground (Figure 4.7). The angulation of the scapula, humerus and fetlock joint and the support of the suspensory apparatus also reduce the concussive effects.

Grip

When the ground is soft the toe cuts in to prevent slipping, but this is not effective on hard or greasy going. When the foot sinks into the ground, the dome shape of the sole

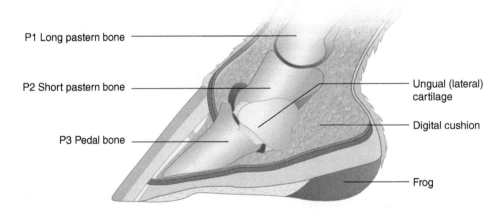

P1 Long pastern bone

P2 Short pastern bone

P3 Pedal bone

Ungual (lateral) cartilage

Digital cushion

Frog

Figure 4.7 Anticoncussive structures of the hoof.

has a suction effect which gives firm grip. This is so effective that the horse will have to work very hard in soft ground. The contact of a properly formed frog with the ground is an important anti-slip device, especially on firm ground. However, shoes tend to raise the frog clear of the ground, depriving the horse of its anti-slip mechanism. This is counteracted by using modifications to the shoe such as studs.

Circulation

As there are no muscles below the horse's knee it cannot rely on muscle massage of veins to promote venous return of blood to the heart, and so the frog is used instead. As the foot comes under pressure the blood in the three venous plexi (i.e. the coronary, dorsal and palmar venous plexus) is squeezed into the digital veins. As the weight comes off the foot, arterial blood enters the foot and venous blood is prevented from flowing back into the foot by valves. Frog pressure is needed for this to work and the theory is probably an oversimplification, as horses that have had the frog pared away do not seem to suffer from bad circulation or concussion. It may be that spreading of the heels and the role of the lateral cartilages is more important. Indeed, one theory poses that as the heels spread when the horse lands, blood is drawn into the foot, and as the heels contract blood is squeezed out of the foot.

The foot or digit of the horse is equivalent to the human middle finger, consisting of three bones known as:

- first, second and third phalanges
- proximal, middle and distal phalanges
- long pastern, short pastern and pedal bone.

These bones give rise to the fetlock, pastern and coffin joints. The joint between the cannon bone and the long pastern bone is the fetlock joint, between the long and short pastern bones is the pastern joint, and between the short pastern bone and the pedal bone is the coffin joint.

The hoof capsule surrounds the pedal bone and the navicular bone and part of the short pastern bone. The hoof is a continuation of modified skin, similar to horns and claws in other animals, and consists of two distinct parts:

- external hoof, which is equivalent to the epidermis
- internal or sensitive hoof, which is equivalent to the corium or dermis.

The External Hoof

The external hoof is insensitive and non-vascular (Figure 4.8a&b), that is, it does not have a blood supply. It consists of three parts: wall, sole and frog.

Wall

The wall is produced by and grows down from the coronary band and is the part that can be seen when the foot is on the ground. It consists of dense horn, and is divided into the toe, quarters and heels. At the heels it is reflected back, inwards and forwards, to form the bars of the hoof. The bars:

- Give strength at the heels and allow the hoof to withstand the weight of the horse. It is difficult to balance a piece of paper on its edge, but if each end of the paper is folded over, like the bars, it will stand quite easily.
- Allow for expansion when the horse's weight lands on the hoof. Except at the walk, when the foot lands virtually level, the hoof is placed heel first, then the frog and finally the toe. Each time this happens the frog is designed to take the weight, force the angle of the bars open and prevent the heels from caving in and contracting.

The bars must be allowed to grow. If they are pared away by the farrier the horse's heels will start to contract. The area of sole between the walls and the bars is sometimes known as the seat of corn.

Two sets of lines can be seen on the smooth glossy outer wall: vertical lines run in the direction of hoof growth and indicate the direction of the tubules which grow down from the papillae of the coronary band; and

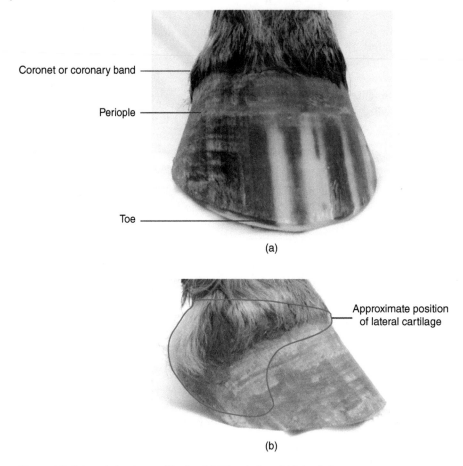

Coronet or coronary band

Periople

Toe

(a)

Approximate position
of lateral cartilage

(b)

Figure 4.8 External structures of the hoof. (a) Front view; (b) lateral view.

rings consisting of alternating ridges and depressions run parallel to the coronary band and indicate the growth rate of the hoof, much the same as the rings within a tree trunk indicate its age. The rings will deviate if the growth rate of the hoof has been abnormal – for example, as seen in some post-laminitic horses. The colour of the hoof wall depends on the colour of the horse's skin at the coronet.

The upper wall is covered by a thin layer of epidermis called the periople which originates from a rim of soft grey horn at the coronary band, the perioplic cushion (Figure 4.9). This rim is thickest at the top of the hoof and at the heels forms a wide cap to blend with the frog. It is best seen when the hoof is wet. The periople is carried down the

hoof by the growth of the wall, dries out and forms the cuticle, which tends to flake off and does not extend much below half-way down the hoof. It is thought that the periople controls the movement of moisture in and out of the foot, and that when the horse is shod the periople should not be rasped away. As the periople extends only a short way down the hoof it is acceptable to rasp the toes, but it is important not to rasp the upper hoof.

The internal surface of the wall carries the insensitive laminae which consist of 500–600 horny leaves, each of which has 100–200 secondary laminae. These dovetail with the sensitive laminae of the sensitive foot to create a very strong bond between the two (see Figure 4.9).

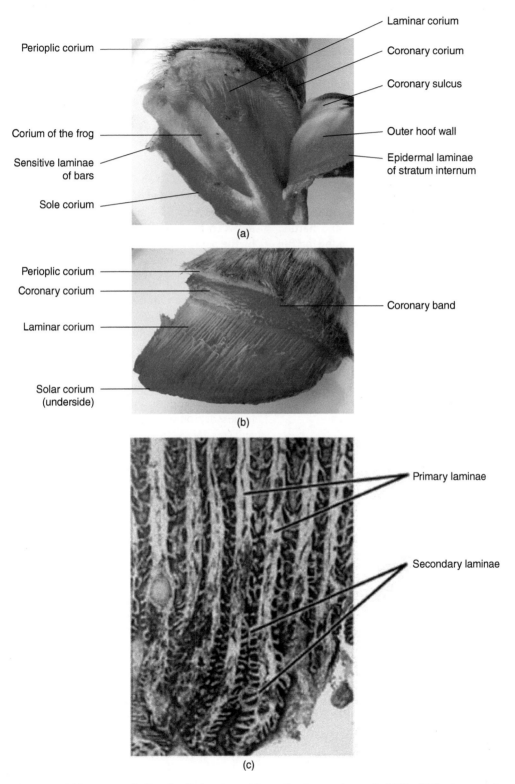

Figure 4.9 (a) Part removal of hoof wall, showing epidermal laminae underneath. (b) Hoof following complete removal of hoof wall, showing the corium. (c) Photomicrograph cross-section of the equine hoof. *Source*: Baxter 2011. Reproduced with permission of John Wiley & Sons.

The junction between the insensitive and sensitive laminae is shown on the underside of the foot by the white line. This indicates the thickness of the wall and determines where the farrier fits the nails. The wall consists of about 25% water and is thicker at the toe than at the heel, enabling the farrier to nail higher up the wall at the toe than at the heel. It grows about 2.5 cm (1 in) in 3 months, so that it takes the toe 9–12 months to grow from coronary band to ground and the heel about 6 months. As the horn grows down from the coronary band it becomes keratinised and compressed, and thus stronger and harder. The toe is harder than the heel, allowing the heel to expand, as described.

The bar is an extension of the hoof wall which runs along the side of the frog, terminating approximately half-way along the frog. Its primary purpose is to control the movement of the back of the hoof, adding strength to the heel area and protecting it from excess distortion. It should have a high ratio of pliable inner wall to ensure it can move correctly as the heel moves.

Sole

The sole is the ground surface of the hoof. It is crescent-shaped and concave so that it arches over the ground, protecting the sensitive structures within the foot (Figure 4.10). It contains more water (33%) than the wall and is thus less dense and resistant. It supports the weight of the body rather than bearing it. Soles are of variable thickness and a horse with relatively flat soles which can be compressed will be more prone to bruising and sore feet. The sole should have natural concavity and not be dependent upon the wall of the hoof.

Frog

The frog is a wedge of soft elastic horn containing about 50% moisture. It is situated between the bars and separated from them by the paracuneal groove or central sulcus of the frog. The frog has several functions:

- shock absorption
- returning venous blood back up the limbs
- balance control
- to aid grip on the ground.

At the rear it becomes the bulbs of the heels, while at the front the dorsal tip of the frog is called the apex. The central groove divides the frog into two crura. If the groove is very deep it means that the digital cushion will be affected beneath it. Figure 4.11 shows the internal surface of the sole and frog.

Collateral grooves are the grooves that run along either side of the frog. The outer wall of the groove is made up of the wall of the

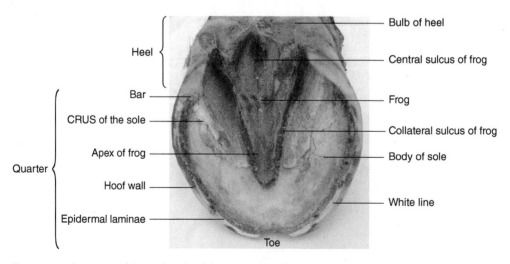

Figure 4.10 Structures of the underside of the external hoof.

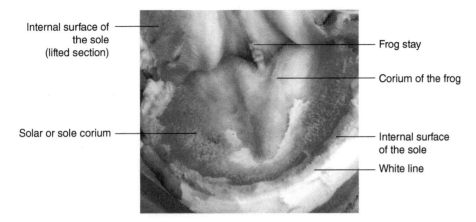

Internal surface of the sole (lifted section)

Frog stay

Corium of the frog

Solar or sole corium

Internal surface of the sole

White line

Figure 4.11 Internal surface of the sole and frog.

bar and sole and the wall on the other side comprises the wall of the frog. In theory, the frog should come below the level of the sole and come into contact with the ground when the horse moves. When the frog hits the ground it is compressed and expands, putting pressure on the digital cushion, which in turn squeezes the lateral cartilages and wall of the foot and the wall expands. If the horse is shod so that the frog does not come into contact with the ground, this cushioning effect is lost and the frog shrinks and the heel contracts.

Two types of mechanoreceptors have been identified in the equine hoof:

- Pacinian corpuscles (Figure 4.12) – sense light pressure or vibrations.
- Ruffini endings – sense light, tactile pressure.

These mechanoreceptors help with proprioception and hoof development. Pacinian corpuscles are located in the bulb of the frog, digital cushions, lateral cartilages and bulbs of the heel. Their distribution is highly localised. They are located close to blood capillaries and may have some function in monitoring changes in local circulation of the hoof. Ruffini endings are located around skin areas and major nerves.

Figure 4.12 This Pacinian corpuscle has a connective tissue receptor surrounding the terminus of the primary afferent neuron. *Source*: Frandson 2009. Reproduced with permission of John Wiley & Sons.

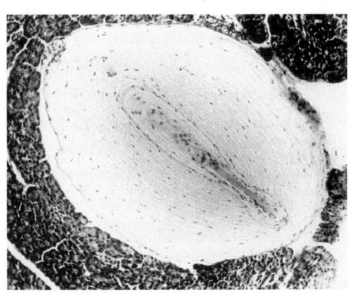

Hoof Horn

The horny or keratin tubules are impregnated with keratin and make up the external hoof structure. These are hollow (approximately 200–300 µm in diameter) and run vertically down the length of the hoof. They are surrounded by intertubular cellular matrix, which lies at right angles relative to the long axis of the tubules. The matrix and horn tubules together provide the viscoelastic properties of it, which means that the hoof wall has both strain and fracture resistance. Hydration has an influence on the stiffness and strain capacity of the intertubular matrix. Highly hydrated hoof horn induces more mobility and greater movement. Hoof wall keratin is extremely strong.

Internal Structures

The corium (dermis) or sensitive laminae of the foot is a specialised vascular continuation of the dermis of the skin and provides nutrition to the foot and an attachment for the insensitive foot. There are five layers of corium:

- perioplic corium
- coronary corium
- laminar corium
- solar corium
- frog corium.

A very thin layer of epidermis covers each corium, which gives rise to the growth of epidermal cells which are keratinised to form the horny components of the hoof.

- The perioplic corium is situated above the coronary corium and separated from it by a small groove; it broadens at the heel to become continuous with the frog corium. The perioplic corium supplies the periople with nutrients.
- The coronary corium is an enlarged band above the laminar corium (sensitive laminae) which produces the wall, much as skin produces hair, and nourishes the wall of the hoof. The coronary corium is pigmented in dark hoof and bears papillae which produce the wall of the hoof.

- The laminar corium consists of the sensitive laminae which attach to the periosteum of the pedal bone and suspend this bone within the hoof by interlocking with the insensitive laminae. The primary laminae have lateral secondary laminae, giving a total surface area of $0.75 \, m^2$ ($8 \, ft^2$), which supports the weight of the horse.
- The solar corium or sensitive sole attaches the sole of the pedal bone to the horny sole and supplies nutrition to the sole.
- The epidermis of the frog corium or sensitive frog produces horny tubules which are flexible and only partly keratinised, hence the soft nature of the frog. It is attached to the digital cushion in the heel of the foot and nourishes the digital cushion.

Digital or Plantar Cushion

The digital cushion is a wedge-shaped fibro-elastic pad situated in the back part of the foot, filling the heels and lying above the frog and below the deep flexor tendon. Fibrous bands run through the digital cushion of the healthy hoof. The digital cushion lies between the lateral (ungual) cartilages and is a collagenous, elastic tissue infiltrated by adipose tissue. At the bulbs of the heel, it is subcutaneous and is soft and loose in texture. The flexible material that forms the digital cushion is produced from the hypodermis of the frog. (The hypodermis is not part of the skin, and lies below the dermis. Its purpose is to attach the frog to underlying bone and muscle, as well as supplying it with blood vessels and nerves. It consists of loose connective tissue and elastin.)

The bulbs of the cushion are soft and fatty, while the rest is more fibrous. It is not well supplied with nerves and a pricked digital cushion may not give the horse any pain but a serious infection may develop. Its role is as a shock absorber. It also has extensive microcirculation and acts as a pump to return venous blood up the limb. The lateral cartilages lie on either side of the digital cushion.

Lateral (Ungual) Cartilages

The medial and lateral cartilages of the distal phalanx extend from the palmar processes of the bone to the coronary region of the hoof (see Figure 4.8b). They can be palpated proximally. They curve towards each other in the heel region and become thicker distally. The cartilages contain several foraminae through which veins pass from the palmar venous plexus to the coronary venous plexus. The lateral or ungual cartilages are held in place by a series of five ligaments going to the medial/lateral surfaces of the three phalanges and distal sesamoid (navicular) bone.

The lateral cartilages are two plates of cartilage which attach to the wings of the pedal bone and curve back inside the wall, reaching just above the coronary band. In young horses the soft cartilage is very flexible, but as the horse ages the cartilage becomes tougher and is less able to withstand distortions of the limb which may occur during exercise. Injury may cause ossification of the lateral cartilages, resulting in sidebone. The palmar venous plexus lies between the cartilage and the digital cushion.

Pedal and Navicular Bones

The pedal and navicular bones are highly vascular and fit closely together. The deep flexor tendon fans out to run over the navicular bone and attach to the undersurface of the pedal bone. The navicular acts as a pulley as the tendon exerts pull on the pedal bone during locomotion.

The Balanced Foot

There is probably no such thing as the 'perfect foot' and when the horse is being shod it is more important that the farrier should match the foot with the leg, so that the shape and proportions of the foot are the most suitable for that limb, rather than making the foot 'ideal'.

Assessment of Foot Balance

Before either barefoot trimming or trimming the foot and then nailing on the shoe the foot balance should be assessed when the horse is (1) stationary (static) and (2) moving (dynamic).

Static Foot Balance

The foot should be looked at from the front (anterior view), underside (solar view) and side (lateral view).

Front (Anterior View)

A vertical axis drawn through the centre of the cannon bone should bisect the hoof into two equal halves (Figure 4.13). A line running across the top of the coronary band should be horizontal, that is, the same distance from the ground on both sides of the hoof, showing that the hoof wall is at the same angle on both sides (Figure 4.14). The wall should not flare out or run under.

Underside (Solar View)

The frog is the best guide to the foot's symmetry. A trimmed frog is shaped like a wedge that starts between the heels and ends in a point (the apex) just in front of the hoof centre. The frog should exactly bisect the foot, and the hoof should be equal in shape

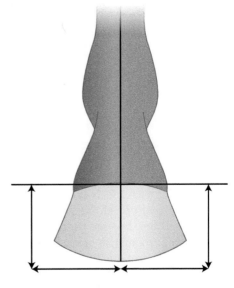

Figure 4.13 A vertical line drawn through the centre of the cannon bone and down through the hoof should bisect the hoof equally.

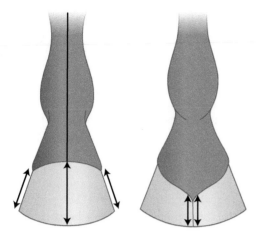

Figure 4.14 A line running along the top of the coronary band should be horizontal, that is, the same distance from the ground on both sides of the hoof.

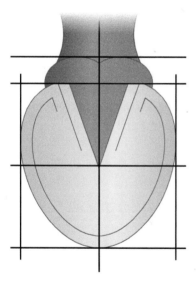

Figure 4.15 Foot balance (solar view).

and proportion on either side of the frog for foot balance (Figure 4.15). If the hoof wall is not evenly proportioned the foot should be reshaped and the shoe set symmetrically around the frog, so that it too is bisected equally by the centre of the limb.

Side (Lateral View)

It is essential that the hoof pastern axis (HPA) is in alignment. Ideally, the hoof wall and angle at the heel should also align (Figure 4.16). If the HPA is broken back (i.e. it has a low hoof angle, where the angle of the dorsal hoof wall is lower than the angle of the dorsal pastern), great strain is thrown upon the stay apparatus and dorsal wall laminae. If the horse has long toes and low heels, the chances of tendon injury are increased and the toe should be dressed back and the horse shod with upright heels and a rolled toe. Long toes delay and prolong the breakover of the leg over the foot, with the heel remaining on the ground longer. This compresses the front of the joints and the navicular bone, contributing to poor stride length, stumbling and forging. A broken forward HPA is not as serious as a broken back HPA but can lead to stumbling and excessive landing on the heels. Poor HPA conformation is usually induced by shoes being left on too long and/or short shoeing. The ideal hoof angle is said to be 45–50° in front and 50–55° for the hind feet. The angle depends on the individual horse's conformation, and in practice tends to be more upright than the 'ideal'.

Dynamic Foot Balance

The horse's movement and soundness are the greatest tests of foot balance. The farrier cannot influence the flight of the horse's foot through the air, but he can influence the way the foot lands and takes off. The hoof has good side-to-side balance if it lands level. This can be judged by standing directly in front of the horse as it is walked towards you. An out-of-balance foot may 'toe out'; as the foot lands, the outside toe (which is usually flared) lands first and as the body-weight passes over the foot the inside heel is snapped down. The weight of the horse is rolled over the inside toe as the foot breaks over and lifts off. This type of movement is liable to cause the inside heel to shunt up higher than the outside heel. At first glance the inside heel appears higher and is often trimmed down to 'level it' with the outside heel, exacerbating the problem. Instead, the shoe should be set wider to support the limb more evenly (Figure 4.17).

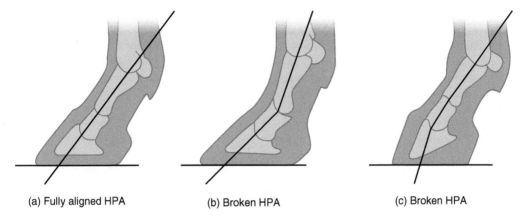

(a) Fully aligned HPA (b) Broken HPA (c) Broken HPA

Figure 4.16 The hoof pastern axis (HPA) should always be aligned.

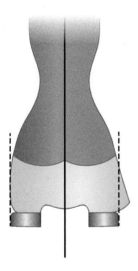

Figure 4.17 An unbalanced foot trimmed to remove flare and shod to support the underrun side.

From the side, the well-balanced foot should land level or slightly heel first. Horses that land toe first are usually showing signs of pain in the rear area of the foot and are prone to stumbling.

Adaptations of Hoof Tissue

Recent research has shown that hoof material can adapt and lay down new tissue, that is, within the frog and digital cushion, as a result of specific external stimuli to the sole. Standing horses recovering from laminitis with a soft boot to remove pain on pea gravel over 5 months showed significantly improved sole tissue and depth. Increased heel tissue and therefore volume may also result following laminitis to help the hoof compensate for laminae damage.

Summary Points

1) The horse has no muscles below the knee. The pull of the muscles is transmitted to the bones of the lower leg and foot via long tendons, which can be easily felt running down the back of the horse's leg.
2) The collagen fibres of tendons have a 'crimped' structure rather than being straight and they bend in a regular zig-zag pattern. This gives the tendon a degree of elasticity, or rather a slight ability to lengthen.
3) It is now thought that the horse's hoof is able to adapt and change to forces applied to it and because of this adaptability it is often thought of as a smart tissue.
4) When the frog hits the ground it is compressed and expands, putting pressure on the digital cushion, which in turn squeezes the lateral cartilages and wall of the foot and the wall expands. If the horse is shod so that the frog does not come into contact with the ground this cushioning effect is lost and the frog shrinks and the heel contracts.

5) Two types of mechanoreceptors have been identified in the equine hoof, namely the Pacinian corpuscles – which sense light pressure or vibration – and the Ruffini endings – which sense light, tactile pressure.

6) Recent research has shown that hoof material can adapt and lay down new tissue, that is, within the frog and digital cushion, as a result of specific external stimuli to the sole; the hoof is now thought of as a smart tissue.

Q + A

Q How does the suspensory ligament differ from other ligaments?

A It is a modified muscle and contains some muscle tissue which gives it considerable elasticity compared to other ligaments.

Q What are the main functions of the hoof?

A Shock absorption, storage of energy, grip, circulation and as a lever for muscles of the upper limb to attach to phalanges.

Q What are the functions of the frog?

A The frog has several functions, namely shock absorption, returning venous blood back up the limbs, balance control and to aid grip on the ground.

Q Describe static foot balance.

A The foot should be looked at from the front (anterior view), underside (solar view) and side (lateral view). A vertical axis drawn through the centre of the cannon bone should bisect the hoof into two equal halves. A line running across the top of the coronary band should be horizontal, that is, the same distance from the ground on both sides of the hoof, showing that the hoof wall is at the same angle on both sides. The wall should not flare out or run under.

5

The Digestive System

The digestive system is the horse's largest sensory organ. The horse evolved as a grazing animal and the anatomy and physiology of the digestive system and feeding behaviour reflects this. Equidae belong to the order Perissodactyla which includes tapirs and rhinoceroses. They are hindgut fermenters. Many horses are stabled for all or part of the time and only have access to limited areas of grazing, preventing them from following their natural feeding patterns. This can lead to digestive and general health problems.

The horse has a large and complex hindgut comprising the caecum and large colon in which digestion (or fermentation) of plant fibre (complex carbohydrates) takes place. The digestive tract is designed to take in small amounts at frequent intervals, with wild horses grazing up to 14–16 hours per day. This is known as trickle feeding and the digestive system has evolved over millions of years to suit this way of feeding. In the wild, the horse is also able to select from a wide variety of grasses, herbs and shrubs. Domestication of horses has led to increased stresses on their digestive systems due to 'abnormal' feeding patterns which are frequently imposed.

The natural diet of herbivores consists of grasses and vegetation containing large amounts of insoluble or complex carbohydrates such as hemicellulose, cellulose, pectins and lignin. These complex carbohydrates are digested in the hindgut by microbiota and do not elevate insulin levels. For horses relying mainly on forage as a large proportion of their diet, these complex carbohydrates provide most of their daily calorie intake. Mammals do not have the ability to secrete the enzyme cellulase, which breaks down cellulose, in their digestive tract and the horse therefore has to rely upon a large number of microbiota formerly known as gut flora in its hindgut to perform this task. This is a symbiotic relationship.

Much research is being undertaken now on the human gut and its effect on the brain. Work published in 2013 showed that taking a specific bacterial cocktail for a month altered the brains of humans, particularly the areas associated with emotions and pain, and that the gut may affect behaviour; this has been shown in mice, for example. This may be an area of future research in horses, as the microbiome of the hindgut is now receiving considerable attention.

The enteric nervous system (ENS) is essential to the function of the horse's digestive tract. The gut is continuously monitored by this complex system, which is often informally referred to as the 'brain' of the digestive tract. The ENS works locally in the gut and also has input from the central nervous system (CNS) via the vagus nerve (parasympathetic) and sympathetic ganglia. The ENS is a complex nervous network supplying the gut, which includes afferent neurons, interneurons and motor neurons.

The entire digestive system is completely unique to the horse and can be split into two parts: the foregut and hindgut. The foregut is similar to that of simple-stomached animals such as humans and pigs and the hindgut is

Equine Science, Third Edition. Zoe Davies and Sarah Pilliner.
© 2018 Zoe Davies and Sarah Pilliner. Published 2018 by John Wiley & Sons Ltd.

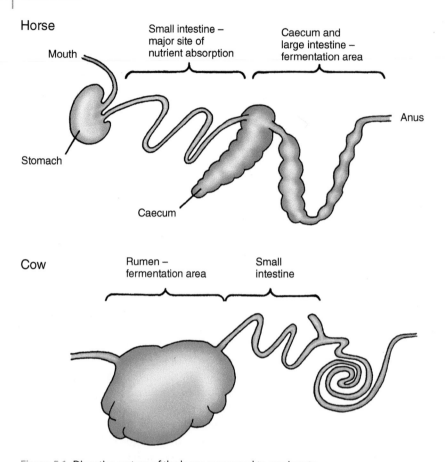

Figure 5.1 Digestive system of the horse compared to ruminants.

somewhat similar to the rumen of the cow (Figure 5.1).

In simple terms, the digestive tract (Figures 5.2 and 5.3) is a tube beginning at the lips and ending at the anus, the role of which is to break down food into substances that can be absorbed into the bloodstream and utilised by the horse. This breakdown is accomplished by the digestive juices which are secreted by glands housed within the tract. The digestive tract is approximately 30 m (100 ft) long and in order to fit into the abdomen it is coiled and looped and loosely held in place by sheets of mesentery tissue. Throughout its length there are several changes in direction and diameter, which partially explains the horse's susceptibility to blockages of the gut which manifest themselves as colic.

Foregut

Mouth

The upper lip is strong, mobile and sensitive, and the horse uses it to sort through food, before manoeuvring between the teeth. The incisor or biting teeth can bite off pieces of food selectively and if necessary, can graze a pasture very closely (Figure 5.4). The tongue then moves the food to the molar teeth for grinding, through a series of up-and-down and side-to-side chewing movements, which pulverise the food into smaller pieces, suitably lubricated by saliva for swallowing. Chewing also breaks open fibre, releasing some soluble nutrients to be digested in the small intestine.

Horses have evolved as forage eaters and rely on their teeth for 'processing' this fibrous

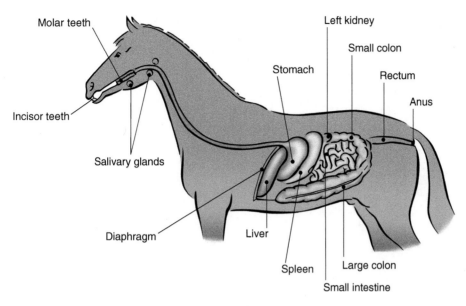

Figure 5.2 Structure of the equine digestive system.

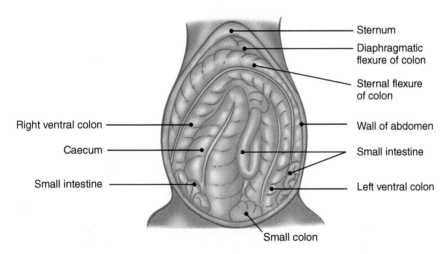

Figure 5.3 Structure of the equine digestive system as seen from beneath.

food. All food has to be ground down to less than 1 mm in length before swallowing – obviously this will take much longer for hay than for concentrates. Indeed, it has been estimated that horses will chew 1 kg of concentrate feed 800–1200 times but need 3000–3500 chews to get through 1 kg of hay. Horses have three distinct phases to the chewing cycle, namely the opening phase, closing phase and power stroke. While saliva has virtually no digestive activity (0.44 U/ml compared with 77 U/ml in humans and 98 U/ml in pigs), it acts to wet and lubricate the food so that it is turned into an easily swallowed 'porridge', which is passed via the pharynx into the oesophagus on its way to the stomach. It also acts as a buffer of gastric acid in the stomach. Concentrations of sodium, chloride and bicarbonate increase with the rate of saliva secretion. As much as 10–12 litres per day of saliva with a pH of 9.6–9.1 may be produced by an adult horse.

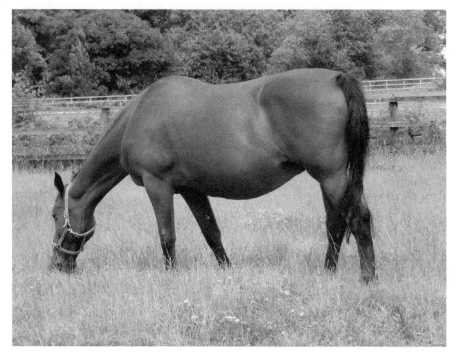

Figure 5.4 Horses can graze pastures closely using their incisors. *Source*: Courtesy of Harthill Stud.

The pharynx helps to guide food into the oesophagus, which is a muscular tube about 1.2–1.5 m (4–5 ft) long. Food or water cannot return to the mouth from the oesophagus because the soft palate blocks its return. The epiglottis (a muscular flap) also closes over the top of the trachea to prevent food going into the lungs.

The horse has three salivary glands (Figure 5.5):

- parotid
- sublingual
- submaxillary.

Equine saliva contains over 99% water. Saliva also contains bicarbonate which is alkaline and helps to neutralise or buffer the acid in the stomach. The rate of saliva production is stimulated by chewing or mastication and ingestion of feed. The dryer the feed, the more saliva is produced.

The bolus of food, after it has been swallowed, moves along the digestive tract by

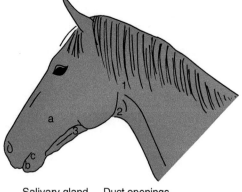

Salivary gland	Duct openings
1. Parotiod	a
2. Submaxillary	b
3. Sublingual	c

Figure 5.5 Position of the three pairs of salivary glands.

waves of muscular contractions known as peristalsis. These waves are usually irreversible. Occasionally, food becomes lodged in the oesophagus and this is known as choke.

Oesophagus

The oesophagus is 1.2–1.5 m in length with sphincters at both ends and is lined with modified stratified squamous epithelium (see Chapter 2). The upper two-thirds of the oesophagus are made up of striated muscle, whereas the proximal one-third is smooth muscle. The striated area has shorter 'squeezes' of peristalsis, leading to faster propulsion of food in this area. The oesophagus does not have any significant secretory activity.

Stomach

The stomach is very motile and is held in place by four folds of peritoneum. A muscular valve called the cardiac sphincter controls the passage of food from the oesophagus into the stomach. This valve (cardiac sphincter) is very powerful and does not allow food to be regurgitated in the horse. The walls of the stomach may burst rather than allow digesta back up the oesophagus.

The presence of food in the nostrils may indicate a ruptured stomach. The oesophagus is long and narrow and lacks the nerves required to move food back up the digestive tract towards the mouth.

The horses stomach is rarely empty given it is a natural trickle feeder and retention time is short in the stomach. The stomach is relatively small compared to the size of the horse and in a 500 kg horse it is around 8–15 litres. The stomach tends to act as a holding area before passage to the small intestine.

There is often confusion regarding the histology of the stomach which does not always accurately relate to the more commonly known areas of the stomach. The oesophageal region contains stratified squamous epithelium and lines the saccus caecus (see Fig 5.6). The saccus caecus is located at the entrance of the stomach and the oesophagus.

The rest of the stomach is glandular and contains columnar epithelium. The change from the stratified squamous epithelium of the oesophageal region to columnar epithelium of the glandular area is the beginning of the cardiac region and is separated by the margo plicatus.

The cardia and pylorus are quite close together creating a shorter side (the lesser curvature) and the J shape of the stomach. The opposite side provides the greater curvature of the stomach.

The body of the stomach expands with food and the rugae help this expansion when required.

The cardiac region gets its name from the cardiac glands in this area which produce mucus and is a relatively small area in horses.

The fundic region contains the tubular shaped fundic or gastric glands that open into gastric pits. Fundic glands line a large part of the glandular are of the stomach lumen i.e. more than just the anatomical part known as the fundus.

The pyloric region contains glands similar to the cardiac glands and secrete mucus and a small amount of protein digesting enzymes. This region does not contain any parietal cells.

In addition there are cells that are found throughout the stomach mucosa which secrete hormones such as gastrin and these are known as Enteroendocrine cells.

The stomach is composed of the same 4 layers as the rest of the digestive tract namely the mucosa, submucosa, tunica muscularis and the serosa. The serosa (external peritoneum) covers the entire stomach.

There are three layers of the tunica muscularis, namely the outer longitudinal, middle circular and inner oblique muscle layers.

Fundic or gastric glands secrete three types of substances from the following exocrine glands, namely mucous neck cells, chief cells and parietal cells.

- Mucous neck cells (found in the neck of gastric pits) – secrete mucus
- Chief (zygomatic) cells – secrete inactive pepsinogen in response to vans nerve stimulation and gastrin release
- Parietal (oxyntic) cells – secrete hydrochloric acid which converts inactive pepsinogen to active pepsin. Also secrete intrinsic factor.

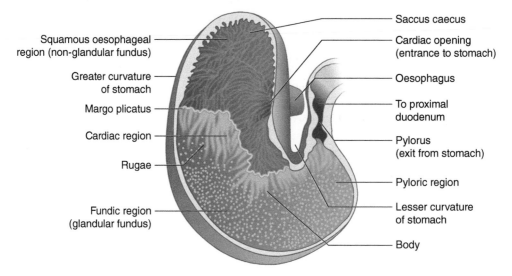

Figure 5.6 Structure of the equine stomach.

Gastrin is also released from pyloric G cells, while somatostatin is released from pyloric D cells which suppresses gastrin release. Histamine is released from enterochromaffin-like (ECL) cells which secrete histamine in response to gastrin. Horses continue to secrete acid at a variable rate even when the stomach is empty. This secretion involves histamine. The amount of acid varies between regions of the stomach and depends upon the food eaten. The higher pH area at the top is from swallowed saliva, which amounts to 10–12 litres per day in an adult horse, and has a bicarbonate concentration roughly twice that of blood. The lower pH areas are the bottom of the stomach.

The distal pyloric region connects to the small intestine via the pyloric sphincter. If the stomach is empty, the mucosa lies in folds called rugae which look like large wrinkles. Equine gastric lipase, which has a peak activity at pH 4.0, is produced by zymogen cells, primarily in the fundic mucosa. Horses produce a large amount of gastric lipase. Gastric pits are deeper in the pylorus than they are in other parts of the stomach (Figure 5.7).

The acid secretions help to kill any bacteria that may have been eaten with the food. As feed arrives in the stomach, the fundic glands in the stomach wall are stimulated to secrete gastric juice, which contains mucus, pepsin and hydrochloric acid. Gastric impaction, food engorgement, excessive water intake after exercise, aerophagia and *Gasterophilus* infestation may lead to gastric rupture. Gastric rupture is always fatal (Figure 5.8).

Foods begin to break down due to enzymic and microbial digestion in the stomach. The stomach also has a small microbial population which allows a small amount of digestion to take place. (VFAs)

Gastric Juice

Some 10–30 litres of gastric juice are produced daily, containing:

- Pepsin – this enzyme is initially secreted as a substance called pepsinogen which is activated to form pepsin by the presence of hydrochloric acid. Pepsin breaks down proteins in the food into peptones and proteoses. Most of the protein digestion takes place later on in the small intestine.
- Hydrochloric acid – produced by parietal cells, it is responsible for the conversion of pepsinogen to pepsin. It also has a strong antibacterial function.

The chewing of food results in large quantities of saliva being produced. This is alkaline and helps to neutralise the acidic

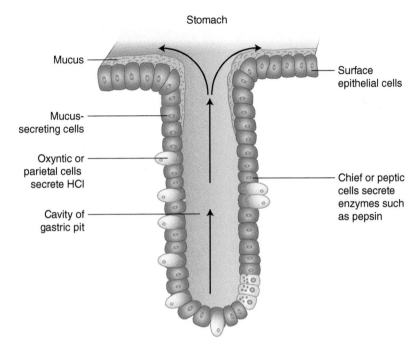

Figure 5.7 Gastric pit showing origins of stomach secretions.

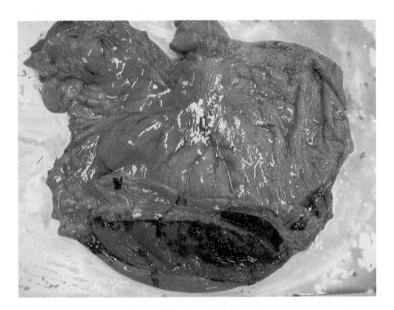

Figure 5.8 Post-mortem image of a spontaneous gastric rupture secondary to gastric impaction in an 18-year-old Quarter-horse mare. The site of rupture is along the greater curvature, with marked reddening and haemorrhage evident from the site of perforation. *Source*: Southwood 2013. Reproduced with permission of John Wiley & Sons.

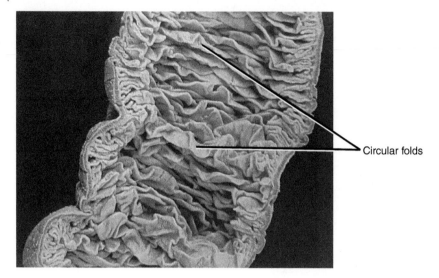

Circular folds

Figure 5.9 Internal anatomy of the jejunum. *Source*: Tortora 2009. Reproduced with permission of John Wiley & Sons.

environment of the stomach, as the saliva is swallowed. This results in marked variations in the acidity of the food in various regions of the stomach. Near the entrance to the stomach – in the oesophageal and cardiac regions – the material is neutral; in the fundic region it is slightly acidic; and in the pyloric region it is highly acidic. This is where protein digestion begins. However, food material is only in the stomach for a short time and this limits the amount of digestion that can take place. It is in the less acidic regions of the stomach that some bacterial breakdown of food (or fermentation) occurs, resulting in a small amount of lactic acid. The secretion of gastric juice in horses is thought to be continuous, but the rate of secretion increases when food is present in the stomach.

The food material produced by the stomach is now known as chyme and is poured into the first part of the small intestine.

Small Intestine

The length of the small intestine in the horse is approximately 20–27 m (65–88 ft) with a capacity of 55–70 litres (12–16 gallons). It runs between the stomach and the caecum. The small intestine is split into three parts:

- duodenum
- jejunum
- ileum.

The duodenum is about 1 m long. It forms an S-shaped bend which contains the pancreas. The pancreatic and bile ducts enter the duodenum approximately 150 mm (6 in) from the pyloric sphincter of the stomach. The jejunum is 20 m (65 ft) long and its internal anatomy is shown in Figure 5.9. The ileum is 1–1.5 m (3–5 ft) long. Both the jejunum and the ileum lie to the left side of the abdomen between the stomach and the pelvis. The small intestine can move quite freely except at its attachment to the stomach and the caecum. It lies in several coils with the small colon. The mesentery is very long to allow movement around the caecum and colon.

The small intestine is the major site of enzymic breakdown of soluble nutrients from forage and other feed such as starch and protein and absorption of the resulting nutrients. The fibre part of the diet is digested mainly in the large intestine. The digestion of some food in the small intestine is similar to that which occurs in simple-stomached animals such as humans and pigs. The digestive enzymes of the horse's stomach and small intestine are shown in Table 5.1.

Table 5.1 Digestive enzymes: origins, substrates and end products.

Substance source	Content	Effect
Saliva from salivary glands	Amylase (very low activity in horses, insufficient to digest starch)	Little if any starch digestion
Gastric juice from glands within stomach	Hydrochloric acid (HCl)	Provides optimum pH for function of stomach enzymes, disinfects, acts on inactive pepsinogen to convert to pepsin, promotes ion absorption
	Pepsinogen	Activated via HCl to pepsin, digests proteins to produce proteoses and peptones
	Pepsin	Acts on proteins to form proteoses and peptones
	Rennin	Only in foals together with calcium ions, it coagulates milk for easier digestion
	Lipase	Acts on triacylglycerols (TAGS) to form diacylglycerols and fatty acids
	Intrinsic factor	Promotes vitamin B_{12} absorption, required for erythrocyte production
Gastric mucosa	Mucus and bicarbonate	Protect stomach lining from HCl
Pancreatic juice from pancreas – in contrast to most species, this is continuous and profuse in the horse	Pancreatic amylase – very low in horses due to natural forage ration	Digests starch to glucose
	Erepsin (a mixture of peptidases)	Acts on peptides, proteoses and peptones to produce amino acids
	Aminopeptidases	Act on peptides to produce amino acids
	Pancreatic lipase	Digests fats to monoglycerides, glycerol and fatty acids
	Trypsinogen – very low in horses	Digests protein to peptides following activation to trypsin which then also activates chymotrypsinogen
	Chymotrypsinogen	Forms chymotrypsin which digests protein to form peptides
	Carboxypeptidase	Digests peptides to constituent amino acids
	Sucrase	Breaks down sucrose to glucose and fructose
	Lactase	Breaks down lactose to glucose and galactose
	Maltase	Breaks down maltose to glucose
	Nucleosidase	Breaks down mononucleotides to nucleosides, pentoses and trypsin
	Enterokinase	Activates only trypsinogen to trypsin
	Trypsin	Catalyses the hydrolysis of peptide bonds, breaking down proteins into smaller peptides

(Continued)

Table 5.1 (Continued)

Substance source	Content	Effect
Bile from liver	Bile salts	Emulsifies fats into 1-μm droplets which increase the surface area for lipase action. Also aids absorption of fats
	Bile pigments, e.g. bilirubin	Produces breakdown products of haemoglobin which are excreted in the faeces
Succus entericus from crypts of Lieberkühn and Brunner's glands – produce Intestinal juice	Aminopeptidase	Digests peptides to form amino acids
	Maltase	Digests maltose to glucose
	Sucrase	Digests sucrose to glucose and fructose
	Lactase	Digests lactose to glucose and galactose
	Enterokinase	Activates trypsinogen to trypsin

In order to increase the contact area with the food and the wall of the intestine (the mucosa) the wall is thrown into folds. Furthermore, the entire mucosa is covered in fine finger-like projections known as villi (similar to a carpet with a fairly close pile). Opening between the bases of the villi are the glands known as the crypts of Lieberkühn. The glands in the duodenum take the form of highly branched and coiled structures. There are three types of gland in the small intestine, which are responsible for the production of many different enzymes:

• intestinal glands (crypts of Lieberkühn)
• duodenal glands (Brunner's glands)
• Peyer's patches.

The intestinal glands or crypts of Lieberkühn and Peyer's patches are found throughout the small intestine, but the duodenal or Brunner's glands are found in the first part of the small intestine. Peyer's patches are accumulations of lymphoid tissue and their function is to control bacterial populations and produce antibodies.

Although the enzymes in the stomach need an acidic environment, the opposite is true of the small intestine. Here the enzymes require alkaline conditions. This alkalinity is produced mainly by the pancreatic juice from the pancreas and bile from the liver.

The small intestine is quite mobile and sometimes a small intestinal (SI) volvulus occurs in horses when the intestine rotates on its mesenteric axis, resulting in strangulation and death of SI tissues (Figure 5.10). This is often seen in foals aged between 2 and 4 months due to changing to solid food from milk.

Pancreas

The pancreas is a diffuse organ situated behind the stomach and is made up of small groups of glandular epithelial cells. In 1869 Paul Langerhans discovered the islets of Langerhans. The pancreas is thought of as an organ gland as it has both endocrine and exocrine functions. Its major homeostatic role is to maintain levels of blood glucose within a limited range. The horse has two pancreatic ducts.

Figure 5.11 shows a diagram of a section of pancreatic tissue. There are more beta cells (65%) than alpha cells (15%). The islets of Langerhans constitute the endocrine portion of the pancreas. The acini constitute the exocrine portion.

Endocrine Functions of the Pancreas

• Alpha cells secrete the hormone glucagon, which effectively raises blood glucose if it becomes too low.

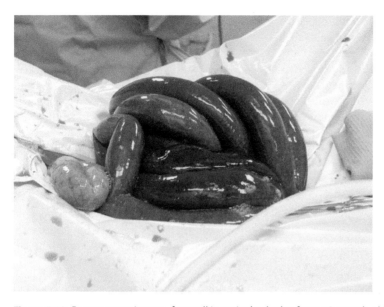

Figure 5.10 Post-mortem image of a small intestinal volvulus from a 2-month-old colt. Note the extensive jejunal dilation and poor viability resulting from this strangulating obstruction. *Source*: Southwood 2013. Reproduced with permission of John Wiley & Sons.

Figure 5.11 Section of pancreatic tissue.

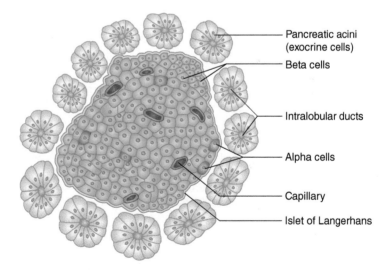

- Beta cells secrete insulin, which lowers blood glucose should it become too high by promoting cellular uptake of glucose around the body.
- Both insulin and glucagon work to keep blood glucose within a stable range.
- Delta cells produce the hormone somatostatin, which has an effect on neurotransmission and the proliferation of cells.

- Epsilon cells produce ghrelin, a hormone that stimulates appetite.
- Pancreatic polypeptide controls self-regulation of pancreatic secretions.

Exocrine Functions of the Pancreas

Enzymes are produced by the pancreatic exocrine cells arranged in clusters known as acini. The cells contain bicarbonate ions in addition to the precursor digestive enzymes. The bicarbonate ions neutralise acidic contents that have arrived from the stomach. This increase in pH is important as it results in the optimal environment for the pancreatic enzymes to function. The acini secrete pancreatic juice into the duodenal area of the small intestine to help digest food. Secretion from the acini occurs via a series of small intralobular ducts (see Figure 5.11). These drain into the pancreatic duct and then the duodenum. The enzymes are as follows:

- trypsin and chymotrypsin
- pancreatic lipase
- pancreatic amylase.

The mechanism of insulin secretion from the beta cells of the islets of Langerhans is a complex process involving the selective entry of glucose into cells and the metabolism of glucose within those cells to trigger the activation of voltage gated calcium channels, enabling the transport of insulin storage granules by exocytosis (see Chapter 2). Insulin is then exported rapidly into an extensive blood vessel network.

Liver

The liver is the largest gland in the body and one of the accessory glands of the digestive system, the others being the pancreas and salivary glands. It is also the largest homeostatic organ in the horse's body. It is situated immediately behind the diaphragm and in front of the stomach, and it is held in position by six ligaments and the pressure of surrounding organs. The liver weighs from 5 to 9 kg (12–20 lb) depending upon the size of the horse. It is reddish-brown in colour and is covered with connective tissue. It has two surfaces and four borders.

The liver is supplied with blood from two sources. The major source (about 75%) is by way of the hepatic portal vein which drains the stomach and small intestine. This blood contains the products of digestion. As the hepatic portal vein enters the liver, it breaks up into a series of branches which supply a capillary bed within the liver tissues. From there the blood drains into the hepatic veins, which eventually discharge into the inferior vena cava, and is taken back to the heart. The blood passing into the hepatic veins has therefore passed through two capillary beds, one in the gut wall and one in the liver tissues. This special arrangement reflects the function of the liver as a regulator of the products of metabolism and also the regulation of the composition of blood. The liver is therefore able to regulate the blood, by assessing the products of digestion and some toxic materials before they enter into the general circulation. The second smaller blood supply (about 25%) to the liver is from the hepatic artery, which delivers oxygenated blood from the dorsal aorta.

The liver tissue is made up of many smaller units known as liver lobules (Figure 5.12). Running through the centre of each lobule is a branch of the hepatic vein, and blood drains across the tissue of the liver lobule from branches of the hepatic portal vein situated around the boundary of the lobule into the central vein. The hepatic portal vein carries nutrient-rich deoxygenated blood from the gut into the liver. As blood drains across the lobule it bathes the liver cells. At the boundary of the lobule, in addition to branches of the hepatic portal vein, are branches of the hepatic artery and accessory branches of the bile duct (bile ductules) which drain away bile produced by the hepatic liver cells.

The tissue of the liver lobule is arranged in vertical rows or sheets, separated by blood spaces (the sinusoids) between rows of hepatocytes (through which blood flows inwards towards the central vein) and small channels through which bile flows known as bile canaliculi. The sinusoids are highly permeable and are lined by special cells, known as phagocytic cells, part of the reticulo-endothelial system which are capable of phagocytosis, that is, they can engulf dead bacteria, blood parasites and cell fragments.

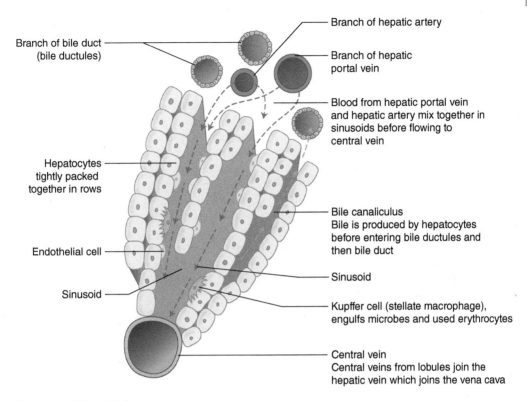

Branch of hepatic artery

Branch of bile duct
(bile ductules)

Branch of hepatic
portal vein

Blood from hepatic portal vein
and hepatic artery mix together in
sinusoids before flowing to
central vein

Hepatocytes
tightly packed
together in rows

Bile canaliculus
Bile is produced by hepatocytes
before entering bile ductules and
then bile duct

Endothelial cell

Sinusoid

Sinusoid

Kupffer cell (stellate macrophage),
engulfs microbes and used erythrocytes

Central vein
Central veins from lobules join the
hepatic vein which joins the vena cava

Figure 5.12 A liver lobule.

Kupffer cells, also known as stellate macrophages and Kupffer–Browicz cells, are specialised macrophages located in the liver lining the walls of the sinusoids (see Figure 5.12). The vertical plates are two cells thick and between these cells run fine canals which drain the bile produced by the liver cells. These are known as bile canaliculi and they drain outwards towards the boundary of the lobule where they join the larger bile ducts.

Functions of the Liver

It is thought that the liver has over a hundred different functions, the most important of which are listed below.

Regulation of Metabolites

When amino acids produced from digestion are absorbed into the body they join the circulating amino acids in the blood. This is known as the amino acid pool and from this tissues take up amino acids in the process of growth and/or repair. The quantity and type of amino acids in this pool will vary depending upon the dietary protein intake by the horse. In well-fed horses, the protein intake may greatly exceed the requirements of the horse. Also, some amino acids can be made by the body itself and these are known as non-essential amino acids. The liver is then able to break down the unwanted excess amino acids and the non-essential amino acids.

Protein Metabolism

Protein metabolism consists of the following:

- Removal of the amino group from amino acids ($-NH_2$), leaving the remainder to be used for adenosine triphosphate (ATP) production or converted to carbohydrates or fats. This is known as the ornithine or urea cycle.

- Conversion of ammonia (which is toxic) to urea (which is less so), before being excreted in the urine.
- Synthesis of plasma proteins, for example globulins, albumin, prothrombin and fibrinogen.

Carbohydrate Metabolism

The liver is especially important in maintaining normal blood glucose levels. When blood glucose is low, the liver breaks down stored glycogen and releases glucose into the blood. It also has the ability to convert certain amino acids and lactic acid to glucose if required. Moreover, it can convert other sugars such as fructose and galactose to glucose. Synthesis of glucose from non-carbohydrate sources is known as gluconeogenesis.

If blood glucose is high, for example owing to excess glucose being absorbed from the intestine, the liver diverts it into storage as either glycogen or triglycerides. The liver cells provide the main storage area for glycogen, although muscles also store glycogen. Liver glycogen is rapidly mobilised and converted to glucose when blood sugar levels become low. The deposition and mobilisation of glycogen in the liver is under the influence of the hormones insulin and adrenaline.

Lipid Metabolism

The liver is also involved in the metabolism of lipids. When the horse is using its fat stores as a major energy source, for example in times of starvation or when energy requirements exceed energy intake, large quantities of triglycerides appear in the liver. Accumulation of fat in the liver is a sign of rapid fat mobilisation to provide the required energy. Hepatocytes are the main functional cells of the liver and undertake a large number of metabolic, endocrine and secretory functions:

- Fatty acids within triglycerides are broken down to ATP.
- Hepatocytes synthesise lipoproteins which then are used to transport fatty acids, cholesterol and triglycerides to and from body cells.
- Hepatocytes make bile salts from cholesterol.
- Cholesterol can be synthesised from acetyl CoA.

Production of Bile

Bile is produced within the cells of the liver and is a product of red cell destruction. It is alkaline and the fluid contains bile salts, bile pigments, cholesterol and salts. The bile pigments biliverdin and bilirubin result from the breakdown of haemoglobin and are excretory products. Gastric and pancreatic lipases require emulsification of the substrate fats for optimal enzymic activity. Bile salts play an essential role in making the products of fat breakdown soluble for absorption because they are amphiphilic (composed of hydrophilic and hydrophobic portions) molecules. Monoacylglycerols (intermediates in lipid breakdown) interact with bile salts, forming mixed micelles enabling the fats to move through the brush border of the intestine where they are absorbed by enterocytes. Once in the enterocyte they are reformed into their original triacylglycerols and moved into the lymphatic system. A micelle is simply a mixture of molecules in a colloidal solution. Emulsification is the breaking down of fat globules which are emulsified to form smaller globules to increase the surface area for action by the fat-digesting lipase enzymes.

After use in the small intestine, the bile salts sodium taurocholate and glycocholate are actively re-absorbed into the hepatic portal vein and taken back to the liver to be re-used in the bile. These pigments are breakdown products of haemoglobin and responsible for the green/yellow colour of bile. Bile does not contain any digestive enzymes.

Bilirubin is derived from the haem group of old red blood cells and is absorbed by the liver before being excreted in the bile juice. Most of this bilirubin in metabolised in the small intestine by bacteria and then excreted in the faeces. Horses do not have a gall bladder as they are almost-continuous trickle feeders. Bile is therefore produced almost continuously.

Detoxification

The liver detoxifies products that have been taken into the body – such as drugs, for example penicillin and sulphonamides – and substances already produced in the body – such as steroid hormones, for example oestrogens – and also thyroid hormones which are then deactivated.

Vitamin Storage

Significant quantities of the fat-soluble vitamins A, D, E and K together with iron and copper are found in the liver. Vitamin B_{12} is also stored here. These are released as required by other parts of the horse's body.

Hindgut

Horses are post-gastric fermenters, unlike ruminants which are pre-gastric fermenters. Fermentation involves huge numbers of microbes which undertake digestion of cellulose and hemicellulose within the hindgut. The microbiome of horses is now receiving considerable interest from researchers following on from research in humans, and this is discussed later in the chapter (see 'Equine Microbiota').

Large Intestine

The large intestine is made up of the caecum, large colon, small colon and rectum. The large intestine is approximately 8m (25ft) long. Although the foregut of the horse is similar to other simple-stomached animals, the hindgut is remarkably different. It is in the horse's hindgut that the complex insoluble carbohydrates (cellulose and hemicellulose) are digested. The horse itself does not have enzymes such as cellulase which could break down these complex substances. Another common component of plant fibrous material ingested by the horse is lignin. This is the woody-type material that

supports the growth of grass stems. Even the microbiota are unable to digest this material and poor-quality forage will be high in lignin. Some microbiota, however, can break down other fibre components by a process of fermentation. The horse has a greatly enlarged large intestine which accommodates a vast number of microbiota and these are able to release the 'locked' energy, providing nutrients to the horse. In return the microbiota are provided with a safe environment in which to live.

More than half the dry weight of faeces produced by the horse is microbiota. The amount of microbes in the digestive tract of the horse is huge and number more than ten times all the tissue cells in the horse's body.

Caecum

The caecum is a large, blind-ended, comma-shaped sac situated at the end of the small intestine. The entrance to the caecum lies near the right hip bone and runs forwards and down 1 m (3 ft) to finish midway along the belly, lying on the floor of the abdomen. The capacity of the caecum is approximately 25–35 litres (6–8 gallons). The caecum acts as a large fermentation vat where plant fibre is mixed with the microbiota. Figures 5.13 and 5.14 show the main anatomical structures of the caecum and colon within the abdomen.

Large Colon

The large colon is approximately 3–4 m (10–13 ft) long and has a capacity of 90–110 litres (20–24 gallons). In order to fit into the abdomen, the large colon is folded into four regions (see Figures 5.11 and 5.12). The first part is known as the right ventral colon and runs forward from the top of the caecum until it reaches the sternal flexure. Here, there is a narrowing of the diameter of the colon and it turns back on itself to continue backwards as the left ventral colon, running along the left side of the horse to the pelvic region. The colon then turns again into the pelvic flexure, the diameter reducing to as little as

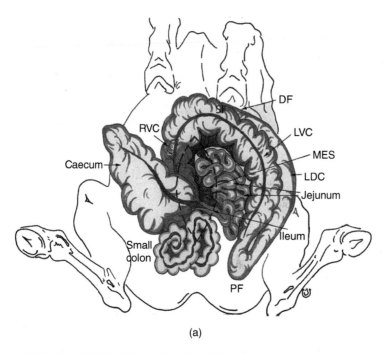

(a)

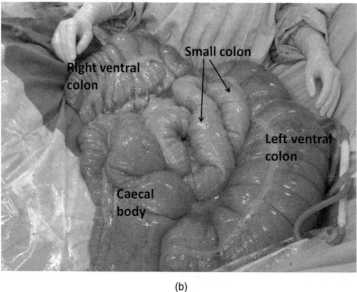

(b)

Figure 5.13 (a) Schematic illustration identifying portions of the gastrointestinal tract accessible from the ventral midline incision. DF, diaphragmatic flexure; LDC, left dorsal colon; LVC, left ventral colon; MES, mesentery of the jejunum with arcuate vessels; PF, pelvic flexure; RVC, right ventral colon. (b) Photograph of exteriorised intestine. The surgeon is standing on the left side of the intestine. *Source*: Southwood 2013. Reproduced with permission of John Wiley & Sons.

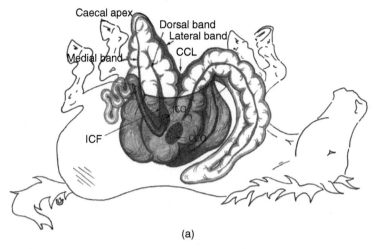

(a)

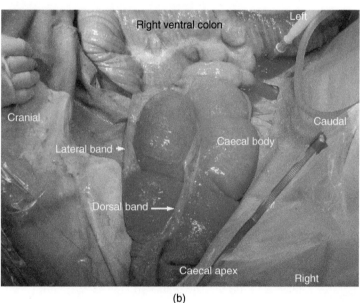

(b)

Figure 5.14 (a) Schematic illustration depicting caecal orientation. Lighter-colored parts of the intestine are able to be exteriorised. CCL, Caecocolic ligament; CCO, caecocolic orifice; ICF, ileocaecal fold; ICO, Ileocaecal orifice. (b) Photograph of exteriorised caecum showing the apex, body and caecal bands. Note that the caecum has been reflected backwards towards the caudal aspect of the horse and the ventral caecal band is not visible. *Source*: Southwood 2013. Reproduced with permission of John Wiley & Sons.

9 cm (2.5 in), before it rapidly expands again to continue towards the diaphragm as the left dorsal colon. The colon makes a final turn at the diaphragmatic flexure and the right dorsal colon runs backwards, narrowing to become the small colon.

The large intestine is only held in place by its bulk. The flexures are points where there is a change in direction and a narrowing of the gut. They are, not surprisingly, vulnerable to blockages. The digesta reaches the caecum approximately 3 hours after a meal and remains in the large intestine for 36–48 hours.

Small Colon

The small colon is 3–4 m (10–13 ft) long but is narrower than the large colon. It lies intermingled with the jejunum, and as it is fairly free to move it can lead to abdominal crises such as a twisted gut.

Rectum

The rectum is a relatively short, straight tube connecting the small colon to the anus. It acts as a storage area for faeces before it is evacuated as dung.

Digestion in the Large Intestine

Water is absorbed from the digesta throughout the large intestine. By the time it reaches the rectum, the waste material is of firm consistency ready to be voided as droppings. The main function of the caecum and large intestine, as already stated, is to provide a safe environment for the millions of microbes which digest cellulose and other plant fibrous material for the horse. The microbes ferment the fibrous part of the diet, but they also synthesise some of the essential amino acids and some of the water-soluble vitamins, namely those of the B vitamin group.

The number and type of microbes in the gut depend to a large extent on the diet being fed to the horse, that is, the substrates available to them. Numbers or densities of specific microbes may change drastically over a 24-hour period if the horse's diet is changed. These changes reflect the changes in availability of nutrients and subsequent changes in pH within the large intestine. A change in the ratio of hay to cereal will have a large effect and will influence the types of microbes that can survive in the large intestine.

The microbes ferment insoluble carbohydrates such as cellulose to energy-producing substances known as volatile fatty acids (VFAs). The principal VFAs produced are acetate, propionate and butyrate. Lactate is also produced, particularly from any soluble carbohydrate entering the hindgut. Horses receiving higher levels of concentrates (cereal-based diets) have higher levels of lactate, resulting in a decrease in pH due to the increased acid, and this reduces concentrations of the fibre-degrading microbes.

VFAs within the colon and caecum are in their ionised forms, but they must be in their non-ionised form to be absorbed by passive diffusion down a concentration gradient across the mucosal wall. This is the principal route of absorption. There is also a net absorption of sodium chloride and water from the lumen of the hindgut into the blood. The pH close to the epithelial wall remains constant even if it is changing in the lumen. VFAs are absorbed into the bloodstream and converted to energy. This allows the horse to thrive on its natural forage diet.

Horses are also able to assimilate dietary nitrogen in the colon, but little is known about how or in what form this is absorbed. There is evidence that horses may absorb ammonia and some amino acids of both dietary and microbial origin into the blood. The large intestine also acts as a large water reservoir in horses. The fermentation process in the gut has a major influence on both plasma and water volume of the gut.

Equine Microbiota

Previously referred to as gut flora, the scientifically correct name used now is microbiota which means 'little life' and refers to the microbes that normally inhabit an environment such as the horse's gut (or skin). Microbiota consist mainly of bacteria, archaeobacteria, protozoa, anaerobic fungi and phages. The microbiome refers to the microbes at a particular site or in a particular habitat, such as the gut microbes and their genes. Microbiota exist throughout the digestive tract, but the majority are found within the hindgut. Protozoal activity is not fully understood, though microbiota appear to have limited cellulolytic activity and can break down pectin. Table 5.2 shows common

Table 5.2 Distribution of bacteria and protozoa in the horse's gut.

Site	Protozoa (per gramme of ingesta)	Total bacteria (per gramme)
Stomach	0	200×10^6
Small intestine	0	36×10^6
Caecum	567	482×10^6
Large intestine	567	363×10^6

bacteria and protozoa that live within the horse's digestive tract.

Colic is one of the most common health problems associated with the gut. It is a leading cause of death in horses and is most often associated with changes in the microbiota in the hindgut due to factors such as dietary disruption, seasonal changes, stress or age. Researchers are now looking at what constitutes a 'normal' gut microbiome for horses; for example, does it vary between good and poor doers and does it change with age and disease?

In humans, it is believed that the intestinal microbiome contains up to 1000 different species and approximately 10^{12} bacteria per gramme of faeces. The gut of many vertebrates is mostly dominated by two groups of bacteria: *Bacteroides* (approximately 20%), formerly known as *Bacteroidetes*, and Firmicutes (approximately 72%). Members of the Firmicutes phylum appear to predominate in horses, yet there are also significant populations of numerous other phyla. Minor populations of *Actinobacteria, Fibrobacteres, Fusobacteria* and *Cyanobacteria* species are also present, as part of a complex microbial community. Recent studies on the equine microbiome of six healthy horses supported the fact that Firmicutes were the major bacterium phylum populating the distal intestine of healthy horses. The predominance of Firmicutes may be related to the feeding habits of horses, which ingest mainly insoluble fibre and use the caecum and large colon for fermentation. In addition, other research has compared the bacterial

component of faeces from horses on two different diets and observed that horses fed supplementary concentrates had ten times more lactic acid-producing bacteria than horses receiving a forage-only diet.

There are marked differences in the microbiome between healthy horses and those with colitis. Colitis may be a disease of gut microbiome dysbiosis, rather than one that occurs simply through overgrowth of an individual pathogen. This new area of research using metagenomic profiling of faecal and distal hindgut microbiota could lead to immense steps forward in the understanding of not only digestion but also its effects on equine health and behaviour. Studies suggest that faecal samples may represent the microbial population of the right dorsal colon but not that of the caecum, indicating that careful consideration is required when planning microbial investigations of the hindgut. In other words, it appears that the microbiome of the caecum is different from that of the dorsal colon. The microbiota and their activity within different parts of the gut depend upon the anatomy and also the substrate or food supplies reaching that part of the gut.

Firmicutes are mostly Gram positive (+ve) and include clostridia such as *Clostridium septicum, Megasphaera, Lactobacillus, Staphylococcus* and *Streptococcus* such as *Streptococcus bovis* and *Streptococcus equinus*. Bacteroides are mainly Gram negative (−ve) and include *Bacteroides* and *Prevotella*. Actinobacteria include *Bifidobacterium* and *Atopobium*. Fibrobacteres is a small bacterial phylum which includes bacteria that can degrade plant-based cellulose in some animals. The genus *Fibrobacter* (the only genus of Fibrobacteres) was removed from the *Bacteroides* a while ago. In addition, the microbiota in the caecum of horses seem more consistent than that in the right dorsal colon and faeces. Table 5.3 shows examples and functions of some common hindgut bacteria.

Each horse will have its own individual microbiota, in terms of numbers and species, and this will depend upon its environment,

Table 5.3 Microbiota – examples of functions of some hindgut bacteria.

Cellulolytic bacteria	Glycolytic and amylolytic bacteria	Lactate-producing bacteria	Lactate-utilising bacteria
Ruminococcus flavefaciens (F)	*Streptococci* (F)	*Streptococcus bovis* (F)	*Megasphaena* sp. (F)
Fibrobacter succinogenes	*Lactobacilli* (F)	*Streptococcus equinus* (F)	*Veillonella* sp. (F)
	Enterococci (F)	*Lactobacilli* (F)	

F, Firmicutes.

diet, stress levels, antibiotic history and so on. There are much smaller numbers of microbiota in the small intestine where the horse is able to digest and absorb the non-fibrous part of the diet quite efficiently.

The Gut and the Immune System

A huge amount of immune cells are located in the gut. The digestive tract mucosal immune system is highly complex. It must be able to respond to potential pathogens but also tolerate food antigens and healthy, beneficial microbiota. The immune system of the intestinal tract is often referred to as gut-associated lymphoid tissue (GALT) and works to protect the horse's body from invasion. Throughout the intestinal tract there are macrophages and lymphocytes, cells of the immune system under the intestinal lining cells. Structures called Peyer's patches are very similar to lymph nodes and are located in the small intestine, as discussed on page 132. Specialised immune cells are also found in the lining of the liver.

Microfold cells, or M cells, are located over collections of lymphoid tissue along the intestinal tract and in Peyer's patches. The M cells reach out to engulf bacteria and other material from the intestinal tract, then pull it inside and present it to immune system cells to deal with. This material is processed through B and T lymphocytes, resulting in the eventual production of immunoglobulin A (IgA) antibodies, which remain in the local tissues to protect them.

The lymphocytes that produce local IgA antibodies are released into the bloodstream before they return to the intestinal lining again. In the process, information is shared with the horse's immune system so that it can produce circulating antibodies (IgG, IgM) to the same organisms. The production of antibodies is only one process in the immune system activity of the gut. Horses with a healthy gut and microbiota are able to support their immune systems far better than those with dysbiosis.

Summary Points

1) The digestive system is the horse's largest sensory organ.
2) The natural diet of herbivores consists of grasses and vegetation containing large amounts of insoluble or complex carbohydrate known as cellulose.
3) Throughout the length of the gut there are several changes in direction and diameter, which partially explains the horse's susceptibility to blockages which manifest themselves as colic.
4) The microbiota ferment insoluble carbohydrates such as cellulose to energy-producing substances known as VFAs. The principal VFAs produced are acetate, propionate and butyrate. Lactate is also produced.
5) VFAs within the colon and caecum are in their ionised forms and must be in their non-ionised form to be absorbed by passive diffusion down a concentration gradient across the mucosal wall.

6) The microbiome of the horse's hindgut is now receiving considerable interest from researchers.

7) Each horse will have its own individual microbiota, in terms of numbers and species, and this will depend upon its environment, diet, stress levels, antibiotic history and so on.

8) This new area of research using metagenomic profiling of faecal and distal hindgut microbiota could lead to great steps forward in the understanding of equine digestion and its effects on equine health and behaviour.

Q + A

Q How long do horses typically spend grazing per 24-hour period?

A 14–16 hours.

Q What is the enteric nervous system?

A The ENS is a complex nervous network supplying the gut, which includes afferent neurons, interneurons and motor neurons.

Q Explain how the diet will affect the amount of chewing movements.

A Horses have evolved as forage eaters and rely on their teeth for 'processing' this fibrous food. All food has to be ground down to less than 1 mm in length before swallowing – obviously this will take much longer for hay than for concentrates. Indeed, it has been estimated that horses will chew 1 kg of concentrate feed 800–1200 times, but need 3000–3500 chews to get through 1 kg of hay.

Q What are rugae?

A These are folds in the mucosa of the gut wall.

Q Which cells of the pancreas produce the hormone somatostatin?

A Delta cells in the pancreatic islets.

6

The Respiratory System

The horse requires a constant supply of oxygen to stay alive. At all times, in all living cells, energy liberation from nutrients to produce adenosine triphosphate (ATP) continues without interruption in the mitochondria. This energy results from the oxidation of complex carbon-containing substances. In simple terms, glucose is broken down in the presence of oxygen to release carbon dioxide (CO_2) and energy. The waste product CO_2 is toxic and must be quickly eliminated from the body. Mitochondria need a steady supply of oxygen to release the potential energy stored in fuels in muscle cells, such as fat and glycogen. However, most mitochondria in muscle cells are a long way from any oxygen in the air. Respiration is the process by which the horse takes oxygen into its body and also rids it of CO_2.

The horse is a relatively large animal and therefore will need to take in more oxygen. In a 5-furlong race, for example, a horse will breathe in approximately 1800 litres of air, of which 378 litres is oxygen and most of the rest is nitrogen. The respiratory system consists of the nose, pharynx, larynx, trachea, bronchi and lungs. The horse does not breathe through its mouth and nose as humans do but breathes through its nares (nostrils) only. Essentially, respiration is the exchange of gases between the horse and its environment. The horse has a system of respiratory organs which are designed to bring oxygen into the cells of the body and to expel CO_2 and water.

There are essentially three steps to the process of gaseous exchange:

- Breathing (pulmonary ventilation) – airflow into and out of the lungs.
- External respiration – exchange of gases at the alveoli/blood interface.
- Internal respiration – exchange of gases at the tissue cells/blood interface in the body.

The primary function of the respiratory system is exchange of CO_2 and oxygen from pulmonary capillaries. The respiratory system has secondary functions too. Secondary functions of the equine respiratory system include:

- phonation (vocalisation)
- containing receptors for the sense of smell
- thermoregulation
- elimination of water
- regulation of acidity of the blood.

If horses are unable to remove excess CO_2 accumulating through metabolism, such as during hard exercise, for example, it will accumulate in the blood, increasing acidity (reducing pH) and this is known as respiratory acidosis. Conversely, if blood CO_2 is lower than normal due to the respiratory system removing too much CO_2 and blood pH rises, then this is known as respiratory alkalosis. These changes in CO_2 and pH are closely linked (see 'Carbon Dioxide Transport').

Equine Science, Third Edition. Zoe Davies and Sarah Pilliner.
© 2018 Zoe Davies and Sarah Pilliner. Published 2018 by John Wiley & Sons Ltd.

Anatomy

The respiratory system consists of the airways of the head, neck and the lungs. It is in essence a series of tubes, starting at the nostrils and ending as a multitude of tiny, thin-walled sacs called alveoli which are in intimate contact with a dense network of blood capillaries. The structures involved are the nasal cavity, pharynx, larynx, trachea, bronchi, lungs, pleurae and thoracic cavity.

Within the Head and Neck

The airways of the head and neck are shown in Figure 6.1. The external nares or nostrils are the entrance to the respiratory system. The horse draws in air only through the nostrils and not through the mouth, and the nostrils can expand in order to take in more air. The lateral wall of the external naris is very flexible, which allows it to expand significantly during peak exercise. During exertion, the lateral wall dilates, creating a wider lower-resistance passageway for the movement of air into the nostril. The nostril is helped by the presence of a short blind-ended diverticulum at the side of the true nasal cavity. This is known as the nasal diverticulum or 'false nostril' and is thought to aid in passive dilation of the nostrils during vigorous breathing.

The nostrils lead to the nasal cavity which is divided into two by the nasal septum. The nasal septum is cartilaginous towards the nose and the back part is bone. Each side contains three delicate bones arising from the lateral wall called conchae, which are scroll-like (also known as turbinates) and covered by a thick, soft mucous membrane which is a yellow-brown colour. The upper (dorsal) and lower (ventral) turbinates are long, rolled up like a scroll and perforated by many holes. Together with the nasal hairs and membrane covering the turbinates this contributes to the accuracy and sensitivity of the horse's sense of smell by providing a large surface area for warming and filtering the air that enters through the nostrils. The nasal cavity is separated from the mouth by the hard and soft palates.

The third turbinate bone (the ethmoid turbinate) is a group of plate-like projections in the back part of the nasal cavity. The surface of the mucous membrane that covers this bone is involved with the sense of smell. It is lined by mucous membrane know as the olfactory epithelium as it contains nerve endings from the olfactory nerve.

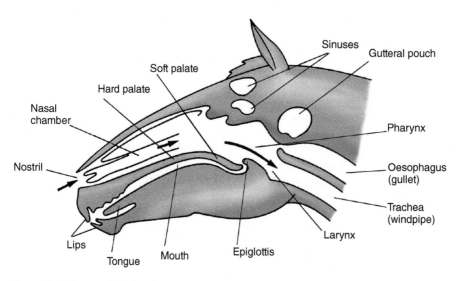

Figure 6.1 Airways of the head.

Each side of the nasal chamber is connected to four air sinuses, the paranasal sinuses. These are pockets in the bone which lie immediately beneath most of the surface bones of the forehead and occupy some space under the facial bones beneath the eyes. Horses have maxillary, frontal, sphenoidal and palatine sinuses in the bones. Also horses have several upper molars which project into the maxillary sinus and these may become infected. Sinuses appear to have no specific purpose other than some protection of the head, rounding out the facial areas and making the skull lighter in weight.

Once warmed and filtered, air passes the pharynx and larynx to go down the trachea (windpipe). The pharynx or throat is situated at the back of the throat and is a funnel-shaped organ involved in both the digestive and respiratory systems as it opens into the mouth and the nasal cavity (Figure 6.2). At the bottom of the pharynx is the soft palate which is overlapped by the

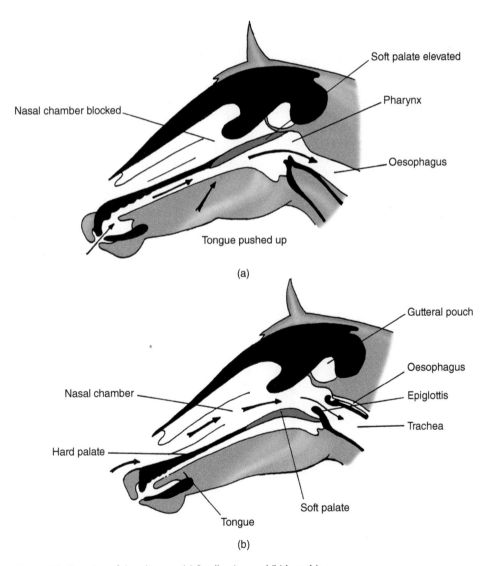

Figure 6.2 Function of the pharynx. (a) Swallowing and (b) breathing.

epiglottis. Most of the time, this overlapping effectively shuts off the mouth and allows the free passage of air into the next part of the respiratory system, namely the larynx. When the horse swallows, however, the epiglottis flips over the opening of the larynx, the soft palate moves up and food is admitted from the mouth into the pharynx and is then swallowed. There are two auditory (eustachian) tubes from the middle ears that also enter into the pharynx. Swallowing (deglutition) and phonation (vocalisation) are achieved by skeletal muscle in the pharynx walls.

The larynx is a short movable framework of cartilage and muscle that connects the pharynx and trachea; it supports the epiglottis and is also known as the voice box because it contains the vocal cords. When muscles in the larynx contract, the elastic ligaments stretched between pieces of rigid cartilage (similar to a stringed instrument) are pulled tight, pushing the true vocal cords into the airway. Air pushing against the vocal cords creates sound and the greater the air pressure, the greater the sound made.

The trachea runs from the larynx to the lungs and consists of a heavily walled tube kept permanently open by closely spaced C-shaped rings of cartilage set in its wall. The trachea passes down and back along the ventral surface of the neck and enters the thoracic cavity at the thoracic inlet.

Within the Chest

The lungs occupy most of the thoracic cavity. The right lung is bigger than the left and has an intermediate lobe (Figure 6.3). The structure of the lungs is shown in Figure 6.4. At the region of the heart the trachea divides

into two primary bronchi, each bronchus entering one lung at the hilus. Within the lung the bronchi divide and subdivide to terminate in the alveoli. The parts of the respiratory system within the lung are as follows:

- trachea
- primary bronchi
- secondary bronchi
- bronchioles – lobular and interlobular
- terminal bronchioles
- respiratory bronchioles
- alveolar sacs
- alveolar ducts
- alveoli.

The C-shaped rings of cartilage become plates in the primary bronchi and disappear completely in the secondary bronchi when these become less than 1 mm in diameter. The secondary bronchioles become bronchioles that continue to branch and reduce in diameter until they become respiratory bronchioles. Respiratory bronchioles have very thin walls and terminate in alveoli. The alveolar sacs are in the middle of a cluster of alveoli that are connected to the sac by delicate alveolar ducts. The lungs have a huge surface area due to the vast number of alveoli, estimated at 3000 million. If all the airways in the horse's lung were opened out and laid flat on the ground, they would occupy a total area equivalent to ten tennis courts. The alveoli are the true respiratory structures. Here the exchange of gases between the inspired air and the bloodstream takes place. Each alveolus is enclosed by a dense network of capillaries (Figure 6.4); the alveolar capillary wall consists of a continuous, extremely thin,

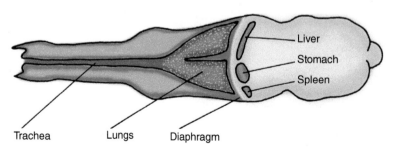

Figure 6.3 Relationship between the stomach, diaphragm and lungs.

Liver

Stomach

Spleen

Trachea   Lungs   Diaphragm

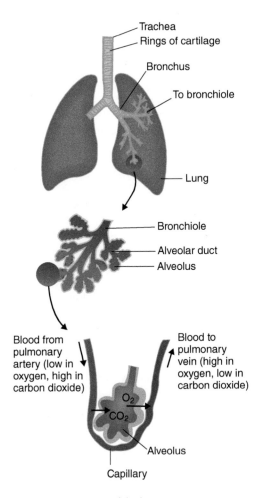

Trachea
Rings of cartilage
Bronchus
To bronchiole
Lung
Bronchiole
Alveolar duct
Alveolus

Blood from pulmonary artery (low in oxygen, high in carbon dioxide)

Blood to pulmonary vein (high in oxygen, low in carbon dioxide)

O_2
CO_2

Alveolus
Capillary

Figure 6.4 Structure of the lungs.

alveolar membrane, a basement membrane and an equally thin capillary endothelium. The air contained within the sacs is in such close contact with the blood that oxygen is able to move from the air in the alveoli into the blood, and CO_2 from the blood diffuses into the air in the alveoli and is removed when the horse exhales.

Air movement in and out of the lungs has little effect on alveolar size; inspiration and exhalation are achieved by the action of smooth muscle dilating and lengthening, and compressing and contracting the bronchial tree. This includes all structures up to the alveoli, with the main breathing activity being in the terminal bronchioles. Ventilation of the alveoli is accomplished by air currents caused by the expansion and contraction of the bronchioles rather than the bellows-like movement of the alveolar walls.

The inner surfaces of the alveoli and terminal bronchioles are coated with a surfactant fluid which reduces the surface tension of the fluids within the lung and helps prevent collapse of the alveoli. The surfactant has low surface tension in small areas and high surface tension in large areas. Without surfactant, therefore, the small alveoli would collapse into larger ones and fail to re-inflate, leading to laboured breathing and poor gaseous exchange.

The respiratory tract is lined and protected by special cells, many of which have frond-like cilia which give the airways a surface resembling a deep-pile carpet. These cilia are highly motile, creating currents which convey tiny bits of debris, carried in mucus, up the tubes to the pharynx, where the horse coughs or swallows. Larger particles are coughed or sneezed out of the system.

Blood Supply

The lung has two separate circulations of blood known as the pulmonary and bronchial circulations. The pulmonary blood system begins with the pulmonary artery which leaves the right ventricle of the heart and carries deoxygenated blood. The pulmonary artery divides to give the right and left pulmonary arteries, and these eventually subdivide to form the capillaries which surround the alveoli. Here gaseous exchange takes place and oxygenated blood is carried back to the heart via the pulmonary vein.

The tissue of the lung itself is nourished by blood carried in the bronchial circulation; the right and left bronchial arteries surround the lung, and the blood returns via the bronchial veins to the anterior vena cava.

Pleurae

The pleurae are membranes that cover the inner wall of the thorax and the organs found within the thorax. They are lubricated to slide over one another as the horse breathes in and out.

Diaphragm

The diaphragm separates the thorax and lungs from the abdomen which contains the digestive organs. It is a strong, dome-shaped sheet of membranous muscle attached to the ribs and involved in breathing.

Physiology of Respiration

Pulmonary Ventilation

Breathing is the obvious and well-known process of bringing air and blood into intimate contact in the lungs and consists of two phases, inhalation and exhalation. Transportation is the carrying of oxygen and CO_2 between the alveoli and the bloodstream. Breathing in (inspiration or inhalation) and out (expiration or exhalation) occurs under muscular effort and elastic recoil, the diaphragm being the main muscle for respiration. The flow of air between the outside environment and into the horse's lungs is due to changes in atmospheric air pressure. Horses breathe in when the pressure inside the lungs is lower than that externally. They breathe out when the pressure in the lungs is higher than atmospheric air pressure.

The diaphragm may contract or relax: when contracted it is flattened and back in the body, effectively lengthening the thorax and increasing the volume of the lungs; when relaxed it is curved into the thorax, reducing the width of the thorax and effectively causing expiration. There is a resting point of respiration which is when the opposing forces are equal. Energy is required to increase or decrease the volume beyond the resting point. This is different to breathing in humans; that is, inspiration and expiration in horses have active phases. Elastic recoil, however, is able to return the chest wall and lungs to the resting point without the use of energy. Elastic recoil of the chest wall and lungs occurs because both have a tendency to want to spring back once stretched.

The breathing cycle is as follows:

- inspiration – passive at first, then followed by diaphragm contraction
- expiration – passive to the resting point, followed by abdominal compression of the rib cage.

The horse draws air in through its nostrils; air passes through the larynx, down the trachea and into the lungs. Here, oxygen passes from the air into the bloodstream and CO_2 passes from the blood into the lungs, a process called gaseous exchange. The alveoli fill with air due to changes in the size and shape of the lungs; as the lungs are held within the thoracic cavity, the lungs change in shape as the thoracic cavity moves. The pleurae hold the lungs so that they conform with the inner walls of the chest. There is no pushing or pulling by the chest wall or diaphragm on the lungs as they inflate and deflate. The lungs are filled by the action of the dome-shaped diaphragm and ribs. When the ribs are pulled forward and outwards, the chest expands; simultaneously, the diaphragm contracts, flattening the dome and thus enlarging the 'box' in which the lungs are contained and drawing in air to fill the available space. As the diaphragm contracts, the abdominal muscles relax, allowing the abdominal organs to move down and back. This process is called inhalation or inspiration.

Breathing out or exhalation is accomplished by the thorax decreasing in size, causing the air to flow out as the elastic lungs contract. There are three groups of muscles that affect exhalation: abdominal muscles, muscles of the chest and smooth muscle around the bronchioles. As the abdominal muscles contract, pressure is put on the organs in the abdomen, which in turn press on the diaphragm and push it forwards to its resting position. The chest muscles rotate the ribs inward and back. The smooth muscle around the bronchioles contracts and forces air out of the lungs.

Table 6.1 Respiratory rate or respiratory frequency (fR) (breaths per minute) of various domestic animals and man.

Animal	Respiratory rate (breaths per minute)
Horse	8–16
Cow	
Dairy cow	18–28
Beef cow	12–20
Sheep	12–24
Goat	12–20
Pig	15–24
Dog	19–30
Cat	24–42
Man	12–30

Source: Adapted from *Duke's Physiology of Domestic Animals*.

The external intercostal muscles and the levatores costarum (very small intercostal muscles) move the ribs outward, upward and forward, thus increasing the size of the chest cavity. The internal intercostals rotate the ribs back to their resting position and the transverse thoracic muscles complete exhalation by compressing the thorax. In quiet breathing the muscles of inhalation do not contract fully and the muscles of exhalation are not used at all; the recoil of the chest wall and the collapse of stretched lung tissue accomplish the movement, as discussed above.

The respiration rate varies between species (Table 6.1). The average resting respiratory rate (fR) for the horse is 8–16 breaths per minute, the rate being higher for young horses. After strenuous exercise the rate can increase up to 150–180 breaths per minute. Table 6.1 shows the resting respiration rates for various domestic animals and man. Respiration rate may also increase due to pain and increased body temperature.

Pressure Changes during Breathing

When the horse's lungs expand, the air molecules inside including the alveoli sit in a larger volume and this reduces the air pressure. This means that atmospheric air pressure outside is now higher than the alveolar pressure inside the lungs and so air moves into the lungs. Conversely, when lung volume decreases on breathing out, gas molecules are squeezed into a smaller area, increasing air pressure inside and so air moves to the now lower atmospheric air pressure outside (see pulmonary ventilation).

Airway Resistance

In respiratory physiology, airway resistance is the resistance of the respiratory tract to airflow during inspiration and expiration and this affects the amount of oxygen reaching the lungs, particularly during maximum exercise by the horse. The horse can reduce this somewhat by dilating the larynx and flaring the nostrils for maximum opening. The horse will also lower its neck and head to create a straighter line for maximising air intake and reducing airway resistance. When horses inhale during exercise, approximately 90% of the airway resistance is in the airways of the head, that is, the nostrils, nasal passages and larynx. However, when horses exhale, the majority of air resistance of around 55% is within the lower airways of the lung.

Lung Air Volumes and Capacities

Horses have a very large lung capacity when accounting for the size of the animal (Figure 6.5). Figure 6.6 shows the position of the lungs externally.

Lung volumes and lung capacities refer to the volume of air associated with different phases of the respiratory cycle. Lung volumes are directly measured, whereas lung capacities are inferred from lung volumes. Table 6.2 shows common factors that may affect the lung volume of horses.

A number of air volumes apply to the breathing process of horses:

- Total lung capacity (TLC) – all the air the lungs can hold (in a 500-kg horse this

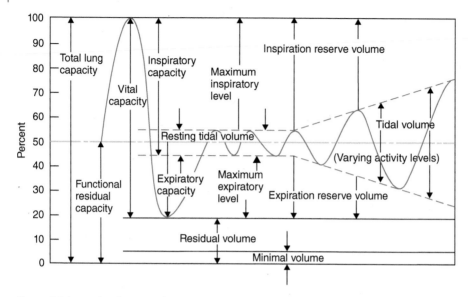

Figure 6.5 Lung air volumes and capacities.

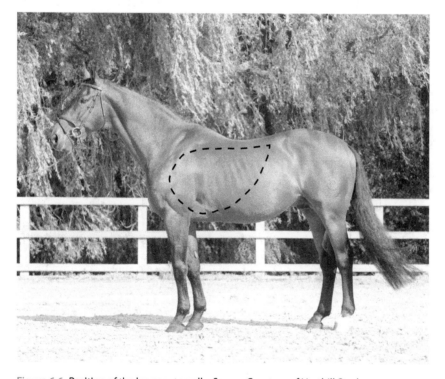

Figure 6.6 Position of the lungs externally. *Source*: Courtesy of Harthill Stud.

is around 40 litres). Total lung capacity of the horse is the amount the horse can hold during the deepest breath in. It is not possible to exhale all of it, as some is left in the airways (see 'Dead Space') and the alveoli cannot completely collapse.

- Vital capacity (VC) – total functional capacity; deepest inhalation followed by

Table 6.2 Some factors affecting the lung volumes of equines.

Larger lung volumes	Smaller lung volumes
Horses	Ponies, Miniatures
Normal bodyweight	Obese
Equines living in lower altitudes	Equines living in higher altitudes

deepest exhalation (about 30 litres). This is the maximum usable lung volume, that is, total lung capacity minus the residual volume.

Vital capacity = Total lung capacity − Residual volume

- Normal capacity – the amount of air remaining in the lungs after a normal quiet exhalation (about 24 litres).
- Tidal volume (VT) – the volume of inhaled or exhaled air in a normal quiet breath (about 4–7 litres at rest, rising to 10 litres per breath at full speed).
- Expiratory reserve volume (ERV) – the maximal volume of air that can be exhaled from the end-expiratory position – that is, air that can be forced out after a normal exhalation (about 12 litres). (ERV is vital when the horse is exercising.)
- Inspiratory reserve volume (IRV) – the volume of air taken in by the deepest possible inhalation after a normal quiet inhalation (about 12 litres). This means that a horse after breathing at rest could inhale an extra volume known as the IRV. (IRV is vital when the horse is exercising.) It can be measured, or determined through VC less the sum of the ERV and VT.
- Residual volume (RV) – air that remains in the lungs even after deep exhalation, as the lungs never collapse completely (about 12 litres).
- Minute ventilation (MV) rate – the amount of air passing in and out of the lungs per minute: $V = V_T \times f$, where V is the minute volume, V_T is the tidal volume and f (or RR) is the respiratory rate.

In a 500-kg horse at rest this equates to approximately 160 litres per minute, and at maximal exercise it rises to 1500 litres per minute. This results from the horse breathing in 6 litres of air ten times per minute. Some of this air will not make contact with the gas exchange surface in the lung due to dead space (see below).

- Oxygen uptake (VO2) – about 5 ml/min/kg, rising to 130–200 maximum during exercise.
- CO_2 production (VCO2) – about 4 ml/min/kg, rising to 140–220.

Dead Space

The anatomical term 'dead space' is used to describe the air passages between the nostrils and alveoli, that is, the nose, pharynx, trachea and bronchi. It is called dead space as there is no gaseous exchange in this area. The percentage of dead space in horses is roughly twice that of humans and dogs. The anatomical dead space amounts to about 60–70% of the tidal volume at rest and 20% of the tidal volume at maximum exercise. The air contained in these passages mixes with the new air taken in at each breath and warms and humidifies it. This helps protect the delicate alveoli from sudden alterations in the temperature and composition of incoming air.

Alveolar dead space exists in those alveoli that are not being used. In resting horses this can be a large percentage of the lungs, but decreases to nearly zero in horses that are working hard. In a healthy resting horse, dead space represents 60% of the volume of a single breath of air. The functional dead space is the anatomical dead space plus the alveolar dead space.

Regulation of Breathing

Breathing is regulated by a coordinated action of the chest muscles, diaphragm and thorax. These actions are controlled by the respiratory centre of the brain which is located in the medulla oblongata. This centre is influenced both by sensory nerves and chemical changes in the blood, and controls the rate and depth of breathing. Motor nerve fibres leave the centre and pass down the spinal cord to emerge as peripheral nerves which pass to the respiratory muscles. The diaphragm is activated by the right and left phrenic nerves which emerge at the level of the seventh cervical vertebrae. Other motor fibres emerge from the spinal cord at the thoracic and abdominal level to go to the muscles that control breathing in and out. Pain can cause the rate and depth of respiration to increase because the respiratory centre has a potential connection to nearly all parts of the body.

The responses of the respiratory centre can be modified by chemicals carried in the bloodstream. An increase in the amount of CO_2 in the blood results in acidity in the brain, and the centre is stimulated to give stronger and more frequent stimulation of the motor nerves so that the CO_2 can be removed from the blood. An exercising horse has elevated levels of CO_2 and lactic acid in the blood due to increased muscle metabolism. This results in the respiratory centre becoming more acidic and it is stimulated to give stronger and more frequent stimulation to the motor nerves, so that the horse breathes more rapidly and deeply, and the CO_2 and lactic acid can be removed from the bloodstream.

During breathing, the rate is influenced by the Hering–Breuer reflex. This is a reflex triggered to prevent overinflation of the lung. Pulmonary stretch receptors present in the smooth muscle of the airways respond to excessive stretching of the lung during large inspirations.

Breathing can be controlled voluntarily, but only within limits. Horses may hold their breath or speed up breathing, but only for a limited time. Vocalisation is a modification of breathing, air being channelled over the vocal cords to result in sound. Breathing can also be controlled to produce abdominal strain; if an animal breathes out with the glottis closed, the tightening of the abdominal muscles causes a rise in pressure inside

the abdomen. This pressure is transferred to the abdominal organs and helps urination, parturition and defecation.

Respiratory–Locomotor Coupling

The respiratory rate is linked to the horse's gait at fast canter and gallop. At walk and trot the horse increases its respiratory rate with small increases in volume of inspired air to meet increased needs. However, at fast canter and gallop only, all air movement comes from movement of the diaphragm. At gallop the stride rate equals the respiratory rate (1:1) about 99.9% of the time and is described as respiratory–locomotor coupling. This means that the muscles of breathing and movement do not work against each other. As the galloping horse lifts the limbs, the head is raised, the gut moves back and the horse breathes in. As the horse lands, the head drops, the gut moves forward and the horse breathes out (Figure 6.7). Increases in respiratory rate at fast canter and gallop are now brought about by increases in volume of air inspired.

There is another theory for this pattern of 1:1 breathing at canter and gallop besides respiratory–locomotor coupling. Some researchers suggest that rather than breathing being passive at canter and gallop and matched to stride linked directly to locomotory forces, the respiratory system itself generates respiratory timing. This is the neuromuscular theory and is based on the findings that horses with lower and upper airway disease may switch from 1:1 to 1:2, that is, two breaths to every stride, some of the time at canter and gallop, depending upon the severity of disease.

The airways of the bronchioles are kept clear by the cilia of the epithelial cells that line them. Coughing is a forcible exhalation made with the glottis closed, which raises pressure within the chest. The glottis then opens, reducing the pressure in the trachea

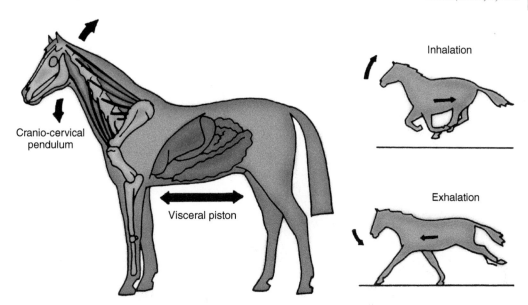

Figure 6.7 Synchronisation of stride and breathing.

and bronchi, while high pressure remains in the deeper air spaces. The sudden drop of pressure in the trachea causes it to collapse inwards; air forced out of the depths of the lung passes through the narrowed trachea at considerable speed, expelling foreign matter. The horse has a poorly developed cough reflex; a horse coughing regularly, if infrequently, is showing signs of respiratory distress. An equine sneeze is an upper respiratory cough, air being expelled through the nostrils with considerable force. Horses are much less likely to cough than humans and therefore coughing in horses must be taken seriously, as it is likely that respiratory disease is present.

External Respiration or Pulmonary Gas Exchange

External respiration converts deoxygenated blood to oxygenated blood and is the diffusion of oxygen from air in the alveoli to blood in the pulmonary capillaries of the horse's lungs. It also includes diffusion of CO_2 in the opposite direction.

Normal atmospheric air has an approximate composition of 78% nitrogen and 21% oxygen, with 1% composed of variable proportions of CO_2, water vapour, argon and a small amount of other gases. Air breathed out of the lungs contains 78% nitrogen, 16% oxygen and 4% CO_2 saturated with water vapour, argon and other gases (Figure 6.8). Four percent of oxygen has been exchanged for CO_2 during the process. The venous blood coming to the lungs is relatively high in CO_2 and low in oxygen. Gaseous exchange takes place across the alveolar membrane, and oxygen is taken into the red blood cells while CO_2 is released from them. Oxygen does not dissolve easily in water and so it is mostly carried in the red blood cells by haemoglobin, or respiratory pigment, which contains iron attached to a polypeptide called globin; 1.5% of oxygen in blood is dissolved in plasma, whereas 98.5% of blood oxygen is bound to haemoglobin. Normal haemoglobin levels vary between species, but the level in the horse is about 11 g per 100 ml of blood. Haemoglobin can combine loosely with oxygen and CO_2. It is part of the blood buffer system which maintains body pH at about 7.4. Haemoglobin can also readily combine with carbon monoxide and become incapable of carrying oxygen. Although this is referred to as gaseous exchange, this is not

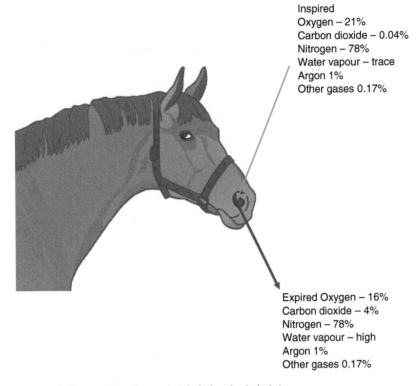

Inspired
Oxygen – 21%
Carbon dioxide – 0.04%
Nitrogen – 78%
Water vapour – trace
Argon 1%
Other gases 0.17%

Expired Oxygen – 16%
Carbon dioxide – 4%
Nitrogen – 78%
Water vapour – high
Argon 1%
Other gases 0.17%

Figure 6.8 Composition of gases in inhaled and exhaled air.

an actual exchange of gases but independent diffusion of gases from an area of high partial pressure to one of low partial pressure. For more information on haemoglobin see 'Oxygen Transport'.

Oxygen diffuses from alveolar air into the blood capillaries lining the alveoli. The partial pressure of oxygen (PO_2) is 105 mmHg in alveolar air, whereas in the pulmonary capillaries it is about 40 mmHg. Diffusion of oxygen occurs until the PO_2 of pulmonary capillaries blood rises to 105 mmHg. While this occurs, CO_2 is also diffusing in the opposite direction. PCO_2 of deoxygenated blood is 45 mmHg compared to 40 mmHg in alveolar air. CO_2 therefore diffuses across into the alveoli until PCO_2 reaches 40 mmHg. Exhalation maintains the PCO_2 at 40 mmHg.

Internal Respiration or Systemic Gas Exchange

Systemic gas exchange is the exchange of oxygen and CO_2 between systemic capillaries and cells throughout the tissues of the horse's body, as opposed to external respiration or pulmonary gas exchange in the lung (see above). As oxygen leaves the blood and enters tissues, the blood becomes deoxygenated. The PO_2 of blood in the systemic capillaries is around 100 mmHg – slightly less than that in the pulmonary capillaries (105 mmHg). The tissue cells PO_2 is about 40 mmHg as cells continuously use oxygen for cellular respiration in making ATP. This pressure difference results in diffusion of oxygen from the systemic blood capillaries into the tissues and PO_2 of the tissues increases. PO_2 returning from muscle tissue following heavy exercise may be as low as 16 mmHg. This increases the driving pressure of oxygen from arterial blood into muscle tissue.

CO_2 also diffuses in the opposite direction. Due to the continuous production of CO_2 by tissue cells, the PCO_2 of cells is 45 mmHg at rest and is higher than the systemic capillary blood supply at 40 mmHg. This results in CO_2 diffusing from the tissue cells via interstitial fluid into the systemic capillaries until PCO$_2$ increases. The deoxygenated blood is then returned to the heart before being pumped to the lungs for another cycle of external respiration. Tissues with higher aerobic needs such as muscle tissue are more highly vascularised.

Transport of Oxygen and Carbon Dioxide Around the Body

Blood transports oxygen inhaled from the lungs around the body to the systemic cells and tissues. It also transports CO$_2$ back to the lungs for removal. Oxygen is not very soluble, whereas CO$_2$ is.

Oxygen Transport

Around 98.5% of oxygen in blood is bound to the haem part of the molecule haemoglobin (Hb) which is found in all erythrocytes (red blood cells) (Figure 6.9). The haem part contains four iron (Fe) ions, each of which can bind to one oxygen molecule.

The structure of haemoglobin is shown in Chapter 1 (Figure 1.8). Oxygen easily binds to deoxyhaemoglobin in the reversible reaction shown below, that is, oxygen is easily attached and unattached as required. Here, aq means aqueous,

Hb(aq) + O$_2$(aq)   → HbO$_2$(aq)
Deoxyhaemoglobin   **Oxyhaemoglobin**

If PO$_2$ (intracellular oxygen tension i.e. amount of oxygen in the cell) is high then Hb will become saturated with oxygen molecules as they attach to all the iron atoms in Hb. This will occur on the capillaries of the lungs. In body tissues, where PO$_2$ is low as oxygen is used up, oxygen is released from the iron atoms in Hb to diffuse into tissue cells of the body.

During exercise, tissue cells, particularly in the muscles, produce more CO$_2$ and more lactic acid which increases acidity, and the temperature increases due to increased metabolism. All these factors increase the amount of oxygen released from haemoglobin; that is, as blood flows through more active tissues, more oxygen is released.

Carbon Dioxide Transport

CO$_2$ is transported in the blood by one of three ways:

- dissolved CO$_2$ in plasma: 7% (CO$_2$ is more soluble in plasma than O$_2$)
- bound to haemoglobin in blood as carbaminohaemoglobin: 23%
- bicarbonate ions (i.e. the bicarbonate buffer system) in plasma: 70%. The bicarbonate buffer system allows little change to the pH of the horse's body system.

The greatest percentage of CO$_2$ (70%) is carried in the blood in bicarbonate ions (HCO$_3^-$) in the plasma. CO$_2$ enters the erythrocytes after diffusing into tissue capillaries from systemic cells and tissues. An enzyme called carbonic anhydrase inside the erythrocytes drives a reaction converting

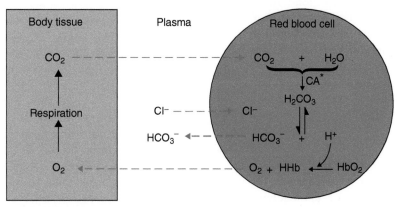

* Carbonic anyhydrase

Figure 6.9 Summary of erythrocyte chemistry related to carriage of respiratory gases.

CO_2 to bicarbonate ions via carbonic acid ($H_2CO_3^-$) within the red blood cells.

$$CO_2 + H_2O \rightarrow H_2CO_3 \rightarrow H^+ + HCO_3^-$$

Thus bicarbonate accumulates inside erythrocytes as blood collects CO_2 from body tissues and cells. Some of this bicarbonate moves out of the erythrocytes down a concentration gradient, and in exchange some chloride ions move the other way, from the plasma into the erythrocytes. This is known as the chloride shift. The net result is that CO_2 is removed from the body cells as waste and transported back to the lungs for removal. As blood passes through the lungs, the above reactions reverse.

- CO_2 dissolved in plasma diffuses into the alveolar air from blood capillaries.
- CO_2 associated with haemoglobin in erythrocytes splits and diffuses into the alveolar air.
- Bicarbonate ions reverse the above reaction to CO_2 and water, with the former leaving erythrocytes and diffusing into alveolar air.

The Oxygen Dissociation Curve

The oxygen dissociation curve is an S-shaped curve (Figure 6.10) which shows the relationship between oxygen tension and haemoglobin saturation and indicates that blood can become almost fully saturated at relatively low oxygen levels. In other words, haemoglobin has a high affinity for oxygen. The steep part of the curve corresponds to the range of oxygen levels found in the tissues; over this part of the curve, a small drop in oxygen level will bring about a relatively large fall in the percentage saturation of the blood. So, if the oxygen level falls as a result of tissues utilising oxygen at a faster rate, haemoglobin will respond by giving up more of its oxygen.

The Bohr Effect

The Bohr effect is the decrease in oxygen affinity of haemoglobin in response to the decreased blood pH which occurs following increased CO_2 concentration in the blood.

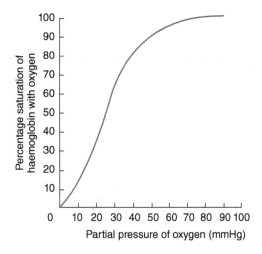

Figure 6.10 Oxygen dissociation curve.

The concentration of CO_2 affects the affinity of haemoglobin for oxygen. With increasing CO_2 levels the haemoglobin must be exposed to higher oxygen levels in order to become fully saturated, but it will also release oxygen at higher oxygen levels. In other words, at high CO_2 levels haemoglobin is less efficient at taking up oxygen but better at releasing it. Release of oxygen is therefore favoured in the tissues where CO_2 concentrations are naturally high due to its release during energy production such as working muscle cells. In the lungs CO_2 tension is lower and this favours oxygen uptake.

Once gaseous exchange has occurred the oxygenated blood passes back to the heart and then to the rest of the body. At the tissues, where oxygenated blood encounters areas of low oxygen and high CO_2 levels, oxygen passes into the tissues while CO_2 diffuses into the blood. The deoxygenated blood returns to the heart and then the lungs.

The respiratory system cannot be trained to work better; in fact, the respiratory system of an unfit horse works as well as that of a fit horse. The use of nasal strips, however, as seen in some competition horses, seems to work well in helping to move more air into the lungs, increasing the amount of oxygen available for working muscles and delaying fatigue.

Cellular Respiration

Horses obtain energy from the process of cellular respiration, a complicated chemical process involving breakdown of simple food molecules such as glucose to produce energy. All mammals mainly respire aerobically, that is, using oxygen absorbed from the lungs, which is then rapidly distributed around the body by the circulatory system via haemoglobin. For aerobic cell respiration to take place, glucose (or other substrates such as amino acids and lipids) and oxygen must be present in the cell. Cellular respiration is therefore the process that releases energy from food such as glucose and lipids. It takes place in every single cell of every living organism every minute of the day and night. To avoid confusion with respiration (i.e. breathing) it is often referred to as cellular respiration or internal respiration. There are two types of cellular respiration:

- Aerobic – respiration with oxygen.
- Anaerobic – respiration without oxygen.

Aerobic respiration releases much more energy in cells than anaerobic. Horses will mostly use aerobic respiration, but during intense exercise muscles may run out of oxygen and muscles then continue for a while using anaerobic respiration.

Although every living cell undergoes respiration, the rate of respiration between tissues varies widely. For example, nervous tissue can exist for more than 4 minutes without oxygen, while bone cells require little oxygen and can survive for hours without it. Oxygen is brought in via the bloodstream, and so hard-working tissues (brain, liver, kidneys, cardiac and skeletal muscle) have a plentiful capillary supply, while relatively inactive tissues (bone, cartilage, tendons, cornea) have a more limited blood supply.

Aerobic Cellular Respiration

Three phases are involved in aerobic cellular respiration:

- transport of oxygen and carbon dioxide to and from the body cells
- exchange of oxygen and waste products between the blood and the body cells
- creation of energy within the cell.

Cells must extract and use chemical energy locked inside the end-products of food digestion, which is mostly glucose. Horses respire glucose with a small amount of fat and amino acids. This balance may change – for example, when horses are not getting enough food, or are on a weight-reducing programme.

When a molecule of glucose is broken down, CO_2, water and energy are released. Some of this energy is released as heat. However, in the cell most energy is captured by transferring the energy lost from glucose directly to another chemical compound called an energy carrier molecule.

$$C_6H_{12}O_6 + 6O_2 \rightarrow 6CO_2$$

| Glucose | Oxygen | Carbon dioxide |

$$+ 6H_2O + Energy$$

| Water | 36 ATP |

The amount of energy contained in the reactants, that is, glucose and oxygen, far exceeds that contained in the products, that is, CO_2 and water, and therefore there is excess energy to be harvested and used. This is the whole basis of cellular respiration.

This is the summary of respiration; in fact, glucose must go through a long series of specialised reactions known as glycolysis and the Krebs cycle to get this end result. The reactions are redox reactions, that is, reduction and oxidation. Redox reactions are two reactions that can occur in the same reaction at the same time. Oxidation involves loss of electrons, while reduction involves gain of electrons. Redox reactions are vital in living systems.

In the process of cellular respiration, oxygen is reduced to form water and glucose is oxidised to form CO_2. The majority of ATP produced is derived from the final stage of the process, that is, the Krebs cycle, which takes place on the inner mitochondrial membrane. If oxygen is fully available then 36ATP may be produced from each glucose molecule.

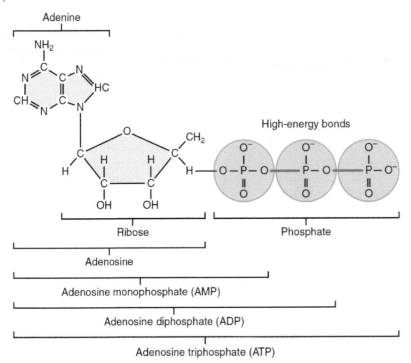

Figure 6.11 Structure of ATP. *Source:* OpenStax College, https://commons .wikimedia.org/wiki/ File:230_Structure_ of_Adenosine_ Triphosphate_(ATP)- 01.jpg. CC BY 3.0.

Labels in figure: Adenine; NH$_2$; High-energy bonds; CH$_2$; Ribose; Phosphate; Adenosine; Adenosine monophosphate (AMP); Adenosine diphosphate (ADP); Adenosine triphosphate (ATP)

These reactions takes place in the power house of the cell – the mitochondria – and is complex, but all life processes utilise energy in the form of a common basic unit. In living cells the major energy carrier molecule is ATP (Figure 6.11). ATP consists of a base adenine and a ribose sugar with three inorganic phosphate attachments. ATP is a relatively small and soluble molecule and so is ideal to diffuse around cells, quickly providing energy where required. It is very useful as an energy carrier mainly because it can quickly give up its terminal phosphate group, releasing energy for powering processes in cells, but without producing excessive heat at the same time.

When ATP is hydrolysed, a large amount of energy is released. This hydrolysis reaction involves ATP reacting with water. During the reaction, one of the phosphates is lost to form adenosine diphosphate (ADP) and energy is released (Figure 6.12). This energy can be used by the cell to perform work such as muscle contraction. The ATP reaction to produce energy is shown below.

$$\text{ATP} + \text{Water} \rightarrow \text{ADP} + \text{Pi}$$

$$\text{Adenosine Triphosphate} + \text{Water} \rightarrow \text{Adensoine Diphosphate} + \text{Inorganic Phosphate}$$

$$+ 30.7 \text{ kJ mol}^{-1}$$
$$+ \textit{Heat Energy}$$

where Pi is inorganic phosphate. In cells, ATP is made by the process of phosphorylation whereby a phosphate is added to ADP. This may be either from a substrate molecule other than ADP, or ATP as occurs in glycolysis and the Krebs cycle, or by another process known as oxidative phosphorylation, from the electron transport chain resulting from the series of redox reactions. The process is called oxidative phosphorylation because ADP is phosphorylated to ATP.

Nicotinamide adenine dinucleotide (NADH) is an important electron carrier in this process. NADH is a coenzyme which collects electrons from glycolysis (via the link

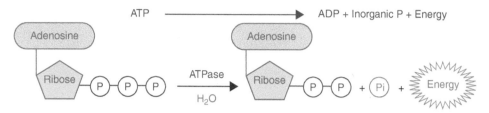

Figure 6.12 **Hydrolysis of ATP.**

reaction and Krebs cycle) and enters the electron transport chain to convert the energy within them to ATP. In fact, the electron transport chain is a series of compounds that transfers electrons from electron donors to electron acceptors via redox reactions, and couples this electron transfer with the transfer of protons (H+ ions) across a membrane. This creates an electrochemical proton gradient that drives the synthesis of ATP. Creatine phosphate is also able to release its inorganic phosphate quickly when reacting with water, releasing energy to make more ATP.

Aerobic Respiration of Glucose

Aerobic respiration of glucose can be summarised in four stages (Figure 6.13):

- Glycolysis – glucose (C6) splits into two pyruvate molecules (each of C3).
- Link reaction – oxidation of pyruvate to acetate (requires oxygen).
- Krebs cycle – strips electrons from acetate.
- Electron transport chain – energy from the electrons is transferred to make ATP via the NADH electron carrier.

Glycolysis

Glycolysis unlike the Krebs cycle takes place in the cytosol of all cells and not in mitochondria. Through a series of ten reactions (Figure 6.14), glucose which contains six carbon atoms is converted to two molecules of pyruvate, each of which contains three carbon atoms. This is a quick process and only releases a small amount of ATP, namely a net two molecules of ATP, and four molecules of reduced NADH, which is later used in the

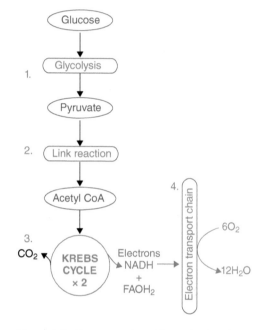

Figure 6.13 **Summary of aerobic respiration of glucose.**

electron transport chain. It actually produces four ATP, but two are used up at the beginning by adding a phosphate group to glucose, making glucose 1,6 diphosphate, which is essential for raising the overall energy level of glucose so there is enough for the second part of the process. This stage also does not need oxygen and so can continue anaerobically, providing a relatively small amount of energy. If oxygen is available pyruvate then enters the link reaction.

Link Reaction

The link reaction (Figure 6.15) links glycolysis to the Krebs cycle. Each molecule of

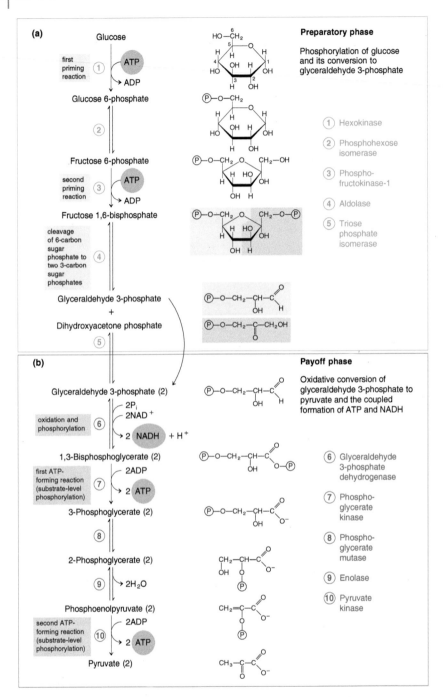

Figure 6.14 The ten steps of glycolysis. *Source*: Nelson, https://commons.wikimedia.org/wiki/File:Glycolysis_pathway.png. CC BY-SA 3.0.

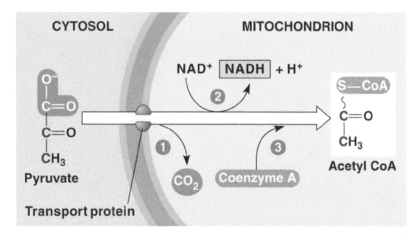

Figure 6.15 The link reaction. *Source*: Campbell and Reece, https://commons.wikimedia.org/wiki/File:09_10PyruvateToAcetylCoA-L.jpg?uselang=en-gb.

pyruvate (three carbons) (there were two for every molecule of glucose) now moves to the matrix of the mitochondria from the cell cytosol and here it is oxidised to acetate (two carbons) and CO_2. Two more molecules of NADH are also produced for later use in the electron chain. Acetate is picked up by a carrier molecule called coenzyme A to make acetyl coenzyme A (CoA).

Krebs Cycle

Otherwise known as the tricarboxylic acid (TCA) cycle or citric acid cycle, the Krebs cycle is named after Sir Hans Kreb. It takes place in the matrix of mitochondria and through a series of reactions provides a supply of electrons for the electron transport chain to ultimately make ATP (Figure 6.16). This cycle occurs twice for each one molecule of glucose, or once for each of the two pyruvate molecules. For each acetate derived from pyruvate and delivered via the link reaction, the Krebs cycle produces:

$1 \times$ ATP from substrate-level

phosphorylation

$3 \times$ NADH (nicotinamide adenine

dinucleotide)

$1 \times FADH_2$ (flavine adenine dinucleotide)

$2 \times CO_2$

It also results in $1 \times$ oxaloacetate, which allows the cycle to turn the second time.

Therefore, as the Krebs cycle turns twice for each glucose molecule, the following are produced:

$6 \times$ NADH

$2 \times FADH_2$

These carry electrons to the electron chain.

Electron Transport Chain

The electron transport chain consists of a series of steps whereby carrier molecules first undergo reduction by accepting an electron and then undergo oxidation by releasing an electron. Each time this happens in the chain some energy is lost. This energy is used to actively transport hydrogen ions or protons (H^+) across the inner membrane to the outer mitochondrial space of the mitochondria. This then produces a concentration gradient, with less H^+ in the inner mitochondrial space. Protons then want to move back to the area of lower H^+ concentration in the inner mitochondrial space, and they can only do this by crossing through structures called stalked particles or inner-membrane spheres which contain ATP-ase, the enzyme required to make ATP. These cover the cristae of mitochondria and are tiny stalked particles, also known

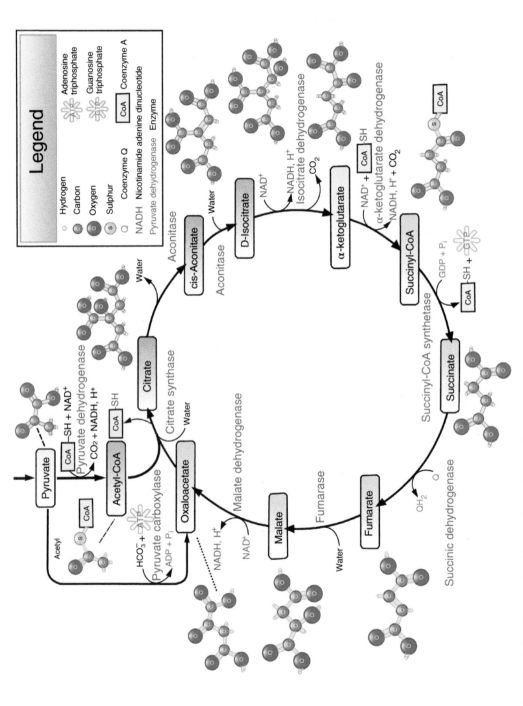

Figure 6.16 The Krebs, TCA or citric acid cycle. *Source*: Baggins, https://en.wikipedia.org/wiki/File:Citric_acid_cycle_with_aconitate.svg. CC BY-SA 3.0.

as knobs or spheres. As the protons pass down the stalk, they lose energy and this is used to convert ADP to ATP. At the other end, low-energy electrons and protons are combined with oxygen to form water. This oxygen is vital for mopping up the electrons and protons, otherwise this series of reactions could not continue. This is the basis for aerobic respiration. A summary of ATP production is shown in Figure 6.17 and Table 6.3.

Total ATP production

= 36 ATP from 1 glucose molecule

Many texts will cite 38 ATP as the total. The difference may come from the shuttle system the electrons use inside the mitochondria. Some electrons choose the

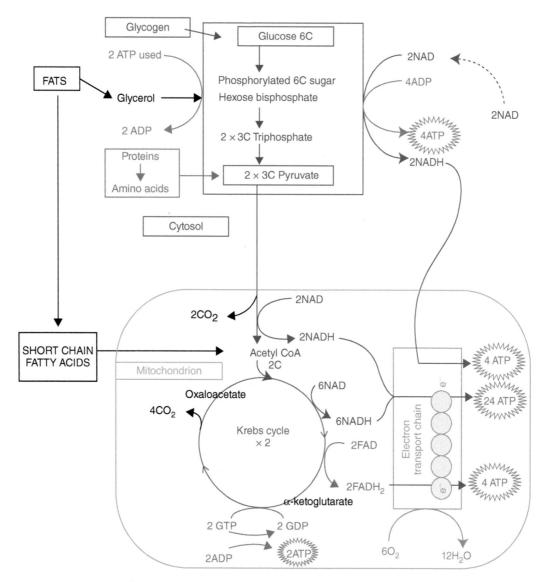

Figure 6.17 Summary of ATP production during cellular respiration.

Table 6.3 Total ATP produced from oxidative phosphorylation in aerobic respiration.

Glycolysis (anaerobic)	Link reaction	Electron transport chain + Krebs cycle (×2)
+ 4 ATP	+ 4 ATP from NADH	+ 24 ATP from NADH
− 2 ATP (used up during a reaction)		+ 4 ATP from FADH$_2$
+ 4 NADH		+ 2 ATP direct from Krebs cycle
Net = + 2 ATP	Net = + 4 ATP	Net = + 30 ATP

NADH route which produces 6 ATPs, while those that choose the FAD$_{2+}$ route produce 4 ATPs.

Although there is a theoretical yield of 36 ATP molecules per glucose molecule during cellular respiration, such conditions are generally not always produced, due to losses. There is an energy cost to moving pyruvate (from glycolysis), phosphate and ADP into the mitochondria. They are all transported by active transport via carriers using the stored energy in the proton gradient. In reality, then, the amount of ATP produced in total and including energy needed for the movement of substrates and so on is more likely to be around 30–32 ATP.

Aerobic Respiration of Other Fuels

Glycogen

Glycogen consists of many molecules of glucose polymerised to form a complex carbohydrate. In glycolysis, successive molecules of glucose in the polymer chain are split off the main body by a process called phosphorylation. The hormones glucagon and adrenalin both activate the enzyme, phosphorylase, which allows the process to take place. Glucose is then available for aerobic respiration.

Lipid Metabolism

Fats or lipids occur in three main forms: triglycerides, phospholipids and cholesterol. All triglycerides and phospholipids contain fatty acids of one type or another, characterised by a long chain of carbon atoms joined to hydrogen atoms.

During digestion in the stomach and small intestine, fats are split into glycerol, monoglycerides and fatty acids, which pass across the intestinal wall. Fat cells or adipocytes are specialised connective tissue cells which are capable of storing triglycerides. When carbohydrate intake is low, stored triglycerides are converted to fatty acids and glycerol. Fatty acids are further broken down by beta oxidation to many two-carbon acetyl fragments, which attach to coenzyme Q and then enter the Krebs cycle as acetyl coenzyme A and eventually supply the electron chain. Glycerol is converted to dihydroxyacetone phosphate via the phosphogluconate pathway and is used for fuel in glycolysis (Figure 6.18).

Horses derive much of their energy from volatile fatty acids (VFAs) produced by microbiota in the hindgut, which ferment fibre or structural carbohydrates such as cellulose and hemicelluloses, lignocellulose, pectins, and soluble and insoluble fibres. Microbes break down structural carbohydrates to short chain fatty acids (SCFAs). SCFAs are saturated organic acids that consist of one to six carbons, of which acetate (C2), propionate (C3) and butyrate (C4) are the most abundant ($\geq$95%). Others include isobutyrate, valerate and lactate. Forage may provide 100% of the horse's energy intake. Fermentation of soluble fibres such as pectin produces mainly acetate, whereas fermentation of starch from feeding high levels results in more lactate produced.

SCFAs (short chain fatty acids) produced by the microbiota in the caecum and the colon can be found in hepatic, portal and

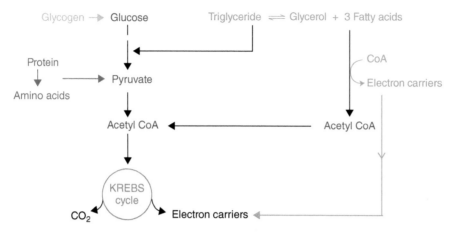

Figure 6.18 Aerobic respiration using lipids, glycogen and protein.

peripheral blood. These SCFAs affect lipid, glucose and cholesterol metabolism in different tissues. SCFAs are readily absorbed, are transported from the intestinal lumen into the blood compartment of the host and are taken up by organs, where they act as substrates.

VFAs are absorbed throughout the caecal and colonic epithelium primarily by diffusion and via a transporter. The rate and absorption of organic acids within the hindgut has large effects on plasma volume due to their osmotic effect, and therefore also on the direction of movement of water across the mucosa wall. The most important VFAs are propionate, butyrate and acetate and these are collected via the hepatic portal system and transferred to the liver. Propionate is converted to glucose in the liver via gluconeogenesis before use in cellular respiration. Acetate enters the peripheral circulation to be metabolised by peripheral tissues such as muscle and areolar tissue. Much of the butyrate is used as fuel by the epithelial cells of the colon named colonocytes.

Protein Metabolism

Horses cannot store excess protein, and so any excess amino acids must be broken down by a process known as deamination in the liver. Here the amine group (NH_2) is removed and the remaining organic acids enter the Krebs cycle via pyruvate. The NH_2 part is used to make urea and excreted via the ornithine cycle. Under normal conditions it is a low-level activity, but during disease or starvation it can become the major source of body energy, hence the wasting away of muscle during starvation.

Anaerobic Respiration

During anaerobic respiration when oxygen is lacking, pyruvate, instead of entering the link reaction to the Krebs cycle, is converted via a reduction reaction to lactate or lactic acid. Anaerobic respiration uses electron acceptors other than oxygen as the final electron acceptor. Lactate builds up in the muscles of hard-working horses and causes fatigue of the muscle and horses will be rapidly tire and stop.

Summary Points

1) Mitochondria need a steady supply of oxygen to release the potential energy stored in fuels in the muscle, such as fat and glycogen. However, most mitochondria in muscle cells are a long way from any oxygen in the air. Respiration is the process by which the horse takes oxygen into its body and also rids it of CO_2.

2) There are essentially three steps to the process of gaseous exchange, namely breathing (pulmonary ventilation) or

airflow into and out of the lungs; external respiration (exchange of gases at the alveoli/blood interface); and internal respiration (exchange of gases at the tissue cells/blood interface in the body).

3) The horse cannot breathe through its mouth as humans can, it can only breathe through the nostrils.

4) The anatomical term 'dead space' is used to describe the air passages between the nostrils and alveoli. It is called dead space as there is no gaseous exchange in this area.

5) The greatest percentage of CO_2 (70%) is carried in the blood in bicarbonate ions (HCO_{3-}) in the plasma.

6) The electron chain is where most of the ATP is produced in aerobic cellular respiration.

7) Oxygen is vital for mopping up the electrons and protons at the end of cellular respiration; otherwise this series of reactions could not continue. This is the basis for aerobic respiration.

Q + A

Q What are the secondary functions of the respiratory system?

A Phonation (vocalisation), sense of smell, thermoregulation, elimination of water vapour and regulation of acidity of the blood.

Q During a 5-furlong race, how much air will a horse take in approximately?

A A horse will breathe in approximately 1800 litres of air, of which 378 litres is oxygen and most of the rest is nitrogen.

Q At what gaits of the horse does respiratory coupling occur?

A Fast or prolonged canter and gallop.

Q Approximately how much oxygen is bound to haemoglobin during oxygen transport round the body?

A Around 98.5% of oxygen in blood is bound to the haem part of the molecule haemoglobin.

Q Describe internal respiration or systemic gas exchange.

A This is the exchange of oxygen and CO_2 between systemic capillaries and cells throughout the tissues of the horse's body, as opposed to external respiration or pulmonary gas exchange in the lung.

Q What is the link reaction?

A This links glycolysis to the Krebs cycle. Each molecule of pyruvate (three carbons) (remember there were two for every molecule of glucose) now moves to the matrix of the mitochondria from the cell cytosol and here it is oxidised to acetate (two carbons) and CO_2. Acetate is picked up by a carrier molecule called coenzyme A to make acetyl coenzyme A.

Q What is the difference between aerobic and anaerobic respiration?

A During anaerobic respiration when oxygen is lacking, pyruvate, instead of entering the link reaction to the Krebs cycle, is converted via a reduction reaction to lactate or lactic acid.

7

The Circulatory System

The main internal transport system of horses is the circulatory system, sometimes known as the vascular system or, if including the heart, the cardiovascular system. Most multicellular animals need a transport system to supply cells with food, oxygen and other materials that cannot reach all cells from diffusion alone. Cells require a constant supply of nutrients and oxygen and also a continuous ability to remove waste.

The circulatory system comprises a four-chambered pump known as the heart and a system of tubes or blood vessels which circulate the transport medium, blood (Figure 7.1). The four chambers consist of two ventricles and two atria, the ventricles being bigger with more muscular walls. Cardiac muscle or myocardium is a specialised tissue of smooth or involuntary muscle.

The basis of the horse's circulation is that blood is pumped from the left side of the heart to the body and limbs, before it returns to the right side, from which it is pumped through the lungs, returning to the left side of the heart and so on. Arterial blood that is pumped away from the heart is under much greater pressure, at around 120 mmHg, because it has to reach the far extents of the horse's body.

The venous system returns blood from the capillaries to the heart, the arterial system carries blood from the heart to the capillaries and the portal systems carry blood between two capillary beds (such as the hepatic portal vein from the digestive tract to the liver).

As a general rule, vessels that carry blood away from the heart are known as arteries, whereas vessels that carry blood back to the heart are veins. The exceptions to this rule are the pulmonary artery which carries deoxygenated blood from the heart to the lungs and the pulmonary vein which carries oxygenated blood from the lungs to the heart.

The pulmonary system carries blood between the heart and lungs, whereas the systemic system carries blood between the heart and the rest of the horse's body. These are anatomically and functionally different from each other. Two important subdivisions of the systemic circulation are the coronary circulation which supplies the heart itself and the hepatic portal circulation which runs from the gut to the liver. In addition there is a system of vessels that carry lymph or tissue fluid to the large veins and these are known as lymph vessels. Functions of the circulatory system include:

- transport of nutrients
- transport of waste products
- transport of respiratory gases oxygen and carbon dioxide
- transport of heat
- transport of hormones, for example insulin, oestrogen
- defence against disease and transport of antibodies and white blood cells
- healing via clotting if required, to prevent catastrophic loss of blood.

Equine Science, Third Edition. Zoe Davies and Sarah Pilliner.
© 2018 Zoe Davies and Sarah Pilliner. Published 2018 by John Wiley & Sons Ltd.

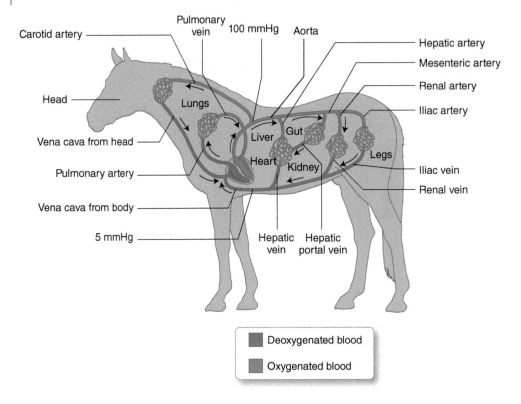

Figure 7.1 The heart and circulation of the horse.

Blood flows in a one-way system around the horse's body in the following consecutive order:

- from the left ventricle of the heart the aorta takes oxygened blood around the body via the arterial system
- body tissues (head, muscles, etc.)
- capillaries
- venous system (takes deoxygenated blood around the body back to the heart)
- vena cava
- right atrium (heart)
- right ventricle (heart)
- pulmonary artery (takes deoxygenated blood to the lungs)
- lungs
- pulmonary vein (takes oxygenated blood back to the heart to be pumped around the body)
- left atrium (heart)
- back to the left ventricle.

Foetal Circulation

In the foetus, two circulations, namely the – systemic and pulmonary are in series and also incorporate the placenta. The foetal heart pumps this entire circulation of blood through the placenta and only a very small proportion through the lungs, which in foetal life in utero do not function (contain no air). Placental circulation sends the blood through vessels in the cord and placenta, extending 2 m or more depending upon the length. This is a remarkable achievement when one considers the small size of the foetal heart and the pressure gradients involved in transporting blood through the capillaries of the placenta. It also passes through the liver, as in the foetal foal there is no bypass to its liver as in other species, that is, no ductus venosus. As a vascular structure, the ductus venosus is present in the foetuses of most mammals;

however, horses and indeed guinea pigs do not have a ductus venosus at term.

In utero, approximately two-thirds of foetal blood bypasses the pulmonary artery and is shunted by the ductus arteriosus directly to the aorta. In late gestation, the ductus arteriosus narrows, and with expansion of the lungs at the first breath postpartum, pulmonary resistance falls and systemic arterial pressure rises, resulting in the reversal of blood flow within the duct until the duct begins to close. Gradually, the ductus arteriosus is replaced by a fibrous band called the ligamentum arteriosum. In normal healthy foals, functional closure of the ductus arteriosus occurs by 320 days of gestation, or within about 3 days of birth.

The Heart

The heart is central to the circulatory system and is a large muscular pump which has the ability to contract and relax, sending blood through a network of vessels which supply the tissues of the body. It is a hollow and highly muscular organ. The heart of the horse is very efficient and is able to adapt to the different conditions imposed upon it, such as fast or prolonged exercise. The external structure of the horse's heart is shown in Figure 7.2. At rest, the heart rate may be as low as 30 beats per minute (bpm), whereas when the horse is galloping this can increase to 230 bpm. This huge range allows horses to pump a phenomenal amount of blood around the body at peak exercise, as much as 250 litres per minute. The horse's blood pressure is on average 120/70, similar to humans. Unlike humans though, horses rarely become hypertensive (high blood pressure), except in cases of severe kidney disease. On the other hand, hypotension (low blood pressure) is commonly seen in cases of dehydration, colic, blood loss and other illnesses associated with sepsis or bacterial infections.

The mucous membranes (gums) are used to aid evaluation of the circulatory system. The membranes should be pink and moist. Pale membranes reflect anaemia, and hyperaemic

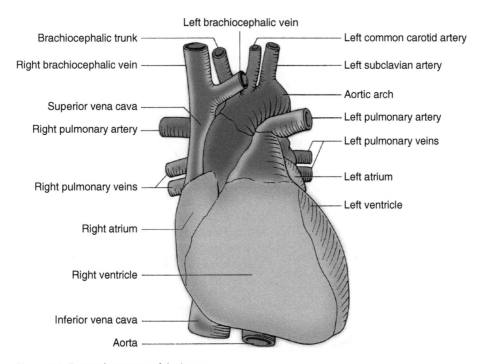

Figure 7.2 External structure of the heart.

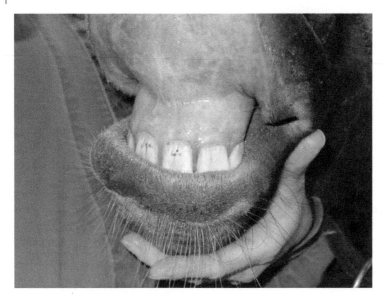

Figure 7.3 Toxic mucous membranes as demonstrated by hyperaemia, with increased discolouration noted at the gum line. *Source*: Southwood 2013. Reproduced with permission of John Wiley & Sons.

(bright pink to red) membranes occur with sepsis and severe inflammation (Figure 7.3).

Capillary refill time (CRT) is used as an estimation of hydration in the horse. To determine this, a finger is placed quite firmly on the gum, pushing the blood out of the capillaries, leaving a blanched print; the time it takes for the pink colour to return to that area is the CRT. Normal CRT is between 1.5 and 2.5 seconds. Prolonged CRT is an indication of dehydration and needs to be addressed.

The heart rate alone is not the only variable. Even the heart beat's rhythm varies substantially in a normal healthy horse. The heart of a 500- to 550-kg horse would weigh approximately 4–5 kg. As the horse gets fitter, the heart size may increase up to about 5.5 kg. A large heart has been associated with great racehorses such as Eclipse, Secretariat and Pharlap. Pharlap's heart weighed 6.4 kg. Heart size was believed to be closely associated with the X chromosome and it was presumed that a larger heart would result in better performance. Thoroughbred (TB) horses have been bred over centuries to move at speed, and consequently they have the genes for the largest and most efficient hearts. This is further improved by training. The TB heart is larger than that of the Quarter-horse, for example.

The horse has a different depolarisation process (as do other hoofed mammals) from small animals and humans because of the wider-spread distribution of the Purkinje fibres. These fibres extend throughout the myocardium and ventricular depolarisation takes place from many sites. As a result, no wavefronts are formed, and the overall effect of the ventricular depolarisation on the electrocardiogram (ECG) was found to be minimal. ECG's therefore provide little information about the size of ventricles and an ECG cannot provide information about heart mass/size. However, heart size may also increase with disease such as a viral infection and can become overly enlarged and less efficient. Many older horses develop leaky heart valves which may ultimately lead to congestive heart failure.

Cardiac Output

Cardiac output (CO), now termed Q, is a measure of the amount of blood (in litres) pumped per minute out of the left-hand side of the heart. It is calculated by multiplying the heart rate (HR) (also known as fc and measured in beats per minute) by stroke volume (SV) (measured in litres):

$$Q = SV \times HR$$

SV is the volume of blood pumped out with each heart beat and is roughly 1.3 litres of blood in the horse and can increase by 20–50% with exercise. At a resting HR of approximately 30 bpm, Q would be 1.3 (SV) × 30 (HR) = 39 litres per minute. This can increase to 1.3 × 240 = 312 litres per minute at maximal exercise in elite equine athletes. The average resting HR of the athletic horse is usually around 30 bpm; this increases with the level of exercise and averages 80 bpm at walk, 130 bpm at trot, 180 bpm at canter and up to 240 bpm at gallop. Compare this to humans with a normal resting HR of 50–60 bpm and a maximum in excess of 220 bpm. In addition to increasing HR with exercise, heart muscle increases the SV, pumping more blood per beat. At lower HR's and at rest, HR is decreased.

Even the heart rhythm can vary substantially in a normal healthy horse. The fact that the horse can increase HR by nearly ten times the resting HR is a contributory factor to the superior athleticism of horses. The heart muscle expends a great deal of energy and so, to conserve energy when required, the heart can:

- decrease its rate
- decrease contraction of the heart muscle
- skip a beat, allowing the heart to rest.

The change in heart rhythm when skipping a beat is known as second-degree atrioventricular (AV) block, which is normal in horses but only occasionally seen in human athletes.

Anatomy of the Heart

The heart is surrounded by a double-layered sac of tough fibrous connective tissue known as the pericardium or pericardial sac which is completely closed, containing a small amount of fluid for lubrication. The pericardium prevents overdistension of the heart and also anchors the heart within the mediastinum, which contains the heart and all other thoracic organs, except for the lungs which are housed within the pleural sacs and the caudal vena cava. The heart wall consists of three layers: the epicardium, the endocardium and the important muscular layer the myocardium.

The heart is divided into four hollow chambers (Figure 7.4). The right-hand side is separate from the left-hand side, so that blood does not mix between the two. The right-hand side of the heart is responsible for moving deoxygenated or venous blood, that is, blood that has had most of its oxygen removed as it travelled around the body. Veins carry this deoxygenated blood via the body's largest vein, the vena cava, to the right atrium of the heart. Once full, the right atrium contracts, pushing blood into the more muscular right ventricle. The tricuspid valve snaps shut to prevent any backflow of blood. This is the first noise of the heart sounds which can be heard using a stethoscope, the 'lub' part of the characteristic 'lub-dup'. The right ventricle then contracts, pushing blood into the pulmonary artery which takes blood to the lungs (Figure 7.4).

Once in the lungs the blood comes into close contact with the alveoli, and the carbon dioxide it is carrying is exchanged for oxygen by a process known as gaseous exchange. The now oxygenated or arterial blood then returns to the heart via the pulmonary vein to the left atrium. Once it is full, blood is forced into the left ventricle and again the bicuspid valves shut to prevent any backflow of blood. Figure 7.5 shows the movement of blood through the horse's circulatory system.

The left ventricle has the thickest muscular wall of any of the four heart chambers because blood from the left ventricle is forced out at great pressure into the aorta, which is the largest artery in the body. Blood from the left ventricle has to travel a greater distance to all parts of the body and not just to the lungs, hence the thicker muscular wall

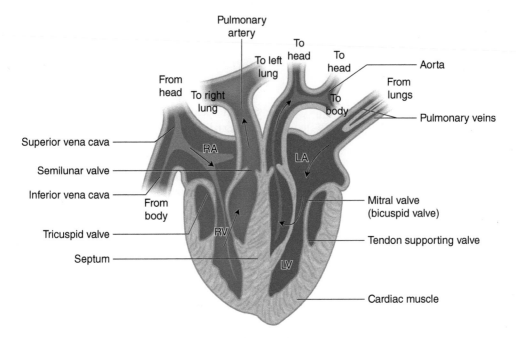

Figure 7.4 Vertical section through the equine heart, showing the flow of blood through it. LA, Left atrium; LV, left ventricle; RA, right atrium; RV, right ventricle.

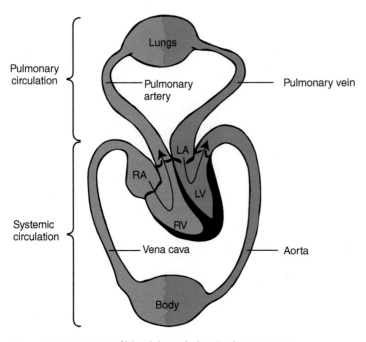

Figure 7.5 Movement of blood through the circulatory system.

(see Figure 7.2). Valves at the entrance of the aorta known as semi-lunar valves prevent backflow and lead to the second sound of the heart beat, the 'dup' part of 'lub-dup'.

The Cardiac Cycle

The cardiac cycle involves all the events of a single heart beat. It consists of a contraction/ejection phase (systole) and a relaxation/filling phase (diastole). The heart beat has four phases involving the filling and contraction of each of its four chambers, but because the atria and ventricles empty almost simultaneously, often only two phases can be heard through an ordinary stethoscope. All four may be heard when the resting heart rate is low. The sounds actually come from the valves snapping shut and not from the heart muscle itself. The first sound ('lub') is a loud sound from the AV valves closing following the start of ventricular systole. The second ('dup') is a short sharp sound from the semi-lunar valves closing at the end of ventricular systole. This is followed by a pause as the heart relaxes. Thus the four sounds with intermittent pauses are:

- lub systolic: S1
- dup diastolic: S2
- pause
- lub systolic
- dup diastolic
- pause.

Occasionally, two other distinct sounds may be heard. S3 represents the sound of blood filling the ventricles and S4 is heard during atrial contraction. Put together, the cycle that repeats itself is S4 → S1 (lub) → S2 → S3 (dup).

Systole is the term that describes the contraction phase, whereas diastole refers to the relaxation phase. At rest, around two-thirds of each cardiac cycle is spent in diastole and one-third in systole. This means that the heart is actively contracting for a third of the time and 'resting' or relaxed for the other two-thirds. As the heart rate increases, the length of systole also increases so that when

the horse is at maximum speed, systole and diastole are of equal duration.

Regulation of the Heart Beat

The heart is essentially a self-contained organ which can carry on working without the direct intervention of the voluntary or involuntary nervous system. This explains why isolated hearts can continue to beat for a long time if kept in the correct environment. The heart rate is controlled by the parasympathetic nervous system, which responds to very small changes in its environment. Variations in heart rate in horses can occur not just minute by minute but also beat by beat. This could be interpreted as an irregular rhythm, but this is rarely significant. The variation from beat to beat is an index of health and could be a sign of ill health. Variations occur as responses to the horse's physiological status. It is more obvious because the athletic horse is often quite fit, which can make the heart rate lower. These large ranges of normal can make it difficult for veterinary surgeons to know when an arrhythmia becomes a problem in the individual horse. For example, long pauses between heart beats are quite common in older horses and in very fit horses with a long history of aerobic training, such as racehorses. An exception to this would be atrial fibrillation (see 'Arrhythmias').

The heart has its own in-built nervous system in the form of a pacemaker otherwise known as the sino-atrial (S-A) node or SAN (Figure 7.6). The SAN is situated in the right atrium. An impulse originates at the SAN and spreads in all directions at a rapid rate, causing contraction of the atria. The muscle fibres of the atria are not continuous with those of the ventricles and so this impulse stops at the AV border.

The cells of cardiac muscle tissue are shorter than those of skeletal muscle tissue and are branched. They also touch end to end, allowing direct electrical connections between neighbouring cells via special regions know as intercalated discs. Intercalated discs are specialised electrical junctions

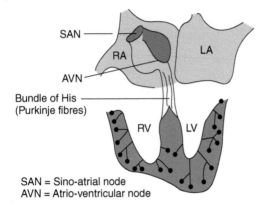

SAN = Sino-atrial node
AVN = Atrio-ventricular node

Figure 7.6 The natural pacemaker of the heart.

that separate the cells. Electrical impulses pass quickly through, as electrical resistance of the cardiac muscle cells is low.

The mass of ventricular tissue is much larger than that of the atrial tissue and so a special conducting system is required. Electrical impulses are mostly prevented from passing directly between the atria and ventricles by a fibrous ring. The exception is the Purkinje fibres in the wall between the left and right ventricles. This system is situated at the base of the septum or wall between the left and right atria. A small area of tissue similar to the SAN but known as the AV node conducts the impulse at a much slower rate, ensuring a pause between the contraction of the atria and the ventricles. From the AV node, the impulse travels through a series of modified cardiac fibres (Purkinje fibres) which are arranged into a special bundle known as the bundle of His. These structures cause the contraction of the ventricles.

The heart does have a nervous supply, but this is not responsible for starting the heart beat. Its role is to modify the rate and force of contraction of the heart according to the needs of the horse at the time. The heart is therefore either filling with blood or contracting to pump it round the body (Figure 7.7).

The Heart and Fittening/Training Horses

The ability of the horse's heart to work efficiently relies on exercise and fitness over a period of time. This increases the strength of the cardiac muscle and improves stroke volume, allowing a quicker return to reduced heart rate and stroke volume at rest. The heart has two initial responses to exercise: a rise in blood volume pumped and dilation of blood vessels. The heart rate increases, and beats stronger per beat. The stroke volume may increase from 20% to 50% above resting rates. Through training of horses the heart becomes more efficient at delivering oxygenated blood to working muscles.

Heart size has been shown to increase with training. This increase in size is due to thickening of the walls of the heart and an increase in size of the heart chambers, especially the left ventricle. Although the effects of training on the heart are not clearly understood, heart mass has been shown to increase up to 33% in 2-year-old horses after only 18 weeks of conventional race training. This increase in heart size results in increased cardiac output. Stroke volume has also been shown to increase by as much as 10% in only 10 weeks of training racehorses.

Stroke volume is influenced by the structural integrity of the various parts of the heart (e.g. valves and septa between chambers), the strength of muscular contraction of the ventricles, the resistance to blood flow faced by the ventricles during systolic ejection, and the ability of the ventricles to fully fill during diastolic relaxation. It is thought that in addition to the strengthening, improved filling capacity of the heart chambers when the heart is relaxed may contribute to the increases shown in stroke volume. Maximal heart rates do not increase with training, and resting heart rates do not decrease with training in horses as it does in humans. Training can improve VO_2 max (see below) from 10% to 20% in the first 6–8 weeks of training, after which further improvement is limited.

Although the heart plays an important role in determining several physiological factors related to performance, it is merely one variable in the whole physiological equation that describes the equine athlete.

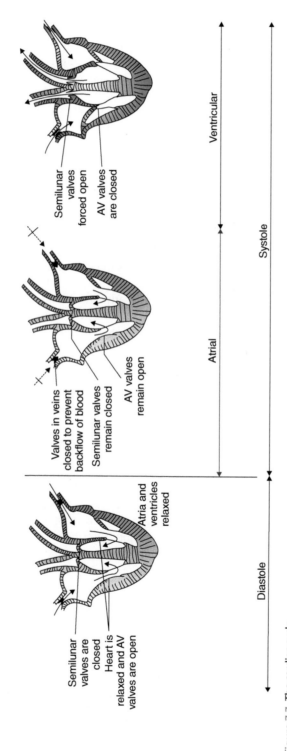

Figure 7.7 The cardiac cycle.

The Heart and VO$_2$ Max

VO$_2$ max is a measure of aerobic capacity and is the maximal rate of oxygen consumption that can be consumed by the horse. It is determined by cardiac output (stroke volume) × heart rate, lung capacity and the ability of muscle cells to take up oxygen from the blood. During exercise the oxygen requirement by muscles increases up to 35 times the resting rate. Research has shown that training can increase a TB's VO$_2$ max by 20% or more, due to the heart's pumping capacity.

VO$_2$ max is expressed in millilitres of oxygen per minute (or second) per kilogram of bodyweight. At rest the horse absorbs 3 ml/min/kg. Maximal rates of oxygen intake vary within breeds and according to training state, but fit TBs have a VO$_2$ max of 160–170 ml/min/kg and elite horses can achieve 200 ml/min/kg. By comparison, human athletes have a VO$_2$ max of about 85 ml/min/kg.

VO$_2$ max is a good indicator of athletic potential, and has been found to be highly correlated with race times in TBs. Horses with a higher VO$_2$ max had faster race times. The ability of the muscles to consume oxygen far exceeds the ability of the heart and lungs to provide oxygenated blood. This means that cardiac output (CO) is actually a limiting factor in performance. Conditions that improve CO will also improve VO$_2$ max.

The relationship between VO$_2$ max and speed is highly correlated, but differences found in the speed and performance of two horses with equal VO$_2$ max can be explained by differences in biomechanics and economy of locomotion.

Heart Murmurs

Heart murmurs are sounds made by the blood circulating through the heart's chambers and valves or through blood vessels near the heart. They may be referred to as 'functional' or 'physiologic' murmurs.

Heart murmurs are without doubt the most common heart abnormalities in horses and they are often found during routine veterinary examinations, for example during the pre-purchase examination. Vascular disease such as atherosclerosis is rare in horses. Where there is no sign of pathology they are referred to as innocent heart murmurs. Acquired degenerative valve disorders are most commonly recognised and these are due to a deformity or defect in the valves. This can lead to disrupted flow or backflow, which further enlarges the heart on the affected side.

Congenital defects are those present from birth, the most common of which is a hole in the heart between the right and left ventricles. A murmur is a disturbance in normal cardiac blood flow which produces an audible sound with a stethoscope. This condition is called valvular regurgitation (heart murmur) or a leaking heart valve. In normal hearts the valve stops the reverse blood flow, but if it becomes thickened, it does not seal properly and blood leaks. As a result, the heart operates less efficiently. A murmur, such as atrial fibrillation, often goes undetected in many horses and never interferes with performance. Mild forms are not necessarily significant and are quite common in racehorses and other sport horses, having very little effect on the horse. Murmurs become more important in older horses which may get age-related scarring in their heart valves, causing leakage of the valves. The condition in older horses tends to progress slowly and often these horses can still be used for light riding activities. There is no cure or treatment for a murmur, but it is important to have horses checked so that appropriate management is undertaken.

Heart or Cardiac Arrhythmia

Cardiac arrhythmia (also called cardiac dysrhythmia or irregular heart beat) is the name for a group of conditions in which the horse's heart beat is irregular – either too fast or too slow. It may result in poor performance and is the third most likely cause of poor performance after musculoskeletal and respiratory causes. Fortunately, cardiac arrhythmia is rare in horses.

Common signs of arrhythmia include exercise intolerance, swelling of the distal limbs, distended veins, general weakness and collapse. This is not surprising as 100% of the horse's blood volume passes through the heart every minute. Arrhythmias include:

- second-degree AV block
- atrial fibrillation.

Second-Degree AV Block

Second-degree AV block is the most common arrhythmia of horses and is basically a dropped beat which seems to resolve itself as the heart rate increases. It may result from an electrolyte imbalance such as hyperkalaemia.

Atrial Fibrillation (AF)

Atrial fibrillation is a more severe arrhythmia resulting from a disorder in the natural electrical stimulation of the heart and this may lead to irregular heart beat, which may even become chaotic. This is the most common arrhythmia associated with poor performance. The atria may flutter as opposed to beating normally, that is, there is no regular rhythm at all. This disorder requires an ECG for accurate diagnosis of the problem and treatment is required to restore normal heart rhythm. Atrial fibrillation is the most common rhythm irregularity that causes poor performance or exercise intolerance in horses. It means that the body is incapable of controlling its cardiac output, leading to affected horses tiring easily during intense athletic efforts such as racing. An estimated 2–3% of horses have atrial fibrillation. A leisure horse might have AF, but, due to low-level exercise only, the owner may never know.

Fortunately, horses do not collapse from atrial fibrillation. Some horses can self-correct the erratic cardiac rhythm, but some require intervention. Atrial fibrillation may be seen in horses with electrolyte imbalances, but it is more commonly caused by enlargement of the atria, often secondary to valvular disease. Treatment protocols involving anti-arrhythmic drugs or electrical stimulation can return the heart to a normal rhythm. The majority of affected horses respond to the drug quinidine sulphate. New treatment also includes electrical cardioversion, or shocking the heart back into rhythm or transvenous electrical cardioversion.

Sudden Cardiac Death

In rare instances horses may collapse and die – a condition known as sudden cardiac death. Typically, the fatal arrhythmia occurs following peak athletic effort as the heart rate is beginning to come down. Also, many apparently healthy horses present with a strange variation in heart rhythm where instead of the rate slowing down smoothly it comes down in sequential steps. In many horses, therefore, during cardiac deceleration, it is quite normal for the heart rate to be irregular as it slows down to normal. Conversely, the probability of sudden cardiac death in pleasure horses is extremely low. In addition, hard-working horses may die because of vascular rupture such as rupture of the aorta, but problems are often identified at post mortem. The horse has a mild species predisposition to degeneration of the walls of the arteries that can result in spontaneous rupture, but it is very rare and does not tend to happen in horses outside of maximal exertion.

Blood Vessels

Arteries

Blood is carried from the heart to the tissues of the body in vessels known as arteries. If an artery is cut, bright red oxygenated blood will spurt from the wound in time with the heart beat. These arteries gradually decrease in size and form branches as they become further away from the heart. This leads to a reduction in blood pressure as blood moves into the tissues. The walls of arteries are thicker than those of veins and contain several layers as do veins (Figure 7.8).

The proportion of elastic to muscle tissue changes from the large vessels to the smaller arteries at the outer limits. This results in two types: elastic and muscular arteries. The elastic arteries are those found closer to the heart and these act as a reservoir of blood.

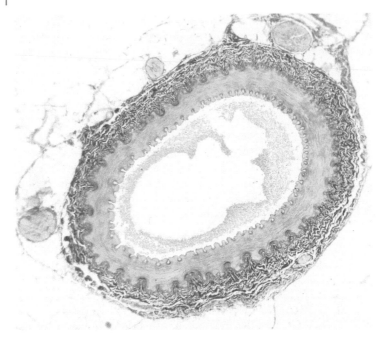

Figure 7.8 Cross-section of a human artery. *Source*: Lord of Konrad, https://commons.wikimedia.org/wiki/File:Artery.png. CC0 1.0.

The arterial wall consists of 3 layers called Tunics.

- Tunica Intima – Inner layer, thin layer of endothelium
- Tunica Media – Thicker middle layer contains more contractile tissue in arteries compared to veins
- Tunica Adventitia – outer layer mostly consists of collagen.

The larger vessels give rise to smaller ones which have smooth muscle in their walls. These are known as arterioles, because they are able to contract and can regulate blood flow to various organs. The arterioles then supply the capillaries with blood. Figure 7.9 shows a photomicrograph of red blood cells squeezing through a capillary. These are very thin-walled vessels whose walls are one cell thick. Here the blood gives up its oxygen, nutrients and hormones, and collects waste products such as carbon dioxide. The capillaries then converge to form very small veins or venules and then progressively larger veins (Figure 7.10).

Arteries have a complex route around the body, often dividing and rejoining to ensure all tissues are supplied with nutrients and so on. Tissues may receive blood from more than one route, and this means that damage to some arteries may not always lead to death of the tissue supplied. Sensors within the arterial system monitor for blood pressure, temperature and biochemical content and give feedback to the brain, so changes can be made when necessary. For example, if oxygen levels fall and carbon dioxide increases, signals will be sent to the brain and action is then taken to increase the breathing rate. High body temperature due to exercise, for example, will result in dilation of blood vessels at the skin to help remove excess body heat.

Veins

Veins have a similar structure to that of arteries, but the walls are much thinner and the proportion of muscular tissue is much less. When several capillaries unite, they form a venule or a small vein. Many veins contain valves which prevent the backflow of blood

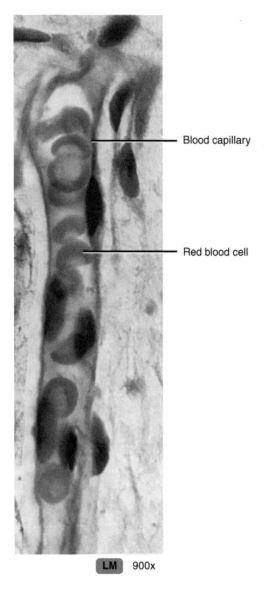

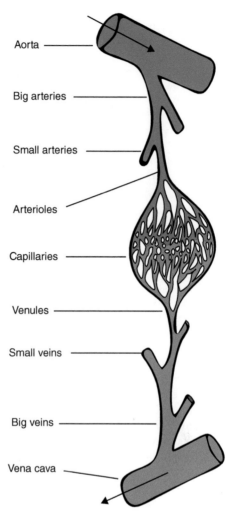

Figure 7.10 Capillary network and direction of blood through it.

LM 900x

Figure 7.9 Photomicrograph showing red blood cells squeezing through a blood capillary. *Source*: Tortora 2005. Reproduced with permission of John Wiley & Sons.

(see Figure 7.11). These large veins become smaller in diameter and turn into venules. The walls of venules have three layers: an inner endothelium composed of squamous endothelial cells that act as a membrane, a middle layer of muscle and elastic tissue, and an outer layer of fibrous connective tissue. The middle layer is poorly developed, compared to arterioles so that venules have thinner walls than arterioles (Figure 7.11).

Muscular contractions of the body help to keep blood moving through the veins towards the heart. This is one reason why horses often develop filled legs when standing in a stable for a long time. This forced inactivity inhibits the venous return to the heart and once the horse starts walking again the swelling should disappear.

Eventually venous blood will enter the great veins or vena cavae and be returned to the right atrium of the heart. If a vein is cut, dark red blood will trickle from the wound.

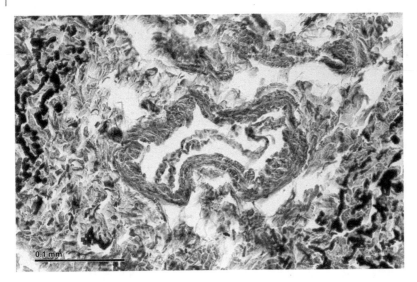

Figure 7.11 Photomicrograph of a venule with a vein valve in cross-section. *Source*: Reischig, https://commons .wikimedia.org/wiki/File:Venule_(238_10A)_With_a_vein_valve;_cross-section;_human.jpg. Used under CC BY-SA 3.0, https://creativecommons.org/licenses/by-sa/3.0/deed.en.

Capillaries

These are the smallest blood vessels making up the micro-circulation and connecting arterioles to veins via capillary beds. They are lined by endothelium which is only one cell thick to allow movement of substances such as oxygen, carbon dioxide, hormones, salts, nutrients etc. to pass between the blood and tissues.

Heart Evaluation and Examination

Ultrasound is now routinely used in evaluation of equine heart health and performance. This is known as electrocardiography (ECG). Ultrasound enables the heart to be evaluated and measured, including heart wall thickness and heart size. Valve function may also be examined in a non-invasive way. Ultrasound emits a high-frequency sound wave through tissues and this information is then interpreted on the ultrasound machine, producing a black-and-white moving picture called a sonogram. The movement can be stopped at any time to take a 'photograph' or take measurements for diagnosis and interpretation by the examiner. The quality of images is determined by the frequency of emitted ultrasound waves.

Ultrasound uses transducers to send high-frequency sound waves into the heart tissue that then bounce back when they hit certain tissue borders, similar to an echo produced in a cave. This echo gets registered by the transducers and transformed into a picture by the computer. Different tissues have different echogenic properties and these change with injury or defects. This allows differentiation of healthy and pathological structures. Doppler ultrasound is another special technique that uses the properties of moving objects to evaluate blood flow.

Electrocardiogram

The conduction of action potentials (electrical signals) through the heart may be picked up by the electrodes of an ECG machine placed in set positions on the horse's skin. The ECG measures the sum of electrical activity in all cardiac muscle cells throughout a heart beat. A recording of the electrical changes that accompany the heart beat is called an ECG and may be printed out for further analysis. In a healthy heart, the ECG will produce a standard trace on the machine known as PQRST complex (Figure 7.12). There are three clearly recognisable waves with each single heart beat. The values for each phase for a mature horse at

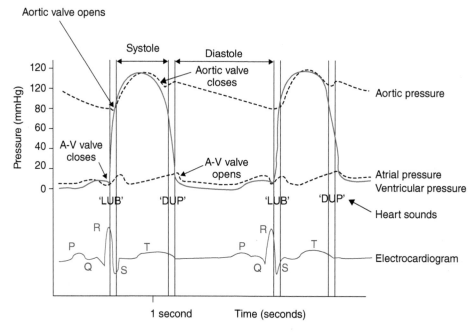

Figure 7.12 Relationship of pressure in the ventricles to the ECG during the cardiac cycle.

rest with a heart rate of around 30 bpm are as follows:

- P wave: 0.12–0.14 seconds – depolarisation of atria.
- PQ interval: 0.35–0.55 seconds – passage of electrical impulses through the AV node, bundles of His and Purkinje fibres.
- QRS complex: 0.1–0.15 seconds – depolarisation of ventricles.
- T wave: repolarisation of ventricles, relaxation.

The SAN pacemaker (see Figure 7.6) creates an impulse which travels over the right atrium and left atrium, leading to contraction of the atria and producing the P wave on the ECG trace. The impulse is then slightly delayed at the AV node, producing the gap between the P wave and the start of the QRS complex. This gap is known as the PQ interval. From the AV node, the impulse passes along the bundle of His to the ventricles to produce ventricular contraction, creating the QRS complex on the trace. The ventricles, having contracted, have to repolarise ready to accept the next contraction of the following heart beat (see Figure 7.12). This repolarisation shows as the T wave on a standard trace. The ECG changes

dramatically when the horse is exercising, with a major change in the T waves.

These traces from an ECG can be used to measure heart rate, rhythm and changes in conduction of impulses where heart problems are suspected. ECG's are also used to monitor horses under anaesthetic. Variation in size and duration of the ECG waves are useful in equine cardiology for the diagnosis of heart arrhythmias and conduction patterns.

Exercise Testing of Horses

Heart rate monitors are now standard equipment. Understanding the heart's function, and its response and adaptation to training, can provide trainers and riders with a great deal of information regarding fitness and ability to compete. Traditionally, trainers relied upon the feel of the horse. Being able to accurately measure the horse's exertion levels during exercise and monitor resting and recovery heart rates is essential in monitoring fitness. Heart meters or cardiotachometers are available which give a read-out of the cardiac cycle at a given time. They have been developed so that they can record the heart beat at fast speed for playback later.

Electrodes are placed in contact with the horse's skin and the machine is attached to the rider by a belt or is strapped to the horse's neck or saddle.

Exercise tests are important in that they can accurately reflect the fitness of the horse and monitor changes throughout the season. They can also be used to assess the effectiveness of the training routine. High-speed tread mills can also be used to help fitten horses. Heart monitors give a basic ECG reading and can be very useful in the training process and can also help to diagnose problems when a horse's performance deteriorates.

Exercise tests are carried out on a treadmill or in the field. Equipment used includes heart rate monitors, on-board ECG's, telemetry ECG's and systems for collecting bloods if required for further analysis. Most trainers use simple heart rate monitors only. Treadmills are preferred for standardised tests. More parameters can be tested, including exercise tolerance, time to fatigue, ventilation, gas exchanges, blood lactate, blood pressure, sweating rate, cardiac output, blood gas analyses and heart beat. They can also be used to find other problems that only surface during work, such as dorsal displacement of the soft palate and obstructive disorders of the upper airway.

Blood

The blood is the body's transport medium and consists of a fluid called plasma, in which are suspended erythrocytes, leucocytes and platelets. It carries gases, nutrients, hormones and salts in solution and acts as a communication system reaching the whole body. The blood volume of a horse is roughly 8% of the body weight in kilograms; that is, an average mature horse of 500 kg will have approximately 40 litres of blood circulating through the body. A summary of blood constituents is shown in Figure 7.13a.

Haematopoiesis is the formation and development of blood cells and platelets. These are developed from pluripotent stem cells known as haematopoietic stem cells (HSC's) or haemocytoblasts. Derived from mesoderm in red bone marrow, these cells give rise to both the myeloid and lymphoid types of blood cells (Figure 7.13b). Haemocytoblasts are self-renewing so as not to deplete the pool of stem cells – a process known as asymmetric division. The daughter cells of HSC's – the myeloid and lymphoid progenitor cells, which cannot self-renew – may follow a number of different pathways, leading to the production of every type of blood cell.

Plasma

Plasma consists mainly of water (about 92%) with many substances dissolved in it, such as glucose, amino acids, hormones, salts, plasma proteins and antibodies (Table 7.1). Plasma proteins are also termed blood proteins or serum proteins and there are many of them. The most common are albumins (around 55% of plasma proteins) and globulins (38%).

Albumins help to maintain the osmotic pressure of plasma and primarily function as carrier proteins for steroids, fatty acids and thyroid hormones. Globulins help to transport ions, hormones and fats. Some globulins are also known as antibodies and they are strongly associated with immunity and resistance to disease (see Chapter 15). They are made in the liver and their production is stimulated by the presence of antigens.

Fibrinogen comprises 7% of blood proteins; conversion of fibrinogen to insoluble fibrin is essential for blood clotting. The remainder of the plasma proteins (1%) are regulatory proteins, such as enzymes, proenzymes and hormones. All blood proteins are synthesised in the liver except for the gamma globulins.

Plasma is often referred to as the 'internal environment' which bathes all the cells of the body. The kidneys are responsible for maintaining a constant level of water and other substances within the plasma. The constituents of cells and plasma can easily be seen if a test tube of blood, which has been prevented from clotting, is left to stand. The heavier particles such as the cells and platelets settle to the bottom, leaving the straw-coloured plasma above. Approximately 45% of blood is made up of cells, the remaining 55% being plasma.

Red Blood Cells (Erythrocytes)

Erythrocytes (Figure 7.14) are specialist cells designed to carry mainly oxygen and a small amount of carbon dioxide. They have lost their nucleus to make room for haemoglobin, an oxygen-carrying protein. The pigment part of haemoglobin molecules requires iron. Haemoglobin is able to form

a reversible combination with oxygen and carbon dioxide:

Haemoglobin + oxygen = oxyhaemoglobin

Haemoglobin + carbon dioxide

= carbaminohaemoglobin

In the lungs, haemoglobin in the erythrocytes combines with oxygen to form oxyhaemoglobin. As blood takes up oxygen it becomes a brighter red colour. This oxygenated blood is returned to the heart and pumped around the body to the various tissues, where some of the oxyhaemoglobin

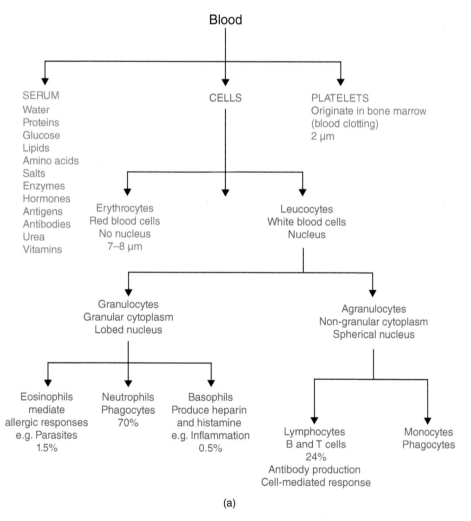

(a)

Figure 7.13 (a) Summary of blood constituents. (b) Origin of blood cells. *Source*: Rad, https://commons.wikimedia.org/wiki/File:Hematopoiesis_simple.svg. CC BY-SA 3.0.

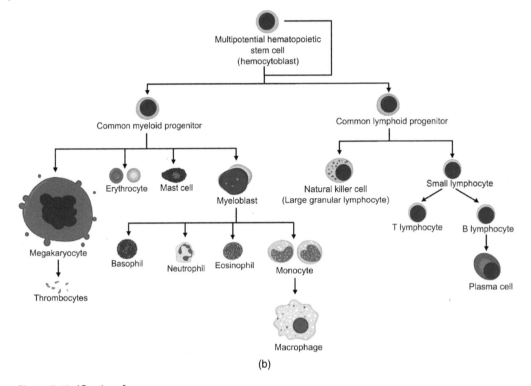

(b)

Figure 7.13 (*Continued*)

gives up its oxygen. When blood gives up its oxygen it becomes a much darker, deeper red colour. In the tissues, the erythrocytes collect some carbon dioxide, forming carbaminohaemoglobin, which is then returned to the lungs via the heart and the carbon dioxide is released and breathed out. However, most carbon dioxide is carried as bicarbonate (HCO^-_3) in plasma (Figure 7.15). Erythrocytes are shaped like a bi-concave disc, which increases the surface area for exchange of oxygen. There are three ways in which carbon dioxide is transported in the blood:

- as dissolved CO_2
- bound to haemoglobin and plasma proteins
- in the form of bicarbonate ions (HCO_3^-): the majority of carbon dioxide is transported in this way.

Because erythrocytes have no nucleus, they have a limited life span of around 3–4 months. They therefore are constantly manufactured in red bone marrow. A large number of these disintegrate and are replaced daily. In the horse, it has been estimated that 35 million erythrocytes are produced every second of the day. Old cells are broken down and the iron-containing part is used to make new ones. The pigment portion is converted to the bile pigments bilirubin and biliverdin which are then excreted via the digestive tract.

White Blood Cells (Leucocytes)

Leucocytes (Figure 7.16) form a major part of the body's defence mechanism, and there are several types, which respond to different types of challenge or infection. They play a vital role in protecting the horse's body from infections and are the cells of the immune system. They are made in bone marrow and lymph nodes and are irregular in shape. They are much lower in number and much larger compared to erythrocytes. Unlike erythrocytes, leucocytes contain a nucleus and this is often quite large and lobed, with the presence of an outer buffer coat. They are capable of

Table 7.1 Components of plasma.

Substance	Source	Destination	Notes
Water	Absorbed in colon	To all cells	Excess removed by kidneys
Plasma proteins, e.g. albumin, globulins and fibrinogen	Albumin – liver	To all cells	Involved in plasma osmotic pressure, transport of steroids and thyroid hormones
	Globulin – liver	To all cells	Immune function; transports hormones and fats
	Fibrinogen made in liver	Remains in the blood	Aids blood clotting
Lipids, including cholesterol and fatty acids	Absorbed from small intestine and also derived from body's fat reserves	To liver for breakdown or adipose tissue for storage	Breakdown of fats yields energy
Carbohydrates, e.g. glucose	Absorbed from small intestine or derived from glycogen breakdown	To all cells for energy, released by process of cellular respiration	Excess glucose is converted to glycogen and stored in liver and muscles
Urea and other excretory substances	Derived from amino acid breakdown in liver (deamination)	To kidneys for excretion	
Mineral ions, e.g. Na, Cl	Absorbed in small intestine and colon	To all cells	Excess excreted by kidneys
Hormones	Secreted into blood by endocrine glands	To all parts of the body	Hormones only have an effect on their target organs; they are broken down in liver and excreted by kidneys
Dissolved gases, e.g. CO_2	CO_2 is released from all cells as a waste product of respiration	To lungs for excretion	Most CO_2 is carried as bicarbonate (HCO_3^-) in plasma

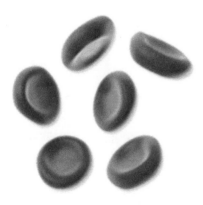

Figure 7.14 Red blood cells. *Source*: Blaus, https://commons.wikimedia.org/wiki/File:Blausen_0761_RedBloodCells.png. CC BY 3.0.

some independent movement, rather like an amoeba, and can squeeze out through the thin walls of blood capillaries into all parts of the body. They are then able to engulf and digest unwanted foreign substances such as invading bacteria.

The horse has approximately 9000 per cubic millimetre of whole blood, compared with 7 million erythrocytes per cubic millimetre. In general, the leucocytes count can vary and will rise to meet specific problems such as disease and infection. However, their number can also increase in response to normal physiological events, such as pregnancy, digestion of food and exercise. Leucocytes are classified as follows:

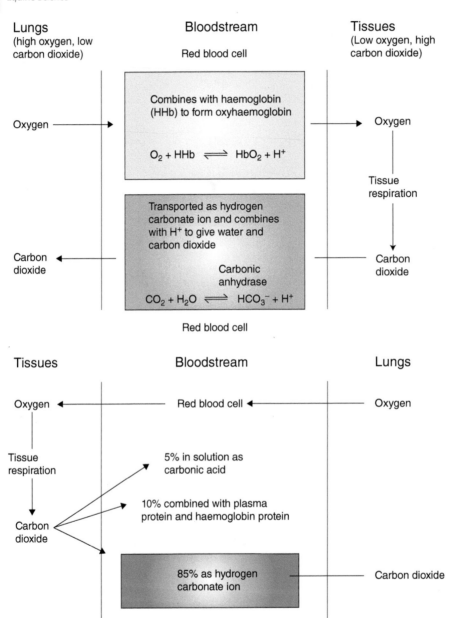

Lungs
(high oxygen, low carbon dioxide)

Bloodstream

Red blood cell

Tissues
(Low oxygen, high carbon dioxide)

Oxygen

Combines with haemoglobin (HHb) to form oxyhaemoglobin

$$O_2 + HHb \rightleftharpoons HbO_2 + H^+$$

Oxygen

Tissue respiration

Carbon dioxide

Transported as hydrogen carbonate ion and combines with H^+ to give water and carbon dioxide

Carbonic anhydrase

$$CO_2 + H_2O \rightleftharpoons HCO_3^- + H^+$$

Carbon dioxide

Red blood cell

Tissues

Bloodstream

Lungs

Oxygen ← Red blood cell ← Oxygen

Tissue respiration

5% in solution as carbonic acid

10% combined with plasma protein and haemoglobin protein

Carbon dioxide

85% as hydrogen carbonate ion

Carbon dioxide

Red blood cell

Figure 7.15 Summary of the transport of oxygen and carbon dioxide.

- Granulocytes – neutrophils, eosinophils, basophils.
- Agranulocytes – monocytes, lymphocytes.

The life span of leucocytes varies considerably. Granulocytes may last only a few hours, whereas monocytes may last for months and lymphocytes for years. Within the blood system itself, the leucocytes tend to be non-functional and are simply being transported to sites within the body where they are required.

Granulocytes

As the name implies, granulocytes contain granules within their cytoplasm, which stain

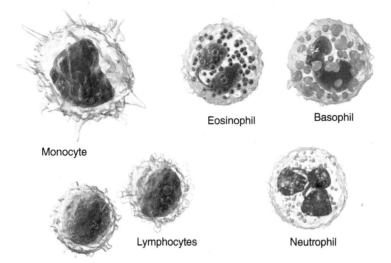

Monocyte

Eosinophil

Basophil

Lymphocytes

Neutrophil

Figure 7.16 White blood cells. *Source*: Blaus, https://commons.wikimedia.org/wiki/File:Blausen_0425_Formed_Elements.png. CC BY 3.0.

with common stains used in blood-staining tests. These stains contain an acid dye, eosin, which is red, or a basic dye, methylene blue, which is blue. The granulocytes are named according to the colour of stain that the granules in their cytoplasm pick up. Thus the eosinophils stain red and the basophils blue. Neutrophils stain indifferently.

Neutrophils

The most common type of granulocyte is the neutrophil which accounts for over 70% of the leucocytes. These neutrophils are actively phagocytic, in other words they engulf bacteria and debris at the site of infection. A localised collection of pus is known as an abscess and the pus contains vast numbers of these neutrophil granulocytes. The neutrophils also degrade dead tissue in the area.

The number of neutrophils in the blood increases rapidly whenever acute infection is present, and this is one of the purposes of taking a blood sample. A blood test may show the presence of infection before the horse starts to show clinical signs. Neutrophils, therefore, constitute the first line of defence against infection by migrating to any area invaded by bacteria, passing through the capillary walls to the site of infection.

Eosinophils

Also known as acidophils, eosinophils are found in much smaller quantities and account for approximately 1.5–2% of all leucocytes. Eosinophils are known to increase in number in certain chronic diseases such as parasite infections. They are also responsible for the detoxification of foreign proteins introduced into the body via the lungs or the gut. Their number also increases in allergic reactions.

Basophils

Basophils are also rare in normal blood, at about 0.5% of leucocytes. Since they contain the anticoagulant heparin, it is thought that they may release this substance in areas of inflammation.

Agranulocytes

As the name implies, agranulocytes show few granules in their rather sparse cytoplasm. These cells include monocytes and lymphocytes.

Monocytes

Monocytes are the largest of the leucocytes and like the neutrophils they engulf foreign matter such as bacteria. However, while neutrophils are active mainly in acute infections, monocytes tend to be called into action for more long-term, chronic infections such as tuberculosis in humans. When monocytes from the blood enter the tissues they develop into larger cells known as macrophages.

Lymphocytes

Lymphocytes include natural killer (NK) cells, T cells and B cells. They are the main type of cell found in lymph, hence the name lymphocyte. They are variable in appearance and size and have a relatively large nucleus surrounded by a small amount of cytoplasm. The major function of lymphocytes is their response to foreign substances or agents otherwise known as antigens. This involves the production of antibodies that circulate in the blood, or the development of cellular immunity, which is discussed in more detail in Chapter 15.

Platelets (Thrombocytes)

In addition to erythrocytes and leucocytes, the blood contains some tiny colourless corpuscles known as platelets or thrombocytes. Each platelet looks like a small rounded or oval disc and there are approximately 400,000 of them per cubic millimetre of blood. They are fragments produced from large cells in the bone marrow called megakaryocytes. Platelets are also relatively short-lived with a life span of between 9 and 11 days.

Platelets are important in the clotting of blood, particularly where blood vessels are damaged. The surface of platelets appears to be quite sticky, and when blood is shed, the platelets tend to stick together in clusters. By adhering together and sticking to the surface of damaged blood vessels, they effectively form a plug or a clot, thereby preventing further blood loss. Platelets are also responsible for the conversion of the element prothrombin, which is present in the blood, to thrombin. Thrombin then assists in the blood clotting process (see below).

Two-thirds of all platelets in a healthy horse are in constant circulation in the blood. The remaining third are held in the spleen, ready for emergency use (see 'The Spleen').

Haemostasis or Blood Clotting

Haemostasis is the body's response to bleeding from a blood vessel, be it large or small. It involves a complicated process between platelets and numerous blood clotting proteins (or factors), resulting in the formation of a blood clot to stop the bleeding.

Whenever blood escapes from the body via a wound or injury, it quickly changes from a fluid to a thick jelly-like material called a clot. The process by which the body stops bleeding and begins healing is called haemostasis. In horses, common diseases such as colic, colitis, endotoxaemia and sepsis are associated with changes to the haemostatic pathway, leading to coagulation abnormalities. Thromboelastometry is a method that allows kinetic observation in real time of clots forming and dissolving and is a relatively new development in equine veterinary care.

This process of clotting (or coagulation) is an essential process that prevents the valuable blood pouring from a wound, which may otherwise result in the horse bleeding to death. Formation of a clot will also prevent the entry of bacteria into the horse's body. The process of clotting is a highly complex one and is dependent upon a large number of factors. The process of clotting (Figure 7.17) depends upon the change in state of a blood protein found in the plasma called fibrinogen. Fibrinogen is normally found dissolved in the blood plasma, but when blood is shed, fibrinogen changes into a long fibrous network of molecules of fibrin. This network gradually contracts to form a clot and within its meshes are trapped various blood constituents such as red and white cells. As the clot shrinks, a clear yellow fluid escapes from the wound and this is serum. It is quite simply plasma without the fibrinogen, which has been converted to fibrin. On the surface of the wound, the clot dries to form a scab and the healing process will take place underneath this mechanical protective covering.

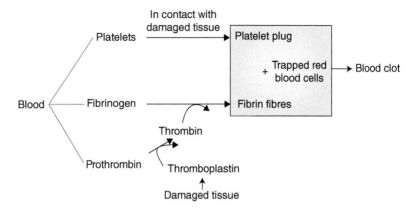

Figure 7.17 Blood clot formation.

Although clotting checks bleeding, it also helps to prevent potential leaks. For example, migrating worm larvae which may damage the lining of blood vessels can result in the formation of clots within the blood vessel which will strengthen the damaged part. These clots when remaining fixed are called thrombi. A thrombus can become so large that it completely blocks the blood vessel, preventing the flow of blood to further parts which may die as a result. The thrombus can also become loose and float freely in the bloodstream, where it may cause a lethal blockage, called an embolus, elsewhere.

Blood Tests

There is no doubt that horses perform at their best when their blood constituents are within a normal range. Blood can change quite rapidly in response to disease, stress and electrolyte imbalances, and regular blood tests will quickly identify problems often before clinical signs are shown by the horse. Changes in the blood also occur as the horse's fitness increases. Moreover, blood parameters vary between individual horses.

Some horses such as racehorses and eventers are routinely blood tested to monitor their health and fitness. Each individual horse may then have the results computerised and an overall picture of the blood profile and patterns can be used to plan training programmes and assess fitness. They

should be used as an aid to diagnosis and to identify health problems. Blood tests help a trainer to decide whether or not a horse should compete. The blood tests generally fall into one of two categories:

- Haematology – the study of blood cells.
- Biochemistry – the study of the chemistry of substances in plasma.

Most blood tests investigate several routine parameters. Often results from one of these routine analyses may suggest whether further tests should be carried out, but this is not always the case. Appendix 2 shows routine haematological and biochemical tests which are carried out on blood samples.

Blood Typing

The process of blood typing includes the mapping of the horse's blood groups, producing a unique identification of an individual horse. Blood typing is carried out by using the genes that have control over the red blood cell antigens found on their surface. These antigens are known as blood factors and vary between groups of red blood cells; hence they can be used to identify blood groups. Because blood typing is genetically determined it remains the same throughout the horse's life and serves as a unique and permanent record of identification.

More than 30 different blood factors have been identified in horses, with around seven being widely recognised. The seven internationally recognised blood groups in horses are A, C, D, K, P, Q and U. There is also an eighth, T, which is mostly used in research. Each blood group has at least two allelic factors. The A blood group has a, b, c, d, e, f and g, all of which can be combined in all combinations, such as Aa, Acg, Abdeg and so on, to make many different alleles. The result of this is that horses can have around 400,000 allelic combinations. This allows accurate blood testing to be used as a method of identifying an individual horse and determining parentage.

Care should be taken when breeding a mare to a stallion with a different blood type – usually Aa or Qa blood – as this may result in the condition neonatal isoerythrolysis if the foal inherits the blood type of the stallion. This can also occur if a mare is bred to a jack donkey, due to donkey factor. This immune-mediated disease is life-threatening and requires a transfusion.

Blood typing can be very useful before giving a transfusion, but because the majority of horses do not have naturally occurring antibodies that could cause a reaction, the first time a horse receives a transfusion it can be done without cross-matching and without risk of reaction. Only two blood types, Aa and Qa, are considered relevant when checking compatibility for blood transfusions.

The Lymphatic or Lymph System

The lymphatic system is basically a system of fine tubes that run through the body in a similar way to blood vessels. The capillaries that carry blood allow leakage of plasma into the tissues. The leucocytes are also able to squeeze through gaps in the capillary wall, but erythrocytes cannot. Lymph or tissue fluid is characteristically a straw-coloured fluid containing leucocytes. The result of this is that leucocytes and plasma continuously move out of the capillaries and bathe all the tissues within the body. This fluid is called tissue fluid and supplies all cells with nutrients and oxygen. Carbon dioxide and waste products then diffuse back into the capillaries. Because each cell is bathed with tissue fluid, it provides a constant environment, that is, a constant temperature and osmotic pressure. This consistency is vital for the health of cells and is known as homeostasis. The main function of the lymphatic system is to help drain away the tissue fluids and eventually return them to the blood via lymph nodes and the venous system.

Lymph makes up 2–3% of the total body fluids of the horse. It absorbs and transports fats from the intestines to the blood, and returns fluid to the anterior vena cava and the subclavian vein. Horses have large groups of lymph nodes, whereas other animals have just one or two.

Within the tissues, alongside the capillaries, are other small vessels called lymphatic capillaries. The tissue fluid slowly drains into these tubes and the fluid once within the lymphatic vessels is known as lymph. The smaller lymphatic vessels link up with larger, blind-ending ones which carry the lymph to the subclavian veins where it rejoins the blood in the horse's chest. The smaller tubes have a thin wall which is one cell thick, whereas the larger vessels have connective tissue in their walls.

The walls of the lymphatic vessels do not contain muscle tissue and therefore they are unable to actively propel the lymph along the vessels. The intermittent pressure of surrounding muscles helps to push lymph along the vessels and valves within the larger lymphatic vessels, prevent backflow and keep the lymph moving in one direction only. Before the lymph drains back into the blood it passes through lymphatic tissue. This consists of lymphocytes and the cells that produce them and macrophages. The function of these is to destroy any bacteria or toxins that may have been drained away from the tissues and so help to reduce the chances of infection. This lymphatic tissue may collect together in groups surrounded by connective tissue and these constitute the lymph nodes (Figure 7.18).

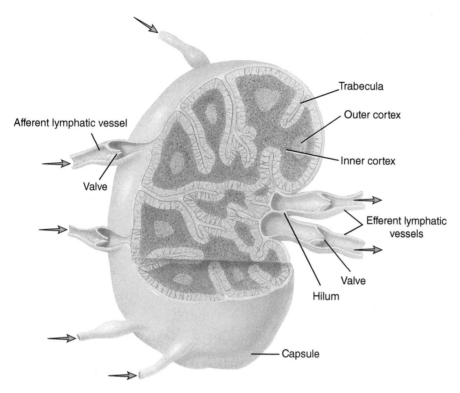

Figure 7.18 Simplified drawing of a lymph node. *Source*: Peate 2011. Reproduced with permission of John Wiley & Sons.

Lymph nodes are found in areas such as the neck, base of the bronchi and along the larger blood vessels in the abdominal cavity. Lymph nodes often become enlarged and tender when the horse has an infection. An example is the mandibular gland which sits between the angles of the lower jaw. This often becomes swollen in young horses as a result of bacteria passing from the lining of the airways of the head to the lymphatic vessels. Strangles is one of the most common equine diseases in the UK. It is a highly contagious infection of the upper respiratory tract caused by the bacteria *Streptococcus equi* (subspecies *equi*). It is prolonged in its course and associated with serious complications, such as 'bastard' strangles. Yards are closed down for considerable periods of time while dealing with an outbreak and disinfecting afterwards. It results in the production of significant abscesses containing pus which

eventually burst through the skin under the jaw (Figure 7.19).

The Spleen

The spleen is an important organ that is involved with the circulatory system. It lies on the left-hand side of the horse against the body wall and plays an important role in the immune system, removing damaged or diseased erythrocytes and leucocytes from the circulation. When the horse is relaxed, the spleen is also relaxed and expanded to its largest size, extending from the ninth rib space back to the point of the hip and covers most of the left side of the abdomen. In this relaxed state it can hold an estimated 30 litres of blood that slowly moves through the spleen, then re-enters the circulation. When the horse is stressed or

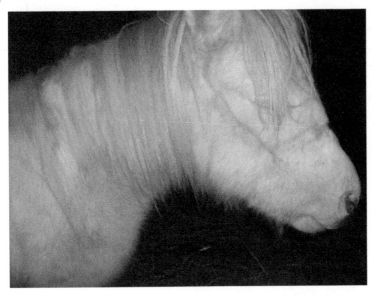

Figure 7.19 Pony with strangles, viewed from the side before abscesses burst. *Source*: AkaEmma, https://commons.wikimedia.org/wiki/File:Odin_strangles_from_the_side.JPG.

excited, for example before a race or any time the 'fight or flight' response kicks in, the spleen contracts, expelling up to 25 litres of stored blood into the circulation, making the extra erythrocytes available to transport a much larger amount of oxygen to the muscles. This can nearly double the oxygen-carrying capacity of the horse's circulation and improve aerobic capability and athletic efficiency within seconds.

Summary Points

1) At rest, the horse's heart rate may be as low as 30 bpm, whereas when it is galloping this can increase to 230 bpm.

Q + A

Q What is the horse's normal blood pressure?
A 120/70 (similar to humans).

Q What is VO_2 max?
A It is a measure of aerobic capacity and is the maximal rate of oxygen consumption that can be consumed by the horse. It

2) It is possible to measure the sum of electrical activity in all cardiac muscle cells throughout a heart beat. A recording of these electrical changes that accompany the heart beat is called an electrocardiogram (ECG) and may be printed out for further analysis.

3) There are seven internationally recognised blood groups in horses, namely A, C, D, K, P, Q and U. There is also an eighth, T, which is mostly used in research.

4) The process by which the horse's body stops bleeding and begins healing is called haemostasis.

is determined by cardiac output (Q) (stroke volume (SV)) × heart rate (HR), lung capacity and the ability of muscle cells to take up oxygen from the blood.

Q What is the most common cause of heart murmurs in horses?

A Acquired degenerative valve disorders are most commonly recognised and these are due to a deformity or defect in the valves. This can lead to disrupted flow or backflow which further enlarges the heart on the affected side.

Q What is thromboelastometry?

A It is a method that allows kinetic observation in real time of clots forming and dissolving and is a relatively new development in equine veterinary care.

Q What is the most common type of granulocyte?

A The neutrophil accounts for over 70% of white blood cells.

8

The Nervous System

The horse's body is extremely complex and consists of many different organs and systems. To ensure these all work together as efficiently as possible there must be a communication system that registers changes in the internal and external environment.

Horses have two coordinating systems, namely the endocrine (hormonal) system and the nervous system, which work together, triggering responses to external stimuli. In horses the flight or fight response to danger is brought about by both nervous and hormonal signals; however, the nervous system is much faster in its reactions and is also responsible for the control of more delicate movements by the body.

The nervous system is made up of highly specialised cells which provide an extremely organised data-processing system and is very complex. It comprises the brain, cranial nerves (Figure 8.1), spinal cord, spinal nerves, ganglia, enteric plexuses and sensory receptors. A cubic centimetre of brain contains several million nerve cells. The skull encloses the brain and 12 pairs of cranial nerves (left and right) which are numbered between I and XII. The hypoglossal nerve is XII.

Cranial nerves may be sensory, motor or both.

- Sensory only: I, II, VIII.
- Motor only: III, IV, VI, XI, XII.
- Both: V, VII, IX, X.

Figure 8.2 shows the major nerves of the horse.

The nervous system as a whole ensures the horse's body responds appropriately to the external and internal conditions at any time. It does this by:

- gathering information from sensor organs or receptors which detect stimuli
- transmitting this sensory information to the central nervous system (CNS) via afferent sensory nerves
- coordinating this information and sending it to the brain via the spinal cord
- the brain then analysing the information and deciding what to do, often based on prior experience
- transmitting this information to the effectors, that is the muscles, glands and so on via motor nerves.

Sensory input is the conduction of signals or messages from the sensory receptors such as the nose, eyes, ears and skin to processing centres in the brain and spinal cord (see Chapter 11). Motor output is the conduction of signals to the effector cells such as muscles which move in direct response to the signal. So, information in the form of signals passes from the receptors to processing centres and from there to the effectors. Figure 8.3 provides a summary of the nervous system.

Information is carried along neurons in the form of electrical signals or nerve impulses. The nerve impulses are known as action potentials, but rather than a flow of electrons or electrical current, the horse experiences a rapid change in the ion balance in the neuron which quickly runs from one end of the neuron to the other, similar to a burning fuse. As the impulse arrives at the end of the neuron, it reaches a small gap or junction between

Equine Science, Third Edition. Zoe Davies and Sarah Pilliner.
© 2018 Zoe Davies and Sarah Pilliner. Published 2018 by John Wiley & Sons Ltd.

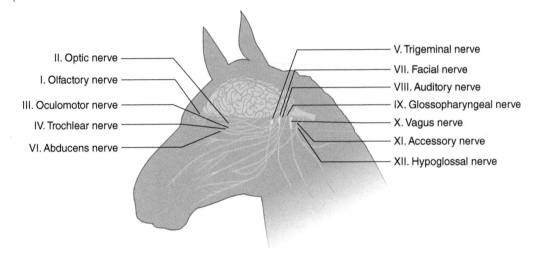

Figure 8.1 Cranial nerves of the horse. *Source*: Functional Anatomy of the Vertebrates. Quiring, Daniel Paul, 1894–1958. https://commons.wikimedia.org/wiki/File:Quiring_1950_146.png.

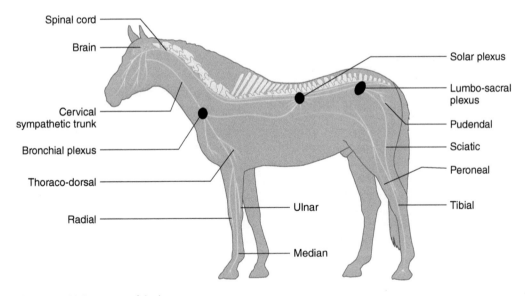

Figure 8.2 Major nerves of the horse.

two neurons known as a synapse. The nerve impulse can cross the synapse via chemical transmitters to the next neuron in the chain. This system allows very rapid transmission of information around the horse's body.

Nerves and Neurons

Neurons are bundled together into larger structures, which may contain hundreds or thousands of axons, to make nerves or nerve

All neurons contain the same basic parts as any animal cell, but they are specially adapted to be able to carry electrical impulses (Figure 8.4). They consist of a cell body containing the nucleus and cell organelles and two types of extensions of the cytoplasm, namely many dendrites and a single axon.

The cell body and shorter 'branch-like' dendrites are the receiving parts of the neuron, whereas the axons are the sending parts of the neuron, taking the signal towards another neuron. The axon joins the cell body at the axon hillock. Nerve impulses often arise from the axon hillock before travelling down the axon. At the end of axons are the axon terminals. Here they will connect either to another neuron or to an effector such as a muscle cell, but either way it will be via a synapse. Most axon terminals therefore end in a synaptic end bulb. The synaptic end bulb contains neurotransmitters stored in synaptic vesicles.

Similar to muscle cells, neurons have electrical excitability, whereby they can convert a stimulus to an action potential. The nervous impulse or action potential travels along the surface of the neuron membrane. Neurons have many different functions and this will affect their structure. The three main types of neuron (Figure 8.5) are:

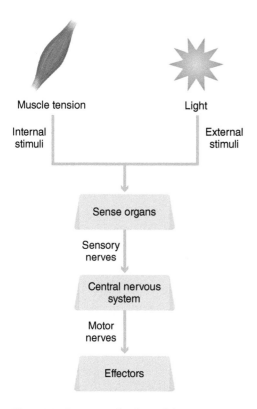

Figure 8.3 Summary of actions of the nervous system.

- Unipolar – for example, myelinated sensory neuron.
- Bipolar – for example, retinal neuron.
- Multipolar – for example, motor neuron.

Nerve fibres of horses are wrapped in a layer of insulating material called myelin which forms a sheath known as the myelin sheath around the nerve fibre. These insulated fibres carry impulses much more quickly than those fibres without a myelin sheath. Neurons are classified according to their function:

- Sensory or afferent neurons.
- Motor or efferent neurons.

Sensory neurons contain sensory receptors at the dendrite end or another neuron which

fibres, some of which are visible to the naked eye. Sensory nerves take information from sense organs and sensory receptors to the brain along afferent fibres, whereas motor nerves carry information usually from the brain to the effectors along efferent fibres such as muscles.

- Sensory fibres – somatic afferent, visceral afferent.
- Motor fibres – somatic efferent, visceral efferent, autonomic (sympathetic and parasympathetic).

Each nerve follows a definite path and serves a specific region of the body. For example, cranial nerve I, the olfactory nerve, carries impulses from the horse's nose to the brain concerning the sense of smell (see Figure 8.1).

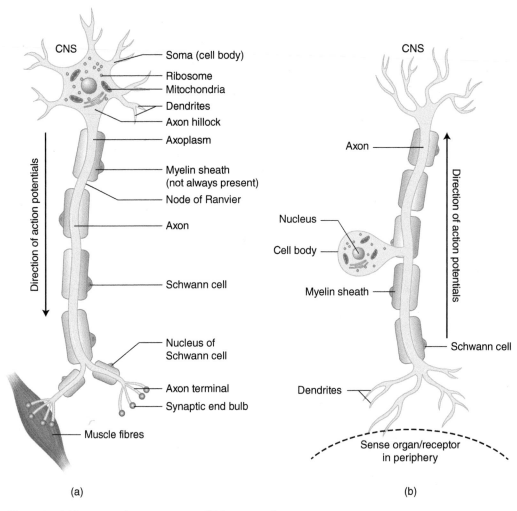

Figure 8.4 (a) Structure of a motor neuron. (b) Structure of a sensory neuron.

originated from a sensory receptor. These take action potentials to the CNS via cranial and spinal nerves along axons. Motor neurons take action potentials away from the CNS to the effectors such as muscle fibres or glands in the periphery or peripheral nervous system (PNS) via the cranial and spinal nerves. Motor neurons have a multipolar structure.

A third category is the interneurons (also called relay neurons, association neurons, connector neurons or local circuit neurons). Interneurons are found exclusively in the CNS and create neural circuits, enabling communication between sensory or motor neurons and the CNS.

Neuroglia or Glial Cells

Neuroglia, sometimes called glial cells or simply glia (Greek for 'glue'), are non-neuronal cells with several functions. They:

- offer mechanical support to neurons
- act as insulators between neurons, preventing neuronal impulses from spreading in unwanted directions
- are involved in phagocytosis of foreign material

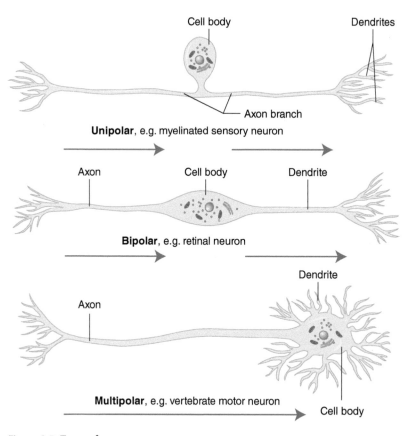

Figure 8.5 Types of neuron.

- repair damaged areas of nervous tissue by proliferation (gliosis) forming a glial scar and filling gaps left by degenerated neurons
- store neurotransmitters released by neighbouring synapses
- are involved in homeostasis of the ionic environment for neurons
- synthesise myelin for the myelin sheath.

Neuroglia make up around half of the CNS and are much smaller than neurons, but far more numerous. Neuroglia do not carry action potentials, that is, they are not excitable, but they do carry on multiplying in the adult horse. There are many different types of glial cells with different functions (see above). Astrocytes are star-shaped glial cells that nourish and support neuroglia, oligodendrites increase speed of the nerve impulse and microglia are phagocytes.

Neuron cell bodies are often found in clusters or groups, known as a ganglion in the CNS and as a nucleus in the PNS. The axons are grouped together to form a nerve in the PNS, whereas this is known as a tract in the CNS. The CNS tracts interconnect neurons in the brain and spinal cord. When the brain is dissected, some regions appear grey whereas others look white.

- White matter is composed mainly of myelinated axons; myelin is white and hence the colour.
- Grey matter is composed mainly of cell bodies, dendrites, neuroglia and unmyelinated axons, appearing grey in colour.

Within the spinal cord the white matter surrounds the grey matter on the inside. A transverse section through the spinal cord (Figure 8.6) shows an H-shaped central grey area comprising cell bodies, dendrites, neuroglia, unmyelinated axons and synapses around a central canal filled

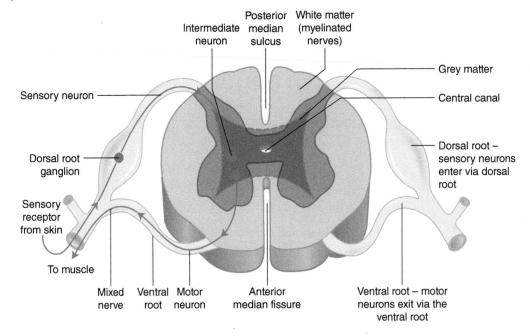

Figure 8.6 Transverse section through the spinal cord.

with cerebrospinal fluid. The area of white matter sits on the outside of the grey matter and contains nerve fibres.

Organisation of the Nervous System

For convenience, the nervous system is divided into two main parts: the CNS and PNS. Figure 8.7 shows the organisation of the nervous system.

CNS

The CNS consists of the brain and spinal cord, which are protected by the skull and spinal column, respectively. The CNS receives input from the sense organs such as

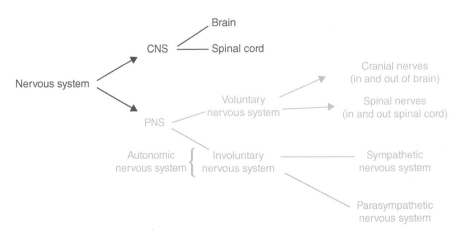

Figure 8.7 Organisation of the nervous system.

the skin, eyes and ears and sends signals to the muscles and glands via the PNS.

PNS

The PNS consists of all the nerves that connect the brain and spinal cord to the rest of the body, that is, all nerves outside of the CNS. The PNS also has ganglia, which are clusters of nerve cell bodies belonging to neurons which make up the nerves. The PNS may be subdivided into:

- the autonomic nervous system (ANS)
- the enteric nervous system (ENS)
- the somatic nervous system (SNS).

The Autonomic Nervous System consists of:

- sensory neurons taking impulses from autonomic sensory receptors in the visceral organs (internal organs of the body within the chest or abdomen), for example the stomach and heart, to the CNS
- motor neurons taking impulses from the CNS to cardiac and smooth muscle tissue and glands.

These motor responses are involuntary, that is, not under conscious control, and the motor part of the ANS further consists of two branches, namely sympathetic and parasympathetic (Table 8.1). Effectors mostly receive impulses from both these divisions of the ANS, but the divisions have opposing actions. In general, the sympathetic division prepares horses for flight or fight and emergency situations, whereas the parasympathetic division supports rest and normal activities.

The Enteric Nervous System is involuntary and supplies the horse's gut. It contains millions of neurons extending almost the entire length of the horse's digestive system. Sensory neurons of the ENS monitor changes to gut contents and changes to dilation of the gut wall (see Chapter 5).

The Somatic Nervous System conveys sensory signals from sensory neurons in the head, body walls and limbs and from the special senses, that is, the eyes, ears and nose, to the CNS. It also takes motor impulses

Table 8.1 Examples of parasympathetic and sympathetic functions.

Parasympathetic division	Sympathetic division
Slows the heart	Accelerates the heart
Dilates arteries	Constricts arteries
Constricts bronchioles	Dilates bronchioles
Constricts pupil	Dilates pupil
Stimulates lacrimal gland	Contracts erector pili muscle
Stimulates saliva flow	Increases sweating
Speeds up gut movement	Slows down gut movement
Relaxes bladder and anal sphincters	Contracts bladder and anal sphincters
Contracts bladder	Relaxes bladder

from the CNS to skeletal muscles only. These motor impulses are under conscious control and are therefore the only motor part of the PNS that is voluntary.

The nerves and ganglia of the PNS form a vast communications network. The nerves that carry signals to and from the brain are known as cranial nerves, whereas those carrying signals to and from the spinal cord are known as the spinal nerves. The horse's eyes, nose, tongue and ears, for example, are served by the cranial nerves, whereas the muscles and skin of the limbs are serviced by the spinal nerves.

All spinal nerves and most of the cranial nerves contain both sensory and motor neurons. Hundreds of thousands of signals, both incoming and outgoing, pass each other within the same nerves all the time.

Action Potential

The function of the neuron is to transmit an electrical impulse along its axon under certain very specific conditions. The electrical impulse triggers the release of a chemical known as a neurotransmitter from the axon terminals. This neurotransmitter, once released, may have one of a series of effects. It may:

- make a muscle cell contract
- make an endocrine gland release a hormone into the blood
- cause an electrical impulse in a neighbouring neuron.

Neurons communicate by sending action potentials. The ability of a neuron to carry an electrical impulse depends upon a small difference in electrical potential between the inside and outside of the cell. Under the direct influence of an excitatory neurotransmitter, a sudden change in electrical potential occurs at one point on the cell's membrane. This change is known as an action potential and it flows along the cell membrane, and therefore along the axon of the cell, at up to 110 m/s (250 miles/hour).

Resting Membrane Potential

When a neuron is resting or inactive, it is polarised, which means that the cytosol inside the cell has a negative charge, whereas the fluid surrounding the cell has a positive charge. The process of moving sodium and potassium ions across the cell membrane is an active transport process involving ATP to provide energy. It also involves an enzyme sodium-potassium adenosine tripsphatase referred to as Na^+/K^+-ATPase and is known as the sodium–potassium pump (Figure 8.8). Extracellular fluid (ECF) has a higher concentration of sodium in it than the intracellular fluid (ICF) and this is due to the sodium–potassium pump which transports $3 \times$ sodium ions out of the cell, in exchange for importing $2 \times$ potassium ions into the cell. Although the sodium–potassium pump works continuously, positively charged sodium ions are constantly 'leaking' into the cell and positively charged potassium ions are leaving it. However, the membrane is more permeable to potassium ions than to sodium ions, so the amount of potassium leaving the cell is greater than the amount of sodium entering it.

An action potential represents a sudden change in the resting polarised state of the neuron cell membrane following a stimulus. During an action potential, the polarity of the membrane reverses and the inside of the cell becomes more electropositive than the outside. This change is brought about by a sudden increase in the permeability of the membrane to sodium ions. There are three steps to an action potential:

- depolarisation
- repolarisation
- return to the resting membrane potential.

An action potential is initiated when a neuron is stimulated, such as from a receptor cell in a sense organ (Figure 8.9).

The sodium and potassium channels in the axon membrane are voltage gated, which means that they can change shape to let more or less ions through depending upon the voltage across the membrane. When the neuron is stimulated, the voltage across the axon membrane changes. A few voltage-gated sodium channels detect this and open to allow sodium ions in by diffusion. If the stimulus is large enough to reach a threshold level of around −50 mV, then the rest of the voltage-gated sodium channels open, allowing Na^+ to rapidly diffuse into the axon, thereby making the inside more positive than the outside now, that is, there is a reversal of the resting state This process is called depolarisation. When the resting potential reaches zero, the potassium channels open, allowing K^+ to rush out, making the inside more negative again. This process is called repolarisation. This is followed by a refractory period, that is, a delay between one action potential and the next. Large nerves can recover very quickly (in around 1 millisecond), whereas smaller nerve fibres take longer (4 milliseconds).

The nerve impulse can only flow in one direction due to this refractory period, as the wave of depolarisation can only move away from the refractory region towards the axon terminal and therefore the next neuron. The diameter of the axon and the presence of a myelin sheath determine the speed of the action potential along the nerve. Wider axons and those with a myelin sheath

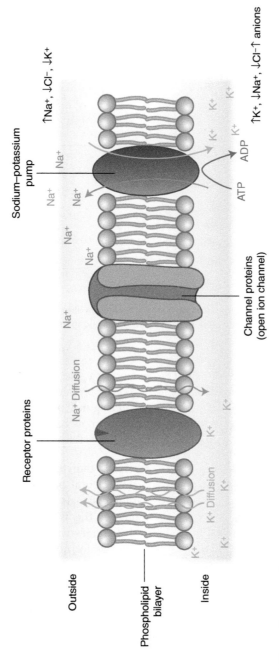

Figure 8.8 The sodium–potassium pump.

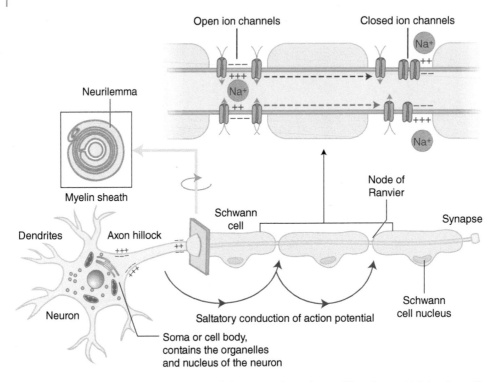

Figure 8.9 Propagation of an action potential along a myelinated nerve fibre. *Source*: Helixitta, https://commons.wikimedia.org/wiki/File:Propagation_of_action_potential_along_myelinated_nerve_fiber_en.svg. CC BY-SA 4.0.

conduct impulses the quickest. The smallest axons are unmyelinated and so conduction of the action potential is continuous.

Pain resulting from tissue damage in horses can be reduced by applying ice or cold treatments, as this also slows conduction of the pain-sensitive neurons. Local anaesthetics such as lidocaine also work by blocking the voltage-gated sodium channels, thereby stopping pain signals from reaching the CNS.

Synapses

Synapses have important roles in the nervous system including:

- passing information between neurons
- ensuring the action potential travels in one direction only
- possibly exciting or inhibiting the next neuron
- possibly amplifying the action potential

- stopping the action potential when the neuron is overstimulated
- filtering out low levels of action potential, for example background noise
- as a basis for memory as modifiable.

Synapses therefore allow the horse to use certain neural pathways and to amplify or dampen signals that may or may not be required. This is a vital part of the learning and therefore training process. This creates memories for horses, such as remembering the aids when they are applied and what movement is required by the horse by the rider. Moreover, recognition of herd members and siblings, and food and water sources and so on is essential for survival.

When an action potential reaches the end of the axon, to be passed to the next neuron or effector cell such as muscle or gland, it must bridge the small gap known as the synapse. A single neuron may have thousands of these connections with neighbouring ones. A typical neuron, as described previously, has one axon that projects from its cell body and this splits into several smaller branches, each ending in a terminal which forms a synapse that is usually close to the cell body of another neuron. At a synapse the two neurons do not actually come into direct contact, because their two surface membranes are separated by a gap known as the synaptic cleft. When an electrical impulse travels along the axon to the synapse, it cannot bridge this gap directly. Instead it causes the release of a neurotransmitter chemical, which then bridges the gap and produces a change in the electrical potential of the membrane of the next neuron. An example of a neurotransmitter is acetylcholine.

The axon terminal of a pre-synaptic neuron is normally swollen and is often known as the synaptic bulb. The gap or synaptic cleft is very small indeed at about 20 nm. The axon membrane from which the neurotransmitter is released is known as the pre-synaptic membrane and the membrane at which the chemical is received is known as the post-synaptic membrane. This is important because signals may pass across a synapse in one direction only, from pre-synaptic to post-synaptic membrane. This is because the

neurotransmitter is produced only by the pre-synaptic membrane. The synaptic bulb contains mitochondria to provide energy to make neurotransmitters; these are small molecules that can diffuse quickly across the synaptic cleft. The synaptic bulb also contains synaptic vesicles which house the neurotransmitters prior to use. The most common neurotransmitter is acetylcholine and synapses that use this are known as cholinergic synapses. Acetylcholine also acts across the brain, modifying activity of other neurotransmitters.

Acetylcholine once released diffuses across the gap and initiates an action potential in the post-synaptic membrane of the receiving neuron. A fast-acting enzyme known as cholinesterase then breaks down acetylcholine into choline and acetic (ethanoic) acid in the synaptic cleft; these are resorbed through the pre-synaptic membrane and ATP is used to resynthesise acetylcholine, which is returned to the storage vesicles. This is so that an impulse is not continuously generated at the synapse. The basic structure of a synapse is shown in Figure 8.10.

Transmission at the Synapse

- The action potential arrives at the pre-synaptic bulb.

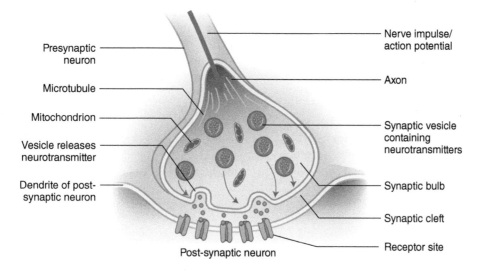

Figure 8.10 Basic structure of a synapse.

- Calcium channels within the pre-synaptic membrane open.
- Calcium ions (Ca^{2+}) rush in.
- Ca^{2+} concentration increases and synaptic vesicles containing neurotransmitters move to the membrane.
- Vesicles fuse with the membrane.
- The neurotransmitter is released into the synaptic cleft.
- The neurotransmitter travels across to the post-synaptic membrane where it binds to receptors.
- The neurotransmitter acts upon the post-synaptic membrane in one of several ways depending upon the neurotransmitter concerned. (Some neurotransmitters open sodium channels, whereas others open potassium and chlorine channels.)
- Once acted, the neurotransmitter is immediately released back into the synaptic cleft.
- The neurotransmitter is immediately broken down by enzymes and the constituent parts diffuse back to the pre-synaptic membrane, where they are resynthesised using ATP for further use.

Some synapses are inhibitory, making it more difficult for action potentials to be generated. These have different neurotransmitters which open the potassium and chlorine channels rather than sodium channels. If a neurotransmitter passes across an excitatory synapse the effect is to excite the post-synaptic membrane, thus producing an electrical impulse in the receiving neuron. Inhibitory synapses have the function of reducing the excitation of the next neuron.

Neuromuscular junctions (see below) always involve acetylcholine, while a synapse only sometimes involves acetylcholine. A synapse is a junction between two neurons, whereas a neuromuscular junction is one between a motor neuron and a skeletal muscle fibre.

Neurotransmitters

There are hundreds of different neurotransmitters within the horse's body. Many neurotransmitters also act as hormones, such as noradrenaline. These are released into the blood where they are taken to their target cells. Noradrenaline is important in the nervous control of blood flow, heart beat and the horse's responses to stress. This hormone is also produced by the adrenal glands as well as the neurons. Neurotransmitters may be excitatory, inhibitory or modulatory, depending upon the receptors concerned.

One of the most important neurotransmitters is acetylcholine, which is released by neurons connected to skeletal muscles, causing these muscles to contract, and also to neurons which are connected to other nerve cells which have an effect on the sweat glands and the heart beat. Acetylcholine is also responsible for transmitting impulses between neurons and the brain and spinal cord.

Dopamine is another neurotransmitter, which plays an important part in the area of the brain that controls movement. Serotonin is another chemical that is found in those parts of the brain that are concerned with conscious activity. Neurotransmitters are synthesised in the nerve cell body and stored in vesicles in the pre-synaptic terminal.

There are four main types of neurotransmitter:

- Cholinergic nerve cells – release acetylcholine.
- Amino acids – for example, glycine, glutamate and gamma-aminobutyric acid (GABA).
- Monoamines – noradrenaline, serotonin and dopamine. Adrenergic neurons release noradrenaline and affect the heart rate, breathing rate and so on, similar to adrenaline.
- Neuropeptides – chains of amino acids with a regulatory effect, for example renin, glucagon, gastrin and somatostatin.

Endorphins and Enkephalins

Endorphins and enkephalins (occasionally spelt encephalins) are secreted by neuroendocrine cells in the brain in response to severe pain or stress (nociception is the sensory nervous system's response to harm). They have a strong analgesic or pain-killing effect and are thought to block pain impulses at specific sites in the spinal cord and brain. Enkephalin (methionine and leucine) is a pentapeptide involved in regulating nociception in the horse's body. Endorphins are thought to block pain principally at the brain stem. Both are morphine-like substances with functions similar to those of opium-based drugs. Endorphin is often used generically to describe both groups of painkillers.

Neuromuscular Junctions

Where a motor neuron terminates on a muscle fibre it is known as a neuromuscular junction. These synapses are wider and are in close contact with the sarcolemma or surface membrane of the muscle fibre and this is known as the motor end plate which contains acetylcholine receptors. When the action potential begins, the sarcolemma, having travelled across the synapse through the motor end plate, starts an impulse that makes the muscle fibre contract.

The pre-synaptic vesicle contains approximately 10,000 molecules of acetylcholine, and around 100 vesicles must be released before an action potential in the motor end plate results in contraction of a muscle fibre.

The Brain

The brain is the control centre of the nervous system. It contains millions of highly organised neurons with a large number of supporting cells, all intricately arranged within the skull or cranium. The structure of the horse's brain is shown in Figure 8.11.

The brain has a jelly-like consistency and is protected by membranous layers known as the meninges. The skull and the meninges have a highly protective function – to prevent injury to the brain. The meninges consist of three layers: the dura mater (thick and tough), arachnoid layer (contains blood-vessels and fluid) and the pia mater (helps to nourish the brain).

The vertebrate brain has evolved from what were originally a group of bulges at the top of the spinal cord. These three ancestral regions, known as the forebrain, midbrain and hindbrain, can still be seen during embryonic development. As the brain evolved further, these three regions became subdivided into specific regions, with particular responsibilities.

Blood supply is via the circle of Willis (also called the cerebral arterial circle). This is a circulatory anastomosis (connections of two parts often found between arteries) that supplies blood to the brain and surrounding structures. It is fed by the internal carotid artery and basilar artery supply in the horse (and humans and dogs). The vertebral artery

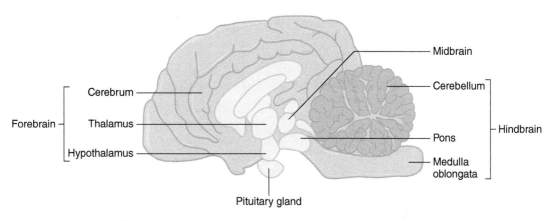

Figure 8.11 Structure of the equine brain.

supplies the rest of the horse's brain. Venous drainage is by the cerebral veins which have no valves.

Forebrain

The most sophisticated information processing occurs in the forebrain. The three main centres are:

- hypothalamus
- thalamus
- cerebrum.

Hypothalamus

The hypothalamus, although small, is important in controlling homeostasis, that is, maintaining the horse's internal environment, such as body temperature and blood chemistry. It also controls the pituitary gland and thus the secretion of many of the body's hormones; and it regulates the fight or flight response which is a strong instinct in horses.

Thalamus

The thalamus contains most of the cell bodies of the neurons that relay information to the cerebrum and is able to exert some control over sensory messages, which receives and then sends, by suppressing some signals and enhancing others.

Cerebrum

The cerebrum is the largest part of the brain. It consists of two halves, the right and left cerebral hemisphere, which are joined together by a thick band of nerve fibres called the corpus callosum. Beneath the corpus callosum are large clusters of nerve cell bodies known as the basal ganglia. These are important in motor coordination. The nerve cell bodies are situated in the outer layer of the cerebrum known as the cerebral cortex, and this area is therefore known as the grey matter, whereas the inner areas which are rich in nerve fibres are known as the white matter. The cerebral cortex stores information with regard to memory, consciousness and sensory perception, and interprets visual and sound signals. It is able to interpret all the sensory information which it receives and then act upon it. The cerebral cortex does not contain any pain-detecting cells.

The cerebrum is folded to increase the surface area, and so the larger the cerebrum and the more folded it is, the better it performs. The horse's cerebrum is highly folded, but it is now thought that it is the brain volume to body size ratio that is the most accurate method of measuring intelligence; the human brain and that of the porpoise are highly folded and these mammals also have the largest brain surface area to body size, making them highly intelligent. The human brain weighs approximately 1.3 kg (3 lb), whereas the horse's brain is relatively small compared with its bodyweight – it weighs approximately 0.65 kg (1.5 lb) or about 1% of its bodyweight. The horse is not considered to be a highly intelligent animal; it is ultimately an animal of instinct and this shows in its behaviour. Reasoning and conscious thought are not abilities that we strongly associate with horses, although there is no doubt that they do have the ability to work things out even if slowly, and do, suffer from depression, which is often brought about by poor management.

Midbrain

The midbrain relays sensory information to the cerebrum, such as sound and touch. In horses, sight is dealt with mainly by the forebrain, with the midbrain coordinating eye reflexes such as blinking. Part of the midbrain is also associated with sleeping and waking.

Hindbrain

The hindbrain consists of three parts:

- medulla oblongata
- pons
- cerebellum.

The medulla oblongata and pons contain all the sensory and motor neurons passing between the spinal cord and the forebrain. These parts are therefore responsible for conducting information. They also control heart

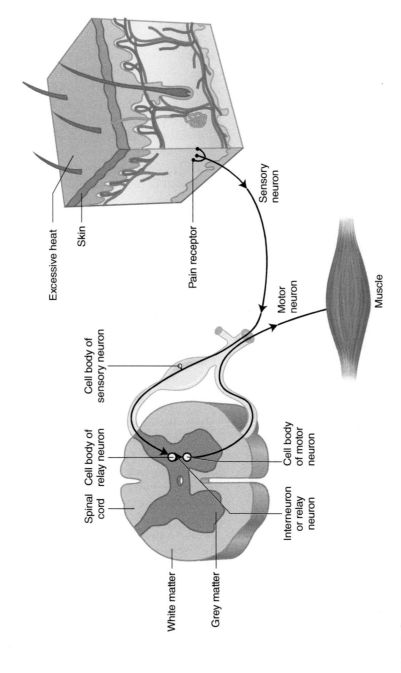

Figure 8.12 Reflex arc.

rate and breathing, and help to coordinate the horse's movements – walking, trotting, cantering and so on.

The cerebellum is mainly responsible for fine tuning and balance of movement. The cerebellum of the horse compared with other species is relatively large. This could be expected due to the horse's ability to move fast over most types of ground.

Spinal Cord

The spinal cord is a cylinder of nerve tissue which is as thick as a thumb and runs down the central canal of the spine. It is an extension of the brain and together with the brain makes up the central nervous system. At the centre of the spinal cord is a region whose cross-section is shaped like a butterfly and this is the grey matter (see earlier and Figure 8.6).

Sprouting from the spinal cord on each side at regular intervals are two nerve bundles, the spinal nerve roots, which contain the nerve fibres of the motor and sensory nerve cells. These join together to form the spinal nerves which connect the spinal cord to all parts of the horse's body and legs.

The cord is capable of handling some of the sensory information itself and of inducing motor responses without involving the brain. These are the reflex actions.

Reflex Actions or Arcs

A reflex is an action that occurs automatically and, more importantly, predictably to a particular stimulus. This reflex action is completely independent of the will of the horse. The stimulus is supplied by one or more senses and an action is initiated by the nervous system in response to the stimulus.

In the simplest reflex, a sensory nerve cell – perhaps at the skin surface of the horse – reacts to a stimulus such as pressure or heat. The sensory cell sends a signal along its axon or nerve fibre to the CNS (brain and spinal cord). Here the fibre connects to a motor neuron which initiates a muscle contraction to move the horse away from the heat or pressure. The passage of the nervous impulse from the source, through the sensory neuron to the motor neuron and finally to the muscle, is known as a reflex arc (Figure 8.12). Often, however, the reflex arcs are more complicated than this example.

Many reflexes are present from birth, such as shivering in response to cold or the emptying of the bladder when it is full. Other examples of reflex actions include sneezing, coughing, swallowing and blinking, and the horse has no voluntary control over these actions. The autonomic nervous system is responsible for these bodily functions, but some autonomic reflexes are under partially voluntary control. For example, an older horse may consciously delay urinating or staling in the field until it is brought in to the stable. Ultimately, however, the reflex is stronger than the will and if the horse is not brought in to the stable until later than normal, it may not be able to hold on as the reflex exerts its control.

Other reflexes are conditioned, having been brought about by experience of the horse through its lifetime. These experiences result in the formation of new pathways and junctions within the nervous system itself. The ways in which these processes are acquired is known as conditioning. Learning is a type of operant conditioning in that once a response to a new situation has been repeated several times, a response becomes automatically initiated next time that stimulus occurs. For example, a horse will learn to move away from the handler when a hand is placed against the horse's side. Eventually this will be done automatically and without conscious will.

Summary Points

1) The nervous system is made up of highly specialised cells which provide a highly organised data-processing system and is very complex.

2) Sensory input is the conduction of signals or messages from the sensory receptors such as the nose, eyes, ears and skin to processing centres in the brain and spinal cord.

3) Motor output is the conduction of signals to the effector cells such as muscles which move in direct response to the signal.

4) Each nerve follows a definite path and serves a specific region of the horse's body. For example, cranial nerve I, the olfactory nerve, carries impulses from the nose to the brain concerning the sense of smell.

5) Learning is a type of operant conditioning in that once a response to a new situation has been repeated several times, a response becomes automatically initiated next time that stimulus occurs.

Q + A

Q What is the most common neurotransmitter in the horse's body?

A Acetylcholine, and synapses that use this are known as cholinergic synapses.

Q What are the four main types of neurotransmitter?

A Cholinergic nerve cells, amino acids, monoamines and neuropeptides.

Q What are the main functions of the hypothalamus?

A The main function is homeostasis, that is, maintaining the horse's internal environment, such as body temperature and blood chemistry. It also controls the pituitary gland and thus secretion of many of the body's hormones; and it regulates the fight or flight response which is a strong instinct in horses.

Q What is the function of the cerebral cortex?

A It stores information with regard to memory, consciousness and sensory perception, and interprets visual and sound signals. It is able to interpret all the sensory information which it receives and then act upon it.

Q Which part of the horse's brain deals with sight?

A In horses, sight is dealt with mainly by the forebrain, with the midbrain coordinating eye reflexes such as blinking.

9

The Endocrine System

Nerves carry electrical messages at high speed from one part of the horse's body to another. However, another much slower messenger system exists and this is the endocrine system. The endocrine system includes glands that secrete hormones into the bloodstream, and the most important endocrine glands in the horse are shown in Figure 9.1. The endocrine system consists of the following:

- Hypothalamus
- Pituitary gland – posterior pituitary (neurohypophysis), anterior pituitary (adenohypophysis)
- Thyroid gland
- Parathyroid glands
- Adrenal glands
- Pancreas
- Ovaries
- Testes
- Pineal gland
- Thymus.

The word 'hormone' is derived from the Greek word 'hormon' which means to activate. Hormones are classified by their molecular structure, as shown in Table 9.1. They are chemical messenger molecules that are made by cells in one part of the body and cause changes in cells in another part of the body. The endocrine system regulates the metabolism and development of most of the horse's body cells and systems through feedback mechanisms. For example, thyrotropin-releasing hormone (TRH) and thyroid-stimulating hormone (TSH) are controlled by a number of negative feedback mechanisms. The endocrine glands release hormones that affect appetite and stress responses, as well as secondary sex characteristics of stallions and mares, controlling puberty, pregnancy and birth, lactation, aggression and so on. The endocrine system has a regulatory effect on other organ systems in the body. In the musculoskeletal system, hormones affect muscle metabolism, energy production and growth. In the nervous system, they affect neural metabolism, regulate fluid and ion concentration and help with reproductive hormones that influence brain development.

An increase or decrease in the hormone level will produce a change in the process it controls. Unlike exocrine glands which pass their secretions through ducts to the target area, for example salivary glands, endocrine glands do not have ducts and they release their hormones directly into the bloodstream to be transported to the target organs. They are therefore often known as ductless glands. All endocrine glands have a good blood supply with capillaries running through them, so that as hormones are synthesised they are released immediately into the blood, where they dissolve in plasma. Each hormone is specific in its effects on its target organs.

There are other differences between the nervous and endocrine systems besides the fact that the nervous system carries messages so much faster. Because hormones are carried in the blood, they are longer lasting than the quick, short-acting impulses carried by the nervous system.

Equine Science, Third Edition. Zoe Davies and Sarah Pilliner.
© 2018 Zoe Davies and Sarah Pilliner. Published 2018 by John Wiley & Sons Ltd.

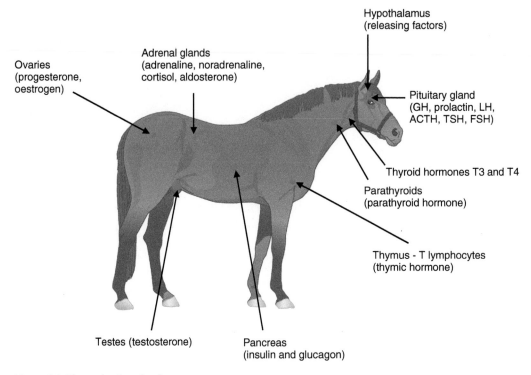

Figure 9.1 The endocrine glands.

Table 9.1 Classification of major hormones.

Molecular structure	Secreted by	Hormone
Polypeptides	Anterior pituitary	Growth hormone, thyroid-stimulating hormone, luteinising hormone, follicle-stimulating hormone, prolactin
	Posterior pituitary	Antidiuretic hormone, oxytocin
	Parathyroid glands	Parathyroid hormone
	Pancreas	Insulin, glucagon
Steroids (derived from cholesterol)	Adrenal cortex	Adrenocortical hormones – aldosterone, cortisol
	Ovaries, placenta, testes	Oestrogen, progesterone, testosterone
Amines (derived from tyrosine)	Thyroid hormones T3 and T4	T3 and T4
	Adrenal medulla	Catecholamines, epinephrine, norepinephrine, dopamine

Hypothalamus

The hypothalamus is a small area in the forebrain and is a functional link between the nervous and endocrine systems, that is, it controls both nervous and endocrine systems. In fact, it controls most of the endocrine glands within the body, largely through stimulation of the pituitary gland by secretion of neurohormones. It secretes releasing hormones which regulate hormones of the anterior pituitary gland and is a vital regulator of homeostasis, including thermoregulation.

The hypothalamus exerts overall control over the sympathetic nervous system and it therefore has nerve connections to most other parts of the nervous system. It has direct contact with the pituitary gland through a short stalk of nerve fibres and can stimulate the pituitary gland in one of two ways: it may release hormones into the blood which will arrive at the pituitary gland, or it may send nerve signals. In this way the hypothalamus can convert nervous signals to hormonal ones.

Pituitary Gland (Hypophysis)

The pituitary gland is an elongated attachment of the brain which lies in a shallow groove. This is unlike humans where it lies within a bony cavity of the sphenoid bone known as the sella turcica. It is sometimes referred to as the master gland as it regulates and controls the operation of other endocrine glands and many of the important body processes of the horse. The pituitary gland is about the size of a pea and is suspended by the thin infundibular stalk ventral to the hypothalamus. It is subdivided into the following:

- Anterior pituitary lobe – adenophysis
- Posterior pituitary lobe – neurophysis

These have different origins from embryonic development and have different functions. See Figure 9.2.

Anterior Pituitary – Adenophysis

The anterior pituitary has an embryonic origin from the growth of epithelium which extends from the mouth cavity of the foetus, known as Rathke's pouch. It consists of the following:

- Pars tuberalis – contains melatonin receptors and regulates reproductive hormones over the reproductive season.
- Pars distalis.

The hormones synthesised, stored and released from here are:

- Growth hormone (GH) – responsible for growth.

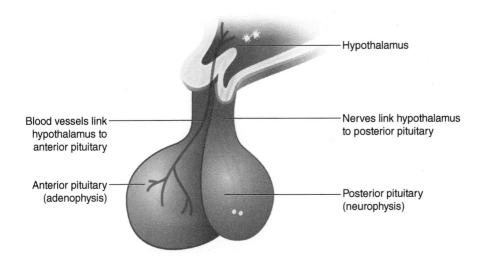

Figure 9.2 The anterior and posterior pituitary gland. *Source*: Southwood 2013. Reproduced with permission of John Wiley & Sons.

- Follicle-stimulating hormone (FSH) – stimulates the ovaries and testes
- Luteinising hormone (LH) – stimulates the ovaries
- Adrenocorticotrophic hormone (ACTH) – stimulates the adrenal glands
- Thyroid-stimulating hormone (TSH) – stimulates the thyroid gland
- Prolactin (PRL) – stimulates milk production from the udder after birth

Hormones are controlled by releasing and inhibiting factors secreted from the hypothalamus via the hypophyseal portal system. There are five different cell types in the pars distalis, which give a guide to their functions, namely lactotropes, corticotropes, thyrotropes, gonadotropes and somatotropes.

Pars Intermedia

The pars intermedia separates the anterior and posterior lobes of the pituitary gland. It contains endocrine cells known as melanotropes which produce melanocyte-stimulating hormone (α-MSH). This area of the pituitary gland is innervated by nervous tissue or dopaminergic neurones which originate in the hypothalamus. This is important in pituitary pars intermedia dysfunction (PPID), which is common in horses and is often referred to as Cushing's syndrome or disease (Figure 9.3).

Posterior Pituitary (Neurophysis)

The posterior pituitary consists of the pars nervosa. Originating in the hypothalamus in the paraventricular and super optic nuclei, it is a down-growth of neural tissue into the neurophysis. It synthesises and releases two hormones:

- Antidiuretic hormone (ADH) otherwise known as Vasopressin or Arginine Vasopressin (AVP) – increases resorption of water by the kidneys and therefore reduces the volume of urine produced (see Chapter 14).
- Oxytocin – produces contractions of the uterus during birth of the foal and stimulates milk secretion from the udder in response to suckling from the foal.

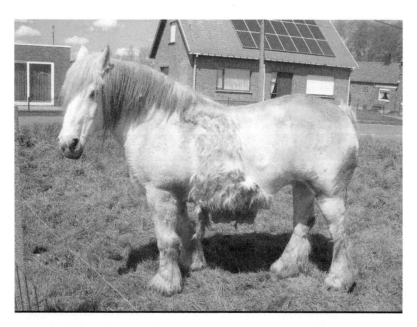

Figure 9.3 Delayed/partial shedding of winter coat is a symptom of PPID (Cushing's syndrome).
Source: Spotter2, https://commons.wikimedia.org/wiki/File:Paard_verliest_wintervacht.jpg. CC BY-SA 3.0.

Thyroid Gland

The thyroid gland is situated in the neck on either side of the trachea (second and third tracheal rings). It consists of two lobes about the size of plums on the left and right which are connected by a string of connective tissue known as the isthmus. Figure 9.4 shows a section through the thyroid gland.

Thyroid tissue is composed of two types of cells:

- Follicular cells – arranged in spherical, hollow follicles, these cells are responsible for the secretion of thyroxine (T4) and tri-iodothyronine (T3) (Figure 9.5). Thyroxine contains iodine. The hollow space is filled with a thick fluid material which is responsible for producing the T3 and T4 hormones.
- Parafollicular cells or C cells – arranged in small groups in the spaces between the hollow follicles, these cells secrete the hormone calcitonin.

The thyroid gland is innervated by both the sympathetic and parasympathetic nervous systems.

Thyroid Hormones

T3 and T4 are responsible for regulating the horse's metabolic rate and are also important in carbohydrate metabolism, temperature control and growth. TSH is released by the pituitary gland and stimulates the thyroid gland. Calcitonin works in conjunction with parathyroid hormone (PTH) secreted by the parathyroid glands to maintain the calcium balance within the horse's body by reducing plasma calcium by the inhibition of calcium removal from bone.

Parathyroid Glands

The parathyroid glands are a group of four small glands around 1–2 mm long located behind the lobes of the thyroid gland in the neck. There are two internal parathyroid glands embedded in the top of the thyroid

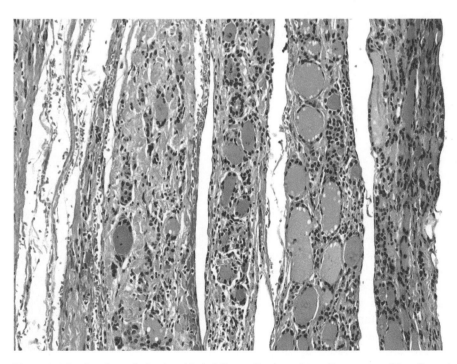

Figure 9.4 Section through the thyroid glad. *Source*: Nephron, https://commons.wikimedia.org/wiki/File:Thyroid_gland_-_high_mag.jpg.

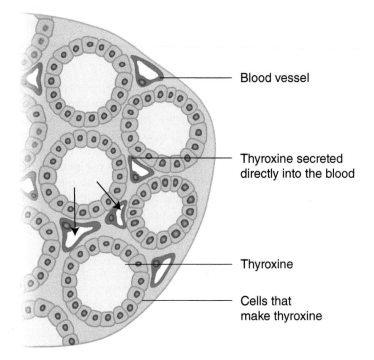

Blood vessel

Thyroxine secreted
directly into the blood

Thyroxine

Cells that
make thyroxine

Figure 9.5 Thyroid follicle cells. *Source*: OpenStax College, https://commons.wikimedia.org/wiki/File:1811_
The_Thyroid_Gland.jpg. CC BY 3.0.

glands and the remaining two lie along the trachea. The parathyroid glands secrete PTH which is released into the bloodstream and regulates calcium and phosphorus levels in the plasma. If the blood level of calcium decreases, then after secretion of PTH the following occurs:

- Bones of the skeleton release more calcium into the blood.
- Calcium absorption from the digestive tract increases.
- The kidneys conserve calcium.

These effects quickly restore the blood calcium level. If the blood calcium level rises, the amount of PTH secreted is reduced and the above effects are reversed, with the body storing more calcium in bone and excreting more calcium in the urine. The parathyroid glands are innervated by the sympathetic and parasympathetic nervous systems.

Adrenal Glands

The adrenal glands lie on top of the kidneys (Figure 9.6). Each adrenal gland is divided into two distinct regions: the adrenal cortex and the adrenal medulla (Figure 9.7).

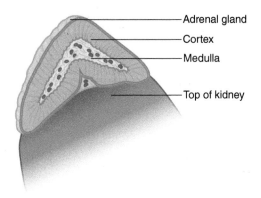

Adrenal gland

Cortex

Medulla

Top of kidney

Figure 9.6 Diagrammatic section through the adrenal gland.

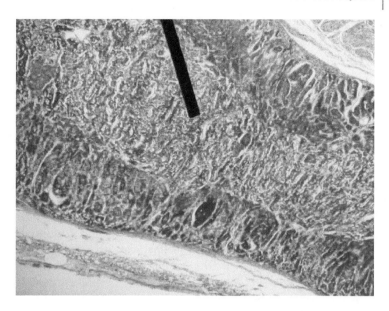

Figure 9.7 Section through the medulla of an adrenal gland (human). The pointer is indicating the medulla. *Source*: Jpogi, https://commons.wikimedia.org/wiki/File:Adrenal_gland_(medulla).JPG.

Adrenal Cortex

The adrenal cortex is responsible for the secretion of a group of hormones known as the corticosteroids and each one has an important effect on the body. The adrenal cortex is red to light brown in colour and comprises 80–90% of the adrenal gland. It is composed of three zones in most species, but the horse is unusual in that it has a small fourth layer – the zona intermedia – all of which synthesise hormones derived from cholesterol, that is, steroid hormones. The layers from outside to inside are as follows:

- Zona glomerulosa – outer zone, secretes mineralocorticoids, the main one being aldosterone
- Zona intermedia – in horses and carnivores only, this layer is very thin and contains mostly small, undifferentiated cells
- Zona fasciculata – middle zone, secretes glucocorticoids, for example cortisol (hydrocortisone), which are involved in the metabolism of carbohydrates, proteins and fats and have anti-inflammatory activity
- Zona reticularis – inner zone, secretes sex steroids or androgens, responsible for the sexual development and function of the male horse

Mineralocorticoids

Aldosterone is the major mineralocorticoid and is important for the regulation of blood pressure, mainly by acting on organs such as the kidney and the colon to increase the amount of sodium reabsorbed into the bloodstream and the amount of potassium and hydrogen ions removed in the urine. This results in a reduction of acids in the blood, which helps prevent acidosis. Aldosterone indirectly regulates blood levels of electrolytes (sodium, potassium and hydrogen) and helps to maintain the blood pH.

Aldosterone is part of a group of linked hormones, which form the renin–angiotensin–aldosterone system. Activation of this system occurs when there is a decrease in blood flow to the kidneys following loss of blood volume or a drop in blood pressure. This may be due to factors such as:

- dehydration
- haemorrhage
- decrease in plasma sodium concentration.

Renin is an enzyme that leads to a series of chemical reactions resulting in the production of angiotensin II, which in turn stimulate aldosterone release. Aldosterone causes an increase in sodium and water reabsorption into the bloodstream from the kidney, thereby increasing the blood volume, restoring sodium levels and blood pressure. Once sodium levels and blood pressure are corrected and the body becomes rehydrated, the level of renin in the bloodstream falls and therefore the amount of aldosterone in the blood also falls, meaning more water is excreted in the urine. The renin–angiotensin–aldosterone system is an example of a negative feedback system.

The other two main regulators of aldosterone secretion are an increase in the plasma potassium concentration and ACTH secreted by the anterior pituitary, which can act via either positive or negative feedback mechanisms, depending on the extent of changes in the levels of these two regulators.

Glucocorticoids

Zona fasciculata cells secrete glucocorticoids, including cortisol, cortisone and corticosterone which control glucose metabolism. Glucocorticoids also have anti-inflammatory effects by inhibiting basophils, the white blood cells that are part of the inflammatory response. Glucocorticoids increase gluconeogenesis in the liver by:

- Glucose synthesis – converting some amino acids or lactic acid to glucose
- Protein breakdown – increasing the rate of protein breakdown mostly in muscle to increase amino acids in the blood for gluconeogenesis
- Triglycerides breakdown – by increasing the rate of triglyceride breakdown in adipose (fat) tissue, fatty acids are used for gluconeogenesis

Glucocorticoids also depress the immune response in high doses and reduce the healing of wounds.

Negative Feedback

Glucocorticoids are controlled by negative feedback, whereby low blood levels stimulate the hypothalamus to secrete corticotropin-releasing hormone (CRH). This is sent to the anterior pituitary via the hypophyseal portal veins, where it stimulates the release of ACTH which then enters the blood and stimulates the production of cortisol from the adrenal cortex. As cortisol levels rise, negative feedback inhibition acts on the hypothalamus to reduce secretion of CRH and the anterior pituitary to reduce secretion of ACTH – both of which result in reduced production of cortisol (Figure 9.8).

In most farm animals, maternal progesterone levels decline and oestrogen levels increase in the last 5–10 days before parturition in response to activation of the foetal hypothalamic–pituitary– adrenal (HPA) axis and increased foetal cortisol concentrations. Foetal cortisol concentrations also rise later in gestation in the horse compared to other species as the adrenal gland has a role in parturition. Very close to term, in association with increasing foetal ACTH levels, the foetal equine adrenals appear to switch to producing cortisol. This late cortisol surge induces a period of rapid foetal maturation.

Adrenal Medulla

The cells of the adrenal medulla secrete hormones which have been converted from the amino acid tyrosine into catecholamines, namely dopamine, epinephrine (adrenaline) and norepinephrine (noradrenaline). These hormones are released at times of stress and produce the fight or flight response. The adrenal medulla represents only 10–20% of the adrenal gland. In the equine foetus, the adrenal medulla plays a role in the autonomic nervous system.

Pancreas

There is a constant secretion of pancreatic juice, which increases after feeding, providing the caecum and colon with a constant supply of buffered solution, which maintains a stable environment vital for

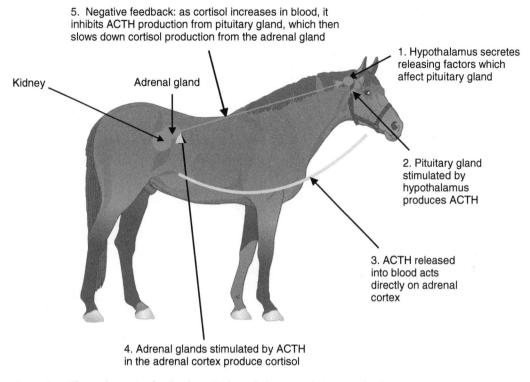

5. Negative feedback: as cortisol increases in blood, it inhibits ACTH production from pituitary gland, which then slows down cortisol production from the adrenal gland

Kidney

Adrenal gland

1. Hypothalamus secretes releasing factors which affect pituitary gland

2. Pituitary gland stimulated by hypothalamus produces ACTH

3. ACTH released into blood acts directly on adrenal cortex

4. Adrenal glands stimulated by ACTH in the adrenal cortex produce cortisol

Figure 9.8 Effects of negative feedback on the hypothalamus and pituitary gland.

important microbe survival in the hindgut. This in turn maintains optimal conditions for fibre digestion and support of the immune system.

The pancreas is both an exocrine and endocrine gland. The exocrine cells secrete digestive enzymes in the form of pancreatic juice through the pancreatic duct directly into the small intestine for the digestion of protein, carbohydrates and fats. The endocrine glands secrete the enzymes glucagon and insulin from small specialised groups of cells known as the islets of Langerhans for regulation of blood glucose concentration, and as such are vital to the health of the horse.

Pancreatic juice discharges into the duodenum through ducts. It is alkaline as it contains bicarbonate and chloride ions. Bicarbonate ions are actively transported into the duct lumen and water passively follows via osmosis. The osmolarity of pancreatic juice is equivalent to the osmolarity of blood. Pancreatic juice is alkaline to neutralise acidic gastric juice which enters the small intestine with food. This is important as it provides an optimal pH for pancreatic enzymes to function and it helps prevent damage by acidic contents flowing in from the stomach to the thin absorptive mucosa of the duodenum. This alkalinity also helps buffer the large intestine, which is important in hindgut fermenters.

Hormones that increase pancreatic secretion include:

- cholecystokinin (CCK)
- secretin
- gastrin.

There is also some negative feedback from somatostatin and enkephalins.

Both insulin and glucagon are responsible for maintaining the blood glucose level within a normal range and diverting glucose to and from tissues. Horses rarely suffer from the common human condition of diabetes mellitus (see Chapter 5 for more information regarding the structure and workings of the pancreas).

Secretion of Glucagon and Insulin

The islets of Langerhans are embedded in exocrine tissue in the pancreas. Each islet is composed of 2000–3000 epithelial cells arranged in a compact structure surrounded by a capillary network. There are four different cell types within the islets of Langerhans that each produce different hormones; they include:

- Alpha cells – produce glucagon, typically located at the periphery of the islet but not present in all islets.
- Beta cells – produce insulin. They are the predominant cell type located in the centre of the islet and contributing around 70% of all cells. Insulin secretion is suppressed during exercise in horses but switched on during recovery after exercise when glycogen repletion is most required.
- Delta cells – produce somatostatin but are present in low numbers in all islets. Somatostatin appears to function locally on the pancreas to alter blood flow during exercise and restrict nutrient absorption.
- PP cells – produce pancreatic polypeptide and again are few in number. They affect digestion and have no effect on insulin or glucagon. Pancreatic polypeptide appears to inhibit bile and pancreatic juice secretion during long-term exercise, when no food is passing through the digestive system, for example during endurance rides.

The main action of glucagon is to increase blood glucose when it falls below normal, whereas the main function of insulin is to reduce blood glucose when it rises above normal. The normal blood glucose value for horses is 80–120 mg/dl. Insulin helps move glucose into cells – mostly skeletal muscle cells – in part by increasing the number of carrier proteins in the cell membrane of these cells.

Beta cells of the islets of Langerhans are sensitive to increases in blood glucose (sugar), such as occur after a feed containing digestible carbohydrates such as grains or coarse mix, and they release insulin in response. Insulin then lowers blood glucose by stimulating the uptake of glucose by many tissues of the body, including skeletal muscle. Insulin also stimulates skeletal muscle and liver cells to synthesise glycogen, the storage form of glucose. Insulin affects the metabolism of amino acids and fats, as it stimulates protein synthesis in skeletal muscle and liver and deposits lipids in adipose tissue. Insulin is the major endocrine stimulus for the state of anabolism that exists after a meal is digested and nutrients are absorbed.

Insulin and glucagon secretion is mostly under negative feedback control. For example, the alpha cells of the islets of Langerhans respond to a fall in blood glucose by secreting glucagon directly into the blood. Only liver cells have the receptors that respond to glucagon by activating the enzyme phosphorylase in the liver which begins gluconeogenesis, that is, it converts glycogen to glucose and amino acids and glycerol to glucose (Figure 9.9).

Secretion of insulin and glucagon is also regulated by the ANS, and the parasympathetic nervous division of the ANS stimulates insulin secretion following a highly soluble carbohydrate meal. The sympathetic part of the ANS, on the other hand, stimulates secretion of glucagon during exercise, for example. Other hormones that can affect blood glucose are epinephrine (adrenaline) and cortisol.

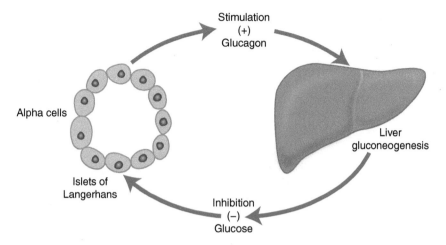

Figure 9.9 Negative feedback of glucose production by glucagon.

Thymus

The thymus is situated just behind the sternum, between the lungs. It is made up of two lobes joined together in front of the trachea and consists of lymphoid tissue made up of fat, epithelium and lymphocytes. In horses, it extends up the neck as far as the thyroid gland. The thymus reaches its maximum weight and size at puberty, and then undergoes involution (shrinking or return to a former size). It is necessary in early life for development and maturation of cell-mediated immunological functions. In horses, the thymus matures earlier and has performed many of its functions well before the foal is born. Removal of the thymus of adult horses has little effect on the immune system.

The thymus produces the hormone thymosin, which stimulates activity of the T lymphocytes which are vital for the horse's defence system in its fight against disease. The thymus is unusual in that it is active until puberty and then starts to lay down more fat and become relatively inactive. It is surrounded by a capsule made of thin connective tissue. Trabeculae from this extend into the thymus, creating thymic 'lobules'.

The cortex of the thymus is dense, consisting of rapidly dividing thymocytes (developing T lymphocytes). Small numbers of dendritic epithelial cells are also present. The medulla has non-dividing, more mature T cells, with dendritic cells at the cortico-medullary junction.

The blood–thymus barrier protects T lymphocytes from exposure to antigens in the blood. It is formed in the capillaries by a continuous endothelium. Macrophages are also present around the capillaries to engulf any antigenic substances that manage to penetrate the barrier.

Ovaries

As well as producing eggs, the ovaries are glands that produce the female hormones progesterone, oestrogen, relaxin, activin and inhibin.

Progesterone is responsible for maintaining pregnancy in the early days after conception. **Oestrogen** is responsible for the behavioural changes in the mare during her oestrus cycle. Oestrogens include oestradiol, oestrone sulphate, oestrone and two other oestrogens which are unique to horses, equilenin and equilin (see Chapter 12). Equilenin is an oestrogenic steroid hormone obtained from the urine of pregnant mares. It was the first complex natural product to be successfully fully synthesised in 1940 by Alfred L. Wilds and is used as one of the components in Premarin™.

During pregnancy, the peptide hormone **relaxin** is produced mainly by the ovaries and placenta in the majority of animals but mostly in the placenta in horses. It acts synergistically with progesterone to maintain pregnancy and to promote loosening of pelvic ligaments at the time of parturition. In horses, relaxin is produced by the foetoplacental unit rather than the corpus luteum. It is detected in mare serum from around day 80 of pregnancy and remains at high levels until parturition. Relaxin accumulates throughout pregnancy and is released in large amounts a few days before parturition. Its target organs are the cervix, vagina, pubic symphysis and related structures. Relaxin is responsible for the softening and relaxation of connective tissues in the cervix, muscles and ligaments in the pelvis prior to parturition, although oestradiol priming is required for this. The relaxation of tissues via relaxin is performed in conjunction with prostaglandin.

Activin is a glycoprotein that is produced within granulosa cells in the ovaries in mares and Sertoli cells in stallions. It is thought to play an almost directly opposite role to that of inhibin and is involved in many physiological functions, including stimulation of FSH synthesis in the pituitary gland, cell proliferation, cell differentiation, apoptosis and homeostasis. The target tissue for activin in the stallion is the epididymis, where it enhances spermatogenesis via increased FSH secretion Activin also enhances the effect of LH on the testes.

In mares, activin has an effect on the anterior pituitary gland, resulting in increased FSH secretion. The increased concentration of activin results in increased FSH binding on the female follicle and increased synthesis of oestrogens. Activin also enhances the action of LH in the ovary.

The ovaries and testes also produce **inhibin** which inhibits secretion of FSH. This may prevent apoptosis (cell suicide) of germ cells in the ovaries and testes.

Equine Chorionic Gonadotropin

Shortly after establishment of pregnancy, high concentrations of the hormone equine chorionic gonadotropin (eCG) appear in the mare's blood. This hormone (also called pregnant mare's serum gonadotropin (PMSG)) has LH (Luteinising hormone) like activity. The source of eCG is the endometrial cups which are found on the placenta but which are derived from the foetus. These form several weeks into pregnancy and are immunologically destroyed 2–3 months later. Foetal production of eCG is highest between 30 and 70 days of pregnancy. The primary target of eCG is the ovaries, where it helps the formation of the accessory corpora lutea to ensure that progesterone production is maintained.

eCG is also thought to stimulate follicular growth and ovulation in the horse. If eCG is given to other species it acts in a similar manner to FSH, and therefore eCG is often used to induce super- ovulation in species where a large number of oocytes are required for embryo transfer.

Testes

The testes are the male gonads and are oval-shaped structures that lie in the scrotal sac. They are responsible for producing the male hormone testosterone which produces the characteristics and specific behaviours of the male horse, such as the Flehmen response (Figure 9.10). Research suggests that the Flehmen response is not an immediate component of sexual behaviour, for example courtship of the stallion, but may be involved in the overall monitoring of a mare's oestrus cycle. The Flehmen response may contribute

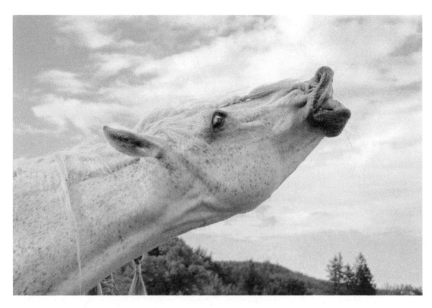

Figure 9.10 Flehmen response shown by an Andalusian stallion. *Source*: Waugsberg, https://commons .wikimedia.org/wiki/File:Flehmendes_Pferd_32_c.jpg. CC BY-SA 3.0.

to the chemosensory priming of a stallion prior to reproduction with the mare.

Testosterone plays a crucial role in the development of male sex organs during foetal growth, where increased production of testosterone causes penis growth and development of accessory sex glands during puberty. Testosterone is responsible for the increased musculature of stallions because it has an anabolic effect (body building). The testes also produce inhibin (see 'Ovaries').

Pineal Gland

The pineal gland or epiphysis is a tiny structure shaped like a pine cone (hence its name), located within the brain itself. It is responsible for the secretion of the hormone melatonin. Melatonin is able to direct biological or circadian rhythms (see 'Circadian Rhythms in Horses') such as sleep–wake cycles and other phenomena showing circadian rhythms. The amount of melatonin secreted varies with the length of the day, as more is produced during darkness.

The pineal gland has light-transducing ability which is why it is often referred to as the 'third eye'. Light exposure to the retina is first relayed to the suprachiasmatic nucleus of the hypothalamus, an area of the brain well known to coordinate circadian rhythms. There is a nerve connection between the hypothalamus and the back part of the pineal gland. Thus, the pineal gland is similar to the adrenal medulla in that it changes signals from the sympathetic nervous system into a hormonal signal. Melatonin's precursor is serotonin, a neurotransmitter derived from the amino acid tryptophan. Synthesis and secretion of melatonin is dramatically affected by light exposure to the horse's eyes. Plasma concentrations of melatonin are low during daylight hours and increase to a peak during the dark.

The pineal gland is known to have an effect on mares in the spring when oestrus activity begins as the days get longer. Melatonin inhibits the secretion of LH and FSH from the anterior pituitary gland. This is due to inhibition of gonadotropin-releasing hormone (GnRH) from the hypothalamus,

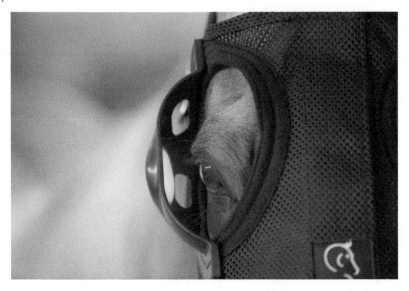

Figure 9.11 The Equilume™ Light Mask is an innovative method of providing light to horses. The automated mask provides the optimum level of blue light to a single eye. *Source*: Courtesy of Equilume Ltd.

which is necessary for secretion of the anterior pituitary hormones.

A practical application of this is found in mares that are seasonal breeders. Thoroughbreds have an artificial breeding season in that mares in the northern hemisphere become reproductively active during late spring and early summer. Thoroughbreds are given a birthday of 1 January no matter when they were born. This means that 2-year-old racehorses will include horses actually born in early January and others born much later in the season, say June, giving the earlier foals an advantage in terms of growth and strength. The industry therefore seeks to breed mares much earlier in the year so foals are born as close to 1 January as possible. To help mares come into season as early as possible, they are now frequently exposed to an artificially lengthened day of approximately 16 hours by providing artificial light or switching on a 100-watt bulb at night in the stable, starting in early December (as the gestation length is 11 months). This can advance the breeding season by as much as 3 months. This extra light suppresses melatonin production which allows GnRH (Gonadotrophin Releasing Hormone) to be

secreted, resulting in successful advancement of reproductive activity to facilitate the early breeding of mares. Recently, a blue light mask for mares kept out in the field for 24 hours a day has been developed. This follows research in humans which shows that release of melatonin is most strongly inhibited by blue light (Figure 9.11). In future, blue light masks may be used for regulating other light-driven circadian rhythms, such as jet lag in travelling horses (see Chapter 12).

The Neuroendocrine System

It was thought that the endocrine and nervous systems worked independently of one another, but it now seems that they are able to work together. It is now known that many neurons can actually produce hormones within the cell itself, and that many endocrine glands act in direct conjunction with the nervous system. The pineal gland and adrenal medulla are examples of this, as seen above. The neuroendocrine system is the mechanism by which the hypothalamus maintains homeostasis, regulating

Table 9.2 Summary of major hormones in the horse's body, their sites of production and effects.

Position	Hormone produced	Effects
Hypothalamus	Releasing factors of hormones	Stimulates pituitary gland to release hormones
Posterior pituitary gland	Oxytocin	Causes uterine contractions during parturition
Anterior pituitary gland	Antidiuretic hormone (ADH)	Reduces urine production by kidneys
	Growth hormone	Stimulates growth
	Adrenocorticotrophic hormone (ACTH)	Stimulates adrenal glands to produce hormones
	Thyroid stimulating hormone (TSH)	Stimulates thyroid gland to produce hormones
	Follicle-stimulating hormone (FSH) and luteinising hormone (LH)	Stimulate ovaries or testes
Brain	Neuropeptides, endorphins and enkephalins	Analgesic effect, pain relief
Thyroid gland	Calcitonin T3 and T4	Maintains plasma Ca levels; affects general metabolism and growth
Parathyroid glands	Parathyroid hormone	Maintains plasma Ca levels
Thymus	Thymosin	Stimulates activity of T lymphocytes
Pancreas	Insulin	Both act to maintain blood sugar
	Glucagon	
Testes	Testosterone	Stimulates male characteristics, development of the testes and sperm production
Ovaries	Oestrogens – include oestradiol, oestrogen sulphate, equilenin and equilin	Controls oestrus cycle and receptive behaviour of the mare
	Progesterone	Maintains pregnancy
Digestive tract	Secretin	Stimulates pancreas to produce digestive fluids rich in bicarbonate; regulates synthesis of some digestive enzymes
	Gastrin	Stimulates secretion of gastric acid (HCl) by parietal cells of the stomach
Placenta	Equine chorionic gonadotropin (eCG) (previously known as pregnant mare serum gonadotropin (PMSG))	Pregnant mares secrete the hormone from their endometrial cups between 40 and 130 days into their gestation; eCG stimulates growth of follicles and ovulation
Adrenal glands		
Adrenal cortex	Corticosteroids:	
	• Glucocorticoids – hydrocortisone	Anti-inflammatory effect; metabolism of carbohydrates, proteins and fats
	• Sex steroids (androgens)	Sexual developments and function
	Mineralocorticoids:	Regulate blood pressure
	• Aldosterone-linked hormones form the rennin–angiotensin–aldosterone system	

(*continued*)

Table 9.2 (Continued)

Position	Hormone produced	Effects
Adrenal medulla	Catecholamines – epinephrine (adrenaline) and norepinephrine (noradrenaline)	Fight or flight response
Kidneys	Erythropoietin	Stimulates erythrocytes production
	Calcitrol	Increases plasma Ca levels
Pineal gland	Melatonin (precursor serotonin)	Directs circadian rhythms

reproduction, metabolism, drinking water and eating, energy utilisation, osmolarity and blood pressure.

Some nerves are able to produce hormones themselves, albeit in smaller quantities than the endocrine glands. For example, the hormone oxytocin is produced as a prohormone in the neurons of specialised areas of the brain. This prohormone is then transported to the pituitary gland where it is stored for future use.

Table 9.2 shows a summary of the major hormones in the horse's body, their sites of production and effects.

Circadian Rhythms in Horses

The circadian system provides horses with a means to adapt their internal physiology to the constantly changing environmental stimuli of light and temperature that exists on a rotating planet such as Earth. The presence of the sun and the continuous rotation of the Earth on its axis results in constantly changing 24-hour cycles of day and night. The study of circadian rhythms is called chronobiology. Circadian rhythms are physical, mental and behavioural changes that follow a roughly 24-hour cycle, responding primarily to light and temperature in the horse's environment. They are even found in microbes.

Over millennia, horses have evolved to take advantage of these cycles, for example for food supply, escape from predation, reproduction and coping with seasonal changes. In other words, the circadian rhythm provides horses with the ability to anticipate periods of activity or inactivity and to time their natural behaviours, such as reproduction, in ways that will optimise survival of their offspring.

Circadian rhythms have a strong genetic component and are now thought to be under the control of genes known as clock genes. The tissues that show constant expression of clock genes are cells from the thymus and testes, and muscle tissues have also shown the presence of clock genes. However, there is also evidence for circadian regulation of immune parameters shown by the rhythmic secretion of the hormone cortisol from the adrenal gland and the pineal hormone melatonin, both of which exhibit diurnal changes in horses (see discussion on melatonin in 'Pineal Gland').

Biological clocks are not the same as circadian rhythms but do control them. A 'master clock' known as the suprachiasmatic nucleus (SCN) in the brain coordinates all the body clocks in the horse's body. The SCN is located in the hypothalamus and is responsible for receiving and transducing light information from the retina to directly drive many rhythms throughout the horse's body via both nervous and hormonal pathways. It is thought that the SCN regulates diverse physiological processes, such as blood pressure, heart rate, sleep and activity cycles, hormone secretion, body temperature, metabolism and immune function.

An example of using the natural circadian rhythms for the management of horses is in racehorses that are trained often very early in the morning but most races actually take place in the afternoon. It may be that the horse's circadian rhythm is more suited to racing in the morning as this is when training takes place, or vice versa – training in the afternoon.

It is clear that research in equine chronobiology will help in the management and training of horses in future.

Sleep Patterns in Horses

Horses can sleep standing up by using the stay apparatus. Historically, this enabled them to escape predators quickly if required, and it was especially useful as they were migratory, moving to new areas regularly. During this

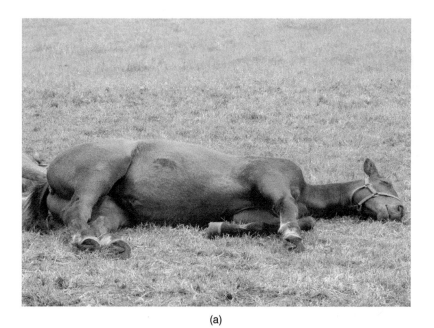

(a)

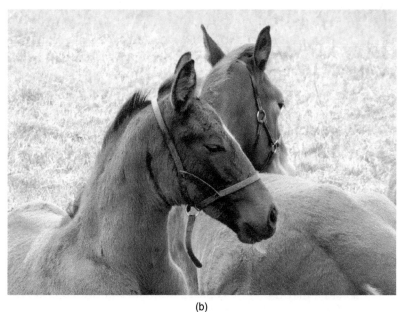

(b)

Figure 9.12 Foals in (a) lateral recumbency, (b) sternal recumbency and (c) paradoxical sleep. *Source:* Courtesy of Harthill Stud.

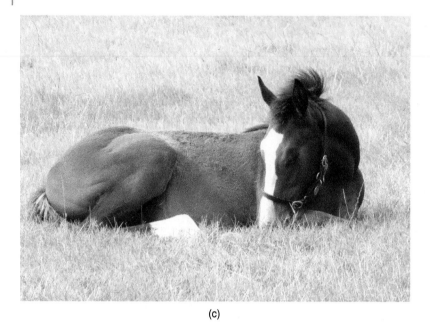

(c)

Figure 9.12 (*Continued*)

sleep standing time they are in slow-wave sleep. During slow-wave sleep, electrical activity in the brain is large and slow. Horses have different types of sleep, namely:

- Two hours of dosing or drowsiness, standing up with full weight on both front legs and one rear leg, while the other rear leg is cocked using the stay apparatus.
- Three hours of slow-wave sleep, at which point the horse is lying down in either lateral or sternal recumbency, that is, lying flat on the side or lying on the chest (Figures 9.12a and b).
- More than 1 hour of paradoxical sleep, during which the horse is commonly positioned on the ground, with forelegs tucked under, but the body is upright with the head tucked to one side, often resting the chin on the ground (Figure 9.12c). This allows for easier breathing than being fully recumbent.

Although researchers agree that rapid eye movement (REM) sleep is important, they do not know what happens to horses if they do not get enough of it. Horses often wait until they have fresh bedding and then lie down, and researchers have found that horses are more likely to lie down and sleep on straw beds compared to shavings beds.

Summary Points

1) Hormones are chemical messenger molecules that are made by cells in one part of the body and cause changes in cells in another part of the body.
2) The endocrine system regulates the metabolism and development of most of the horse's body cells and systems through feedback mechanisms.
3) The hypothalamus is a small area in the forebrain and is a functional link between the nervous and endocrine systems; that is, it controls both nervous and endocrine systems.
4) The anterior pituitary (adenophysis) consists of the pars tuberalis and the pars distalis.
5) Oestrogens include oestradiol, oestrone sulphate, oestrone and two other oestrogens which are unique to horses, equilenin and equilin.

Q + A

Q How does the hypothalamus communicate with the pituitary gland?

A The hypothalamus has direct contact with the pituitary gland through a short stalk of nerve fibres. It can therefore stimulate the pituitary gland in one of two ways. It may release hormones into the blood which will arrive at the pituitary gland or it may send nerve signals. In this way the hypothalamus can convert nervous signals to hormonal ones.

Q What is the precursor of melatonin?

A Serotonin, a neurotransmitter derived from the amino acid tryptophan.

Q What is the main action of glucagon?

A To increase blood glucose when it falls below normal, whereas the main function of insulin is to reduce blood glucose when it rises above.

Q What is the function of the pineal gland?

A It is responsible for secretion of the hormone melatonin.

Q What are circadian rhythms?

A Circadian rhythms are physical, mental and behavioural changes in horses that follow a roughly 24-hour cycle, responding primarily to light and temperature in the horse's environment.

10

The Skin

The skin (sometimes called the cutaneous membrane) is part of the integumentary system, and although only a few millimetres thick (this varies depending upon how exposed the skin is) it is the largest single organ of the horse's body and is an important defence mechanism. The integumentary system includes:

- skin
- hair – including the mane and tail
- hooves
- chestnuts/ergots
- exocrine glands (e.g. sweat glands, sebaceous oil glands)
- associated nerves and muscles (e.g. arrector pili muscle).

In addition for horses, skin is an important organ of thermoregulation through sweating or perspiration and control of blood flow through the skin. Horses are also able to moult the hair as the ambient temperature gets warmer and day length gets longer. Modifications of the skin are used to provide a tough covering to the feet, that is, hooves.

Thus skin acts as a protective envelope, as a secretory and excretory organ, as a sense organ and as a temperature-regulating device. The functions of the skin and coat include:

- protection against wear and tear by providing a covering of cells which are constantly being replaced

- maintenance of shape (the elasticity of the skin restores its shape when bent joints are straightened, for example)
- protection from uncontrolled loss or entry of water
- protection from entry of harmful organisms, and thus immunity
- protection from harmful effects of ultraviolet (UV) light
- production of vitamin D
- receiving sensations from the environment, temperature, pain, touch and pressure
- temperature regulation.

Structure of the Skin

The skin is tough, resilient and highly elastic. It is attached to underlying tissues by fibrous connective tissue (fascia) and fatty tissue. The skin consists of two main parts:

- Epidermis — thinner outer layer.
- Dermis – thicker inner layer.

Under the dermis but not part of the skin is the subcutaneous layer consisting of areolar and adipose tissue. Fibres attach the dermis to the subcutaneous layer, which in turn attaches to the tissues underneath. The subcutaneous layer is where fat is stored and blood vessels which supply the dermis run through this layer. This layer also contains nerve endings such as Pacinian corpuscles

Equine Science, Third Edition. Zoe Davies and Sarah Pilliner.
© 2018 Zoe Davies and Sarah Pilliner. Published 2018 by John Wiley & Sons Ltd.

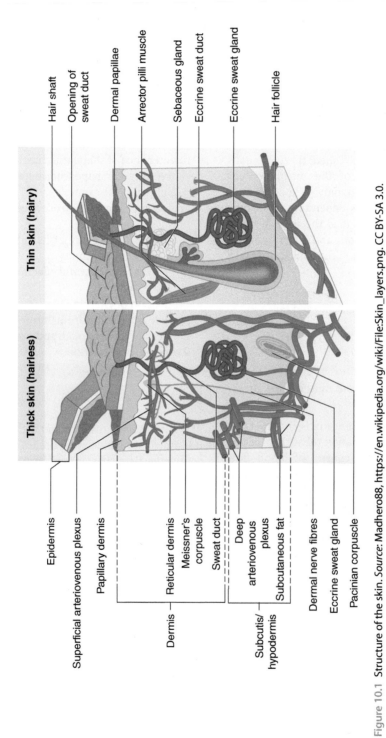

Figure 10.1 Structure of the skin. *Source:* Madhero88, https://en.wikipedia.org/wiki/File:Skin_layers.png. CC BY-SA 3.0.

which are pressure sensitive (see Chapter 4). Figure 10.1 shows the structure of the skin.

Epidermis

Cells of the epidermis include:

- Langerhans cells – derived from bone marrow, these dendritic cells are antigen-presenting cells (APCs) (see Chapter 15) and are an important part of the immune system.
- Melanocytes – also dendritic cells, they are closely associated with keratinocytes, forming an epidermal–melanin unit for transferring melanin to the keratinocytes. They control skin and hair colour and also absorb damaging UV light in exposed hairless areas of skin.

- Merkel cells – part of the sensory apparatus of the skin and located within the stratum basale of the epidermis, where they act as slow-adapting mechanoreceptors detecting touch.

In most regions of the horse's body the epidermis has four layers and is known as thin skin (Figure 10.2). These layers are:

- stratum basale
- stratum spinosum
- stratum granulosum
- stratum corneum.

Thick skin, however, has an additional fifth layer, namely the stratum lucidum between the stratum granulosum and stratum corneum and the stratum corneum is slightly thicker (see Figure 10.1). Thick skin

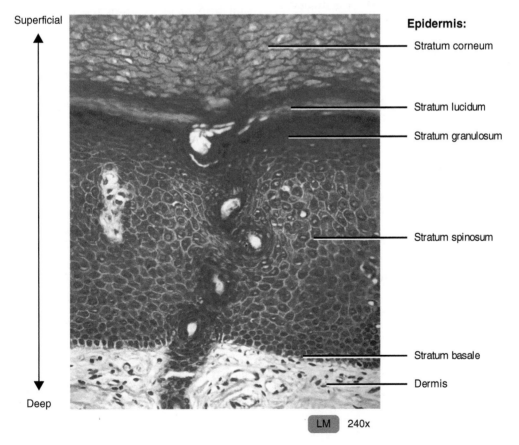

Figure 10.2 Layers of the epidermis – photomicrograph of a portion of skin. *Source*: Tortora 2009. Reproduced with permission of John Wiley & Sons.

is found where there is heavier wear or exposure. Researchers found that the thickness of equine skin varies from around 1.5 mm in the thinnest areas to 4.6 mm on the back of the hindlimbs. Horse's skin on the back is the thickest and the skin on the head, neck and abdomen is the thinnest. The skin on the legs at around 3 mm is not as thin as originally thought.

Stratum Basale

The stratum basale is the deepest layer and follows the contours of the underlying dermis. It is composed of a single layer of cells called keratinocytes. Nutrition is supplied from the underlying capillaries of the dermis. Migration of cells towards the surface begins here. Some of the cells are stem cells, actively dividing to continuously produce new keratinocytes. Keratinocytes may be columnar or cuboidal in shape.

Stratum Spinosum

The stratum spinosum consists of eight to ten layers of many different shaped keratinocytes fitted together, providing flexibility and strength to the skin. It is also called the spinous or 'prickle' layer because of the appearance of the cells. Spinous cells are large polygonal cells with prominent desmosomal intercellular filaments, which act like bridges between the cells. Cells of the upper layers of the stratum spinosum are flatter.

Stratum Granulosum

Consisting of three to five layers of flattened keratinocytes, the stratum granulosum contains lamellar bodies. Keratinocytes migrate from the underlying stratum spinosum to become known as granular cells in this layer. These cells contain keratohyalin granules, which are filled with histidine- and cysteine-rich proteins which appear to bind the keratin filaments together. Also, at the transition between the stratum granulosum and the stratum corneum, cells secrete lamellar bodies which contain lipids and proteins. This forms a hydrophobic (water-hating) lipid envelope which helps waterproof the

skin. At the same time, cells lose their nuclei and organelles, causing the granular cells to become non-viable corneocytes in the stratum corneum.

Stratum Lucidum

Found in thicker areas of skin, the stratum lucidum contains three to five layers of flattened, dead keratinocytes which contain a large amount of keratin.

Stratum Corneum

Consisting of 25–30 layers of flattened, dead keratinocytes, for the stratum corneum to maintain a constant thickness there is a constant turnover of exfoliated corneocytes, being replaced by new corneocytes from the stratum granulosum below. Enzymes in the lamellar bodies from the stratum granulosum help to break down the intercellular lipid 'glue' that holds the cells in place.

Newly formed cells in the stratum basale are pushed upwards through the layers, becoming flattened and eventually dead and containing more and more keratin before they are eventually sloughed off or shed. These layers provide protection to the deeper layers, retain moisture and prevent entry by microbes.

Dermis

The dermis (also known as the corium when associated with the hooves) consists of dense fibrous connective tissue composed of collagen type I, III and V, with some elastin fibres. The mixture of collagen and elastic fibres makes the skin stretchy so it may stretch, for example, during pregnancy as the mare's abdomen increases in size. It provides a supporting framework for blood and lymphatic vessels, nerves and sensory receptors, hair follicles, sebaceous and sweat glands and contains circulating white cells. The superficial part of the dermis makes up roughly 20% of the total thickness of this layer. The surface area is significantly increased by dermal papillae, finger-like projections which project into the undersurface of the epidermis. Sympathetic nerves provide motor innervation to blood vessels, glands and arrector pili muscles of hair follicles in the dermis. In addition some dermal papillae contain tactile receptors, sensitive to touch and known as Meissner's corpuscles. Other free nerve endings are associated with feelings of warmth, itching, pain and tickling, such as when flies land on the horse's skin. The skin around the muzzle is very sensitive and, in conjunction with the whiskers, is used like fingertips.

Sensation

Pain-detecting nerves require greater pressure or injury before they are stimulated. However, the horse is particularly sensitive over the ribs where the rider applies the aids. Sensitive horses are likely to respond to subtle movements, resulting in anticipation of the rider's demands. Before giving an intramuscular injection the vet may bang the horse's neck and this discharges the nerve endings, making the injection less painful. Touch is an important means of communication to the horse and it often indulges in mutual grooming with other horses.

Melanin

The epidermis produces a skin pigment called melanin which acts as a filter for UV light. This is an important function of melanin and absence of pigment will mean greater sensitivity to UV damage. Thus horses with black skin are not liable to sunburn, whereas horses with pink skin can become sunburned, especially on the face. Melanin can migrate to form tumours known as melanomas. They are most common in grey horses and tend to be found on the underside of the dock, around the anus, vulva or sheath, or on the head (see Chapter 13, 'Coat Colour and Genetics'). Melanocytes produce pigment in melanosome structures which are membrane-bound structures involved

in the transfer of pigment to keratinocytes. Albinism is the inherited condition whereby the individual horse cannot produce melanin in its coat, eyes and skin.

Sudoriferous Glands (Sweat Glands)

Apocrine sweat glands are the sole effective sweat glands in hoofed animals, such as the horse, as eccrine glands are lacking. They are simple coiled tubular glands and their secretory portion is found many in the subcutaneous layer (see 'Thermoregulation'). Sweat glands empty into the hair follicles – typical of apocrine sweat glands and in contrast to eccrine sweat glands which open on to the skin surface. Horses are different from other domestic animals in their abundant production of sweat (Figure 10.3).

Sebaceous Glands

The sebaceous glands are oil glands which surround each hair follicle at a point about one-third of its length beneath the skin's surface. Each gland is composed of numerous acini attached to an excretory duct through which they discharge the oily secretions (sebum) onto the hair shaft and epidermis. The secreting portion lies in the dermis. Sebum prevents hair from drying out, prevents excess water loss from the skin and keeps skin supple. Sebum may inhibit the growth of some bacteria.

Hair

Hair is an epidermal structure despite the fact that it penetrates the dermis. Each hair is a thread of fused dead keratinised epidermal cells composed into a visible shaft, set at an oblique angle to the surface of the skin, and with a root which lies in the hair follicle projecting into the dermis and sometimes the subcutaneous layer. At the base of the hair is a bulb of living tissue which is continuous with

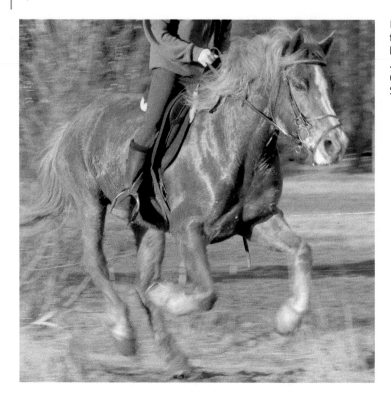

Figure 10.3 Horse sweating freely. *Source*: Wright, https://commons.wikimedia .org/wiki/File:Teppo_works_ up_a_sweat_in_early_ Spring.jpg. CC BY 2.0.

the dermis; here cell division and growth take place, along with the incorporation of the pigment cells which give the hair its colour.

The amount and type of melanin in cortical cells determine the colour of hair, that is, black, brown or red. The medulla may contain pigment, which has little effect on hair colour, but air spaces between medullary cells are believed to give a white or silver colour to the hair if the cortex lacks pigment. Wool hairs lack a medulla or have only a very small one, accounting for their fine structure.

Hair Follicles

Surrounding the root is the hair follicle which is made up of two layers of epidermal cells, namely the internal and external root sheaths. All horse hair has a similar structure of an outer cuticle, a cortex containing pigments, an inner medulla and a root or bulb from which the hair grows out of the follicle to form the shaft. All these parts are basically composed of compressed, keratinised epithelial cells. Each hair follicle also

has a sudoriferous (sebaceous) gland and an arrector pili muscle associated with it. Each hair follicle is surrounded by nerve endings or hair root plexuses which are sensitive to touch. The papilla of the hair follicle contains blood vessels to supply nutrients to the growing hair. Another part of the bulb produces new hairs when old ones are shed or lost, in cells from the hair matrix. From the hair cone at the base of the follicle, the cells keratinise and form a hair. As the hair grows up through the epidermis to the skin's surface, the cells at the point of the cone die, forming a channel, that is, the hair follicle.

Connected to each hair follicle is a sebaceous gland which produces an oily secretion called sebum. The sebum keeps the hair supple and resistant to wetting. The bundle of smooth muscle fibres known as the arrector pili is associated with the hair follicles. The arrestor pili attaches from the dermis to the side of the hair follicle. When it is cold nerve endings cause the smooth muscle of the arrector pili to contract which makes the hair shaft stand up vertically, trapping air more effectively in the coat to produce extra insulation.

The Coat

The coat is the horse's first line of defence against injury and the environment, and it covers the majority of the body surface. More hair is found on the parts of the skin exposed to direct sunlight than on less exposed areas such as the inner thigh and the perineal areas. The skin carries several types of hair:

- Tactile hairs – long stiff hairs of the muzzle and eyes, innervated to touch.
- Guard hairs – smooth, stiff and straight hairs forming the outer coat; modifications of the guard hairs in horses include the coarse hair of the mane, tail, eyelashes and feathers of the lower legs. These long hairs are designed and positioned to help shed rain water.
- Wool hairs – make up the bulk of the undercoat. They are more wavy and more numerous than the tough guard hairs and usually shorter. Their number increases in winter, when they form the thick winter undercoat to help keep the body warm.

The coat is shed and changed for a new growth in the spring and autumn (Figure 10.4). The change of coat is associated with changes in daylight and external temperature (i.e. circadian rhythms). There are clear differences between breeds, and Thoroughbreds have a finer coat than draught breeds and donkeys. A thick coat reduces the horse's winter feed requirement because the horse keeps warmer. The response to longer days and higher temperatures is greater on a higher plane of nutrition

Thermoregulation

In order for horses to survive, internal body temperature must be kept within a very narrow range, to sustain metabolism and maintain optimum conditions for enzymes to function. If the temperature exceeds these limits either above or below, these chemical reactions at cellular level begin to fail and not function. As the body temperature increases or decreases even more, cellular reactions may stop altogether and cells will die. The horse's body can cope with relatively small fluctuations in internal body temperature, as it has to adapt to ambient weather conditions. Exercise and hard work increase the rate of metabolism particularly within the muscle masses and excess heat is a by-product of these reactions; the horse's body systems have to work quickly to remove

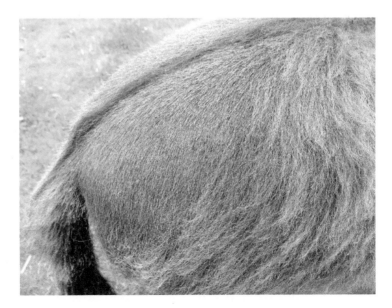

Figure 10.4 A donkey shedding its winter coat, revealing the shorter summer coat underneath.

this excessive internal heat. Infections and illness can also increase body temperature. Horses have evolved methods to maintain their core temperature even when external conditions are harsh, such as in winter or extremes such as in desert conditions.

The mature horse's body temperature is maintained at 37.3–38.2°C; foals have a higher normal temperature. Temperature receptors in the skin sense the external temperature, and there are also thermoreceptors in the hypothalamus which monitor the temperature of blood flowing through it. If the temperature of blood is too high, steps are taken to lose heat; if the temperature is too low, heat is conserved.

For the body to maintain a constant temperature, heat loss must equal heat gain. Heat exchange between the horse and the environment (Figure 10.5) occurs through the following ways:

- Conduction – direct heat transfer; a very small amount is lost from horses unless lying down on a cold surface.
- Radiation – indirect heat transfer; solar radiation from the sun as heat or reflected heat from the ground is transferred to the horse, or heat is lost from a hot horse to cooler air surrounding it.
- Convection – forced convection with air as the horse moves; higher losses in windy weather.
- Evaporation – respiration and sweating; loss of heat by water evaporating from surfaces such as the skin or respiratory tract.

Water has an excellent capacity for transferring heat away from the horse. Its cooling

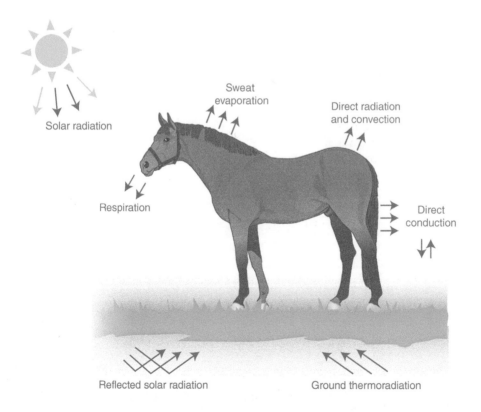

Figure 10.5 Heat exchange between horses and their environment.

power can be up to 20 × that of air. Larger body sizes in horses reduce heat loss due to the lower surface area to volume ratio.

The temperature regulation centre is the hypothalamus. The hypothalamus will react to changes in core body temperature and also to nerve receptors in the skin and then it will coordinate the appropriate responses; these are both nervous and hormonal responses to restore normal temperature. Thus the hypothalamus acts like a thermostat (Figure 10.6).

Heat Conservation

If the body temperature falls too low (the horse becomes hypothermic), body heat is conserved by:

- constriction of the superficial blood vessels, reducing the heat lost from radiation and diverting blood to the core
- the erector pili muscles contracti ng so that the coat rises and traps a layer of warm air next to the skin. Air is a poor conductor of heat, so losses from the surface of the skin are further reduced
- reduced sweating
- shivering, caused by involuntary contraction of the skeletal muscles and resulting in heat production
- (long term) seasonal coat changes.

Heat Loss

If the body temperature rises to too high a level (the horse becomes hyperthermic), excess heat is lost by:

- dilation of the superficial blood vessels and capillaries in the dermis, allowing more blood to come close to the surface and lose more heat to the atmosphere by radiation
- the hairs of the coat lying flat to the skin, so trapping the minimum amount of air
- increased sweating
- slowing down the rate of metabolism.

Horses that are very hot and sweating, following exercise for example, rely on sweating for heat loss (around 85%), as they do not pant similar to dogs and other animals. They also lose some heat from the respiratory system (around 15%). This may change depending upon environmental conditions such as temperature and humidity. For sweating and evaporation to be effective air needs to move over the skin, removing water-saturated air. Sweating is most effective for heat loss in hot and dry, low-humidity conditions. It is least effective in hot and humid conditions. The cardiovascular system plays an important role in transferring heat from the sites of production, such as the muscles, to sites where dissipation can occur, such as the skin and respiratory tract. During exercise, blood flow to the skin increases in order for evaporation of sweat to occur. The amount of heat dissipated by 1 litre of sweat is equivalent to 1–2 minutes of high-intensity exercise or 5–6 minutes of sub-maximal endurance exercise. Although horses do not normally pant, the respiratory tract is able to dissipate heat through air exchange via breathing changes. It is thought that much of the blowing undertaken by horses after racing or extreme exercise is not to replace the oxygen debt but actually to restore core body temperature by removing air heated by capillaries in the lungs.

Horses often struggle to remove excess heat from sweating when the air temperature is more than 25°C and the humidity is high at 80–90%. They may then become hyperthermic, where the body temperature rises to 42°C or more. Hyperthermia may also result from working horses hard in the following conditions:

- with winter coats
- where the horse is unfit
- carrying too much condition
- in the hottest time of day
- young untrained horses
- during endurance rides and three-day events, in hot and humid conditions.

Hyperthermia or heat stroke is a life-threatening condition in horses – they can collapse if this is severe. It should be treated by a veterinary surgeon as soon as possible and intensive attempts to cool the horse

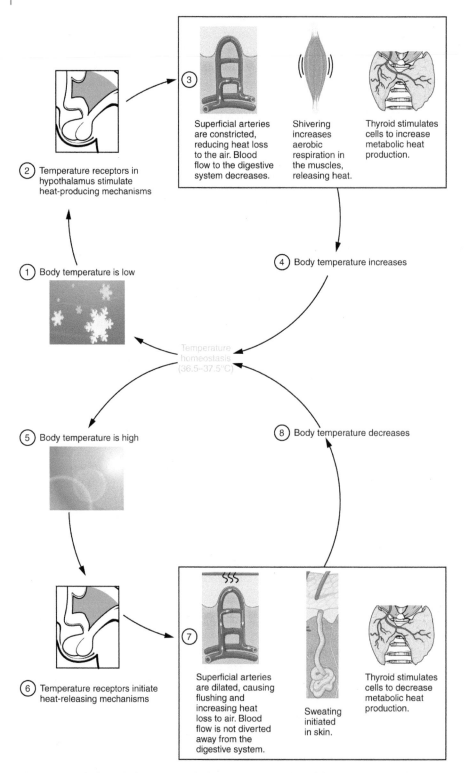

Figure 10.6 The hypothalamus controls thermoregulation (homeostasis). *Source*: OpenStax College, https://commons.wikimedia.org/wiki/File:2523_The_Hypothalamus_Controls_Thermoregulation.jpg. CC BY 3.0.

should be undertaken at the same time. Symptoms of hyperthermia include:

- an unwillingness to move/ataxic if severe, collapse and death
- increased rectal temperature
- fatigue, with depression and distress
- persistently elevated heart rate
- elevated respiratory rate or it may appear slow
- congested mucous membranes and increased capillary refill time
- lack of thirst despite provision of adequate water and apparent dehydration
- thumps – synchronous diaphragmatic flutter.

Sweating

The horse's sweat glands are not under the influence of the hormone aldosterone and so do not conserve sodium as do human sweat glands. In fact, the horse's sweat glands act like a funnel from the interstitial space in skin to the surface, allowing free-flowing movement of a hypertonic fluid containing electrolytes. This means that the sweat fluid contains more salts than the blood from which it is derived. Human sweat, on the other hand, is hypotonic, that is, it contains less salt than the blood due to the conservation action of aldosterone on sodium (Table 10.1).

Horse sweat is very rich in electrolytes, which are mineral salts contained in blood plasma. Electrolytes must be present in the body in the correct proportions so that normal metabolism can continue. Thus it is vital to ensure that the sweating horse is given both water and electrolytes to replace losses during exertion.

The rate of sweat production depends upon many factors, including exercise intensity, ambient conditions, state of hydration, and the training or heat acclimatisation of the individual horse. Sweating rates will increase with a high ambient temperature or humidity which reduces evaporative efficiency, thereby resulting in a rise in core body temperature.

Proteins leave the coat matted and contribute to lathering up. Proteins have detergent-like properties, allowing the sweat to spread along the hair and encouraging more effective evaporation. Excess salts and the protein such as latherin also change the evaporation point of sweat in horses, making evaporation easier. Sweat is considered to be a result of apoptosis or cell death, releasing cell contents into the sweat glands together with secretions and cellular debris, and includes inorganic ions, water, glycoproteins, such as latherin and albumin, and amino acids and waste products including urea and lactic acid. These proteins cause the sweat to froth excessively and the horse is said to have 'lathered up'– notably between the hind legs, on the neck and under the saddle.

The horse's sweat glands are also sensitive to epinephrine (adrenaline) and so nervous horses or those in pain will often break into a sweat. Sweating in the horse is under dual control from a combination of hormonal and neural mechanisms. The horse can sweat freely compared to other domestic animals and has sweat glands over the entire body except for the legs. Some areas, such as the base of the ears, the flanks and the neck, are densely populated with glands. A horse grazing in summer can normally lose 6 litres of fluid a day without any visible dampness of the skin and coat.

Table 10.1 Composition of sweat.

	Sodium (Na) (g/l)	Potassium (K) (g/l)	Chloride (Cl) (g/l)
Plasma	140	3.5–4.5	100
Human sweat	10–60	4–5	10–60
Horse sweat	130–190	20–50	160–190

Table 10.2 Heat loss ability at different effective temperatures.

Ambient temperature	Effective cooling
Less than 54°C (130°F)	No problem
More than 60°C (140°F)	Increased sweating
More than 66°C (150°F)	Effective sweating lowered
More than 82°C (180°F)	Cooling from skin ineffective, horse blows

When looking at the weather conditions, it is the effective temperature that is important, that is, the combination of ambient temperature and relative humidity (how much water the air contains). Table 10.2 shows heat loss ability (effective cooling) at different effective temperatures.

Breaking Out

A horse may sweat when it is cold due to stress or fatigue. There is nervous stimulation of the adrenal glands causing increased epinephrine production which stimulates the areas of the brain controlling sweat production. Thus horses can sweat up in anticipation when being transported to a competition. This is known as 'breaking out'.

Dry Coat or Anhydrosis

Horses reared in temperate climates and then exported to much hotter and humid countries may lose the ability to sweat, a condition known as dry coat or anhydrosis. This malfunction can occur in small patches or produce a near-total inability to sweat. The condition rarely develops in horses native to hot climates. The horse is unable to lose heat and will develop heat stroke if exerted. The signs usually appear within 12 months of the horse's arrival in the new environment and include:

- (initially) excessive sweating
- distressed breathing
- decreased ability to sweat, which may be confined to small areas
- frequent urination
- fever.

Research has now shown that the sweat glands of anhydrotic horses secrete chloride ions differently than normal horses and that these chloride ions underpin the formation of sweat in equine sweat glands.

Skin and Coat Colour

Skin and coat colour relies on the presence of pigment called melanin. Mast cells give rise to melanoblasts which wander throughout the body until the animal matures and eventually migrate to the dermis where they give rise to melanocytes. The cells multiply throughout this migration and eventually reach the epidermis. Here the pigment cells produce pigment (melanin). The horse has two types of pigment:

- eumelanin – black/brown
- phaeomelanin – red/yellow.

Melanoblasts form a continuous layer at the junction of the dermis and epidermis. In the foetus the development of the hair follicle begins as a thickening of epithelial cells, resulting in the hair bulb. Cells migrate from the mesenchyma to the hair bulb and form the follicle. Some melanocytes also migrate to the hair bulb and as differentiation takes place they are incorporated into the hair shaft, to give the birth coat of the foal. Melanocytes within the follicle produce pigment granules, but this process does not take place in albinos. Melanin production requires the amino acid tyrosine and is controlled by the enzyme tyrosinase. Once formed, the melanin moves along the dendrites and is injected into the adjoining tissues and cells to give colouration. Normally this is a continuing process, but it may be interrupted if the surface tissue of the body is damaged. Horses with saddle sores and poorly fitting rugs often develop white areas where pigmentation of the hair is not possible.

Summary Points

1) Skin acts as a protective envelope, as a secretory and excretory organ, as a sense organ and as a temperature-regulating device.
2) In addition for horses, skin is an important organ of thermoregulation through sweating or perspiration and control of blood flow through the skin.
3) The epidermis produces a skin pigment called melanin which acts as a filter for UV light. This is an important function of melanin and absence of pigment will mean greater sensitivity to UV damage.
4) The horse's sweat glands are not under the influence of the hormone aldosterone and so do not conserve sodium as do human sweat glands, making their sweat salty and hypertonic.
5) The horse's sweat glands are sensitive to epinephrine (adrenaline) and so nervous horses or those in pain will often break out into a sweat.

Q + A

Q Which layer of the epidermis is 'extra' in thick skin?

A The stratum lucidum, between the stratum granulosum and stratum corneum.

Q Does the horse have apocrine or eccrine sweat glands or both?

A The horse has apocrine sweat glands – they are the sole effective sweat glands in hoofed animals such as horses. Eccrine glands are lacking in horses.

Q Why is it important to maintain a constant body temperature?

A In order for horses to survive, internal body temperature must be kept within a very narrow range, to sustain metabolism and maintain optimum conditions for enzymes to function. If the temperature exceeds these limits either above or below, these chemical reactions at cellular level begin to fail and not function.

Q What is the normal core body temperature of mature horses at rest?

A 37.3–38.2°C.

Q What substances cause horse sweat to become frothy or lathered?

A Proteins such as latherin.

11

The Senses

All mammals have certain specialised structures that help to give them an awareness of their environment. Horses must be able to make sense of their immediate surroundings and to process this information quickly in order to survive. This is done by the central nervous system (CNS) and sensory receptors which give horses the ability to see, hear, taste, smell, touch, feel pain, respond to changes in temperature and determine the position of their body. Sensory receptors also provide unconscious information regarding blood pressure and volume, and chemical balance such as salts and nutrients in the blood. Sensory receptors are specialised cells adapted for the detection of changes to the internal and external environment. They are either neurons or connected to other neurons and may be enclosed in sense organs. Others are nerve fibre endings in skin, bones, tendon tissue and so on or within organs. There are also sensory receptors that are neurons in the brain that are stimulated by changes in temperature, dissolved blood gases, salts, acids/bases and so on in the fluid surrounding the sensory neurons.

Transduction

All sensory experiences begin at specialised nerve endings called receptors that detect a change in the internal or external environment. Transduction is the changing of heat, pressure or light signals, for example, into electrical signals in neurons. This sequence of reactions results in the initiation of action potentials (nerve impulses) being transmitted along nerve fibres to the CNS. The essential step of transduction is the activation of the receptor molecules, which involves the opening or closing of tiny pores (ion channels) in the cell membrane which creates a change in the movement of charged ions (usually sodium ions), altering the voltage inside the receptor cell. The size of the receptor potential varies with the intensity of the stimulus received. This results in firing of nerve impulses, either in the sensory cell itself or in an adjacent nerve cell.

Adaptation

The sensitivity of sensory receptors mostly depends on how much, how often and how recently they have been stimulated. For example, if a sensory receptor in the skin is repeatedly exposed to a stimulus (such as pressure on the skin, when the rider applies leg, for example) the rate of nerve impulses falls to a lower level, and may stop altogether. This is called adaptation, and means receptors are more sensitive to changes in stimulation as opposed to steady stimulation. This means that the sensory receptors are sensitive to small changes in signal strength but tune out constant signals; thus the sensory nerves are not being constantly stimulated when they are not required.

Some receptors adapt much faster than others, such as touch, smell and pressure, compared to slower adapting receptors responsible for proprioception, pain and

Equine Science, Third Edition. Zoe Davies and Sarah Pilliner.
© 2018 Zoe Davies and Sarah Pilliner. Published 2018 by John Wiley & Sons Ltd.

receptors responsible for chemical changes in the blood such as osmoreceptors. Sensory receptors provide information on both the internal and external environments. Sensory information or nerve impulses from various parts of the body arrive in specific areas of the cerebral cortex in the brain. These sensory nerve impulses are carried by specific sensory neurons which respond only to a particular stimulus. In other words, neurons responsible for pain will not also carry information regarding pressure, heat or pain, and so on.

There are five 'special senses' and their organs:

- sight – eyes
- hearing – ears
- balance – eyes and ears
- smell – nose
- taste – tongue.

These five senses are essential for survival. Sense organs may be considered as extensions of the brain and are directly connected to it by nerve trunks. These special sense organs all differ tremendously in both structure and function.

There are also other senses known as 'general senses' which include:

- Somatic senses – touch, pressure, vibration, heat and cold, pain, proprioceptors (position of the body and limbs).
- Visceral senses – internal organs, bladder, colon and so on.

There are several types of sensory receptors, grouped according to morphology:

- Free nerve endings, for example dendrites, include receptors in the dermis and epidermis of the skin, touch receptors, nociceptors, thermoreceptors.
- Encapsulated nerve endings – visceral and somatic receptors where the dendrites are enclosed by a capsule of connective tissue.
- Specialised separate cells – connect to sensory neurons via synapses.

Sensory receptors may also be grouped according to their functions:

- Mechanoreceptors – respond to stretching of tissue, mechanical strain or stress, hearing.
- Chemoreceptors – detect chemicals in body fluids, and taste and smell receptors.
- Thermoreceptors – detect changes in temperature.
- Osmoreceptors – detect changes in osmotic pressure.
- Proprioceptors – sense of position of self.
- Nociceptors – respond to tissue damage, and may result in pain, but not always.
- Baroreceptors – detect changes in blood pressure.
- Photoreceptors – contain specialised proteins such as rhodopsin to transduce light energy into electrical signals.

The sensory receptors are the first part of a sensory system.

Somatic Receptors

Somatic receptors are receptors 'of the body' and so include those receptors in the skin, such as mechanoreceptors, thermoreceptors and nociceptors, and those in muscles, joints, tendons, ligaments and so on. The resulting sensations from somatic receptors being stimulated are not always even, as some parts of the body have more receptors and others have less. The horse's tongue has a particularly high number of chemoreceptors, for example (Figure 11.1).

There are two different types of sensory nerve fibres. The A delta fibres (Aδ fibre) carry cold, pressure and some pain signals. Because Aδ fibres are thinly myelinated, they send impulses faster. The second type is unmyelinated C fibres, which act much more slowly than the more thickly myelinated 'A' delta fibres.

Thermal Sensations

Thermal sensations arise from thermoreceptors giving two distinct thermal sensations

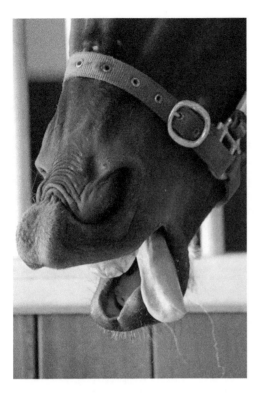

Figure 11.1 The horse's tongue contains a high number of chemoreceptors.

of hot and cold. Thermoreceptors are free nerve endings, some of which are stimulated by hot temperatures and others by cold. Cold thermoreceptors – located in the epidermis – respond to cooler temperatures below 35.8°C. Hot thermoreceptors – located in the dermis – respond to higher temperatures above 37.5°C. When temperatures are very high or very low then often nociceptors producing pain sensations are stimulated.

Pain Sensations

Pain sensations arise from nociceptors and are found in most tissues in the horse's body, with the exception of the brain. They are also free nerve endings. Pain sensation may continue after the original stimulation has gone due to reduced adaptation in nociceptors and also pain-producing chemicals leaking around damaged tissues. Nociceptors produce two types of pain, namely slow and fast. Slow pain begins following a short delay in the original stimulus and gradually increases in intensity to a chronic burning, throbbing or aching pain, whereas fast pain produces a very fast acute sharp pain.

Tactile Sensations

Tactile sensations arise from mechanoreceptors and include touch, pressure, vibration and itching sensations. The follicles from which the whiskers grow on the horse's muzzle are surrounded by nerve endings. Each time the whiskers come into contact with an object, the nerves send electrical messages to the brain, enabling it to determine what the horse is touching.

The whiskers help them to estimate the distance between the muzzle and objects around them. A horse cannot see areas immediately below its head, so whiskers help guide the horse in this effectively blind area and so are very important (Figure 11.2). The muzzle whiskers also help protect the nose and lips from touching things that may harm the horse.

There are four main mechanoreceptors found in the dermis and epidermis of horses:

- Ruffini cells – also known as bulbous corpuscles, these are slow adapters, found

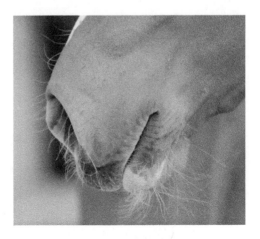

Figure 11.2 Sensory hairs on the muzzle.

in the hoof; maintained pressure gives the horse a sense of position. They are located in the dermis and are sensitive to skin stretch. They are also found in joints, where they respond to mechanical deformation due to angle change in the joint. In skin they also act as thermoreceptors.

- Merkel's discs – slow adapters, found in hair follicles, these sense pressure, deep static touch, for example sharp edges or objects, and position.
- Pacinian corpuscles – also known as lamellar corpuscles, these are fast adapters, found deep in skin layers and in ligaments and joints, which sense vibration and pressure. These receptors are larger than other receptors and in joints they are activated under compression through angle change in the joint capsule. They are also found in the horse's frog (Figure 11.3).
- Lanceolate endings – detect hair movement and respond to mechanical deformation and distortion by generating an action potential. In hairy skin such as that of horses, these are the equivalent

of Meissner's corpuscles – also known as tactile corpuscles – which sense vibration and are fast adapters, but meissner's corpuscles are absent in horses.

Itch Sensation

The itch sensation comes from free nerve endings in the skin. The itch originates following the activation of peripheral sensory nerve endings in the skin owing to damage or exposure to inflammatory mediators such as bradykinin and then ascends to the brain.

Pruriceptive itch (from the Latin word *prurere* meaning to itch) is a sensation of itch that begins following activation of primary afferent nerves. This type of itch is associated with insect bites, such as sweet itch which affects some horses and ponies.

Proprioceptor Sensation

Proprioceptor sensation enables horses to know where their limbs and heads are so that

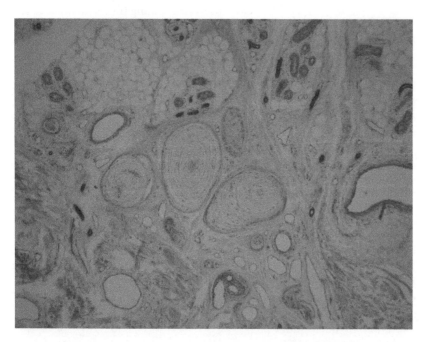

Figure 11.3 Pacinian corpuscle. *Source*: Wbensmith, https://commons.wikimedia.org/wiki/File:WVSOM_Pacinian_Corpuscle.JPG. CC BY 3.0.

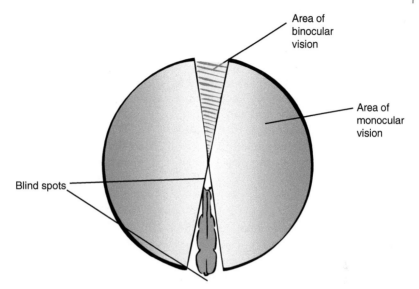

Figure 11.4 The horse's field of vision.

Area of binocular vision

Area of monocular vision

Blind spots

they can move, often referred to as the position of self. This sensation arises in specific nerve receptors known as proprioceptors and these are located in skeletal muscles, tendons and synovial joints and in the inner ear of the horse. The brain integrates information from proprioception and from the vestibular system into the horse's overall sense of body position, movement and acceleration. Proprioception may be conscious or unconscious. Unconscious proprioception is organised by the cerebellum, whereas conscious proprioception is mediated by the cerebral cortex.

Special Senses

Sight

The horse's eye is the largest of all land mammals and is able to make an image on the retina 50% larger than the human eye. Horses have both binocular and monocular vision. The horse's eye also has a bulging contour which allows for a wide monocular field of vision. Like most prey animals, the horse's eyes are set on the sides of its head. This means horses have a range of vision of about 350°, with approximately 65–80° being binocular vision and the remaining

146° on either side being monocular vision (Figure 11.4). The horse's visual acuity is relatively poor compared to humans and is thought to lie between 20/30 and 20/60 (slightly worse than the usual 20/20 in humans).

Visual Streak of the Eye

The horse has an area within the retina which is linear in shape. This area has a high concentration of ganglion cells and is known as the visual streak. The pupils of the horse's eyes are oblique in shape and positioned horizontally within the eye, which optimises their ability to scan horizons. There are up to 6100 cells/mm^2 in the visual streak compared to 150 and 200 cells/mm^2 in the peripheral area. Horses have better acuity when the objects they are looking at fall in the visual streak region, and so they will tilt or raise their heads to help move objects they are looking at to within this region.

Horses are very sensitive to motion in their peripheral vision, and due to the poor visual acuity in this area they tend to react by spooking and then turn their heads to place the distant object in the visual streak area. In bright conditions where the pupil is constricted this allows for maximum horizontal vision of around 350°, with the blind spot just in front of the nose and a couple of metres behind the tail. When the horse lowers its head to graze, the binocular field is directed towards the ground and the horizontal monocular vision is used to scan the horizon. When a horse is ridden and the head is reined in too far behind the vertical, that is, it is over-bent, it cannot see directly ahead. Horses must be able to raise their head and nose before taking off for jumping so they can use their binocular vision.

Colour Vision

Horses are not colour blind but have dichromatic vision with a reduced cone density, meaning they can see washed-out versions of colours including green, yellow, blue and grey. Horses are not thought to be able to see red colour. Dichromatic vision means horses see two of the basic three wavelengths of visible light, compared to the three-color (trichromatic vision) of most humans. In other words, horses naturally see the blue and green colours of the spectrum and the colour variations based upon them, but cannot distinguish red. It seems they find it especially difficult to distinguish between the colours green and yellow. Dichromatic vision is the result of horses having two types of cones in their eyes:

- Short wavelength sensitive cone (S) which is optimal at 428 nm.
- Mid to long wavelength-sensitive cone (M/L) which is optimal at 539 nm.

Night Vision

The horse's eye also has a light-intensifying device called the tapetum lucidum, which consists of a layer within the eye which reflects light back on to the retina, allowing the horse to see in dim light. This layer will reflect back the light of a torch at night, in the same way that a cat's eye reflects the glare of car headlights. This is a modification of the choroid layer.

The retina of horses also has more rods than that of humans, giving a higher proportion of rods to cones of about 20:1. This again gives them improved night vision; it also gives them better vision on slightly cloudy days compared to very sunny days. The ability to see in conditions of poor light indicates that the horse is a nocturnal animal; indeed, studies of feral horses show them to be most active at dawn and dusk.

If horses become alerted by something in the distance they will stand with their heads held very high and their nose back, so that they can focus on the object of interest. In horses, ciliary muscles which help focus the lens and fix images on to the retina are underdeveloped. The horse therefore has to move its head up or down to bring the image on to the part of the retina at the correct distance to focus the image sharply. The ciliary muscles do provide, however, some assistance to the focusing process. Therefore the horse should be allowed to move its head when approaching obstacles so that it can obtain a sharp image of the fence before it jumps.

Horses also have the added problem of their own muzzles obscuring their view. For this reason a horse's view is indistinct below eye level. By the time the horse is 1.5 m (4–5 ft) away from a fence, it can no longer see it, and all horses therefore are jumping blind from this point. In fact, many show jumpers can be seen to ask the horse to move its head from side to side when approaching a fence to improve the horse's vision. Horses that race over fences are less likely to suffer from this problem because they have a longer take-off distance and can see the fence before jumping.

Anatomy of the Eye

The eyes are situated in bony sockets or orbits which are positioned in the skull for maximum protection. The orbit is surrounded by a ridged arch of particularly strong bone known as the supraorbital process. The orbit also contains a large pad of fat which lies behind the eye and acts as a cushion if the eye should receive a blow. Horses have excellent reflexes which is why they rarely injure their eyes (Figure 11.5).

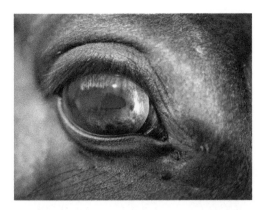

Figure 11.5 The eye of the horse. *Source*: Kallerna, https://commons.wikimedia.org/wiki/File:Hepan_silm%C3%A4.JPG. CC BY 3.0.

Chambers of the Eye

The lens and ciliary body form a partition, dividing the cavity in the eye into two parts known as the anterior and posterior chambers. The anterior chamber contains a watery fluid which is known as the aqueous humour, whereas the posterior chamber contains a thicker, jelly-like fluid known as the vitreous humour. Aqueous humour provides nutrients for the lens and cornea and maintains intraocular pressure. It is replaced several times a day. It is secreted by the ciliary body to the posterior chamber and then the anterior chamber through the canal of Schlemm.

The eyeball of the horse is not perfectly spherical as is the human eye, but rather is flattened anterior to posterior (Figure 11.6). It does not have a ramped retina, as previously thought. The eye consists of the eyeball or globe, the optic nerve and accessory structures such as the eyelids, conjunctiva, cornea, lacrimal apparatus (which makes tears) and the muscles that move the eye (ocular muscles).

The horse's eye is made up of three layers:

- Nervous or internal tunic – retina.
- Vascular tunic – uvea, made up of the choroid, ciliary body and iris.
- Fibrous tunic – cornea and sclera.

Nervous Tunic – Retina

The retina is made up of cells that extend to the brain via the optic nerve. The receptors are photosensitive and include:

- Cones – allow the eye to see colour and provide visual acuity.
- Rods – more light-sensitive than cones and provide night vision.

Since only two-thirds of the eye can receive light, the receptor cells do not need to cover the entire interior of the eye, and line only the area from the pupil to the optic disk. The part of the retina covered by light-sensitive cells is therefore termed the pars-optica retinae and the blind part of the eye is termed the pars-caeca retinae. The optic disk does not contain any rods or cones as this is where the optic nerve leaves to the brain and this area is effectively a blind spot.

The optic nerve enters the eye from behind, passing through the sclera and the choroid, and spreading out nerve fibres over the surface of the retina which they penetrate by turning back on themselves. The nerve fibres themselves are not sensitive to light. The image that the horse sees is caught on the retina, where it is converted to nervous messages which are then sent via the optic nerve to the brain for translation.

Vascular Tunic – Uvea

The uvea is made up of the choroid, ciliary body and iris. The choroid contains pigment and is mostly made up of blood vessels. It forms the tapetum lucidum when it crosses over the fundus of the eye, causing the yellowish-green eye shine when light is directed into the animal's eyes at night. The iris lies between the cornea and the lens and gives the eye its colour. It also allows varying amounts of light to pass through the hole in its centre known as the pupil.

The iris itself contains both circular and radial muscles which make the size of the pupil larger or smaller depending upon the amount of light entering the eye. When light is bright, the pupil becomes narrower and more oblong shaped (in the horizontal

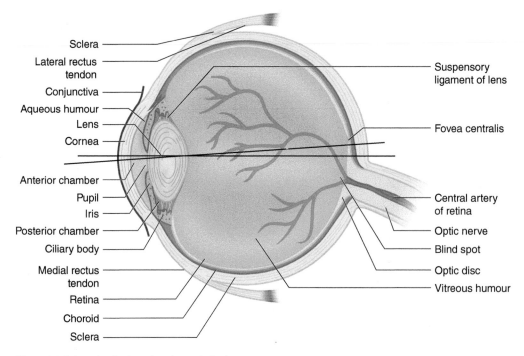

Sclera
Lateral rectus tendon
Conjunctiva
Aqueous humour
Lens
Cornea
Anterior chamber
Pupil
Iris
Posterior chamber
Ciliary body
Medial rectus tendon
Retina
Choroid
Sclera

Suspensory ligament of lens
Fovea centralis
Central artery of retina
Optic nerve
Blind spot
Optic disc
Vitreous humour

Figure 11.6 Longitudinal section through the human eye.

plane). When dull, the pupil becomes dilated and is more round in shape. The edges of the iris in the horse are irregular and are not smooth as in the human eye. Projections of dark-coloured pigment can easily be seen, particularly lining the upper edge of the iris.

Fibrous Tunic

Made up of the sclera and cornea, the fibrous tunic protects the eye. The sclera is the white of the eye and is composed of elastin and collagen. The cornea is the clear covering on the front of the eye and is also composed of connective tissue. The cornea has five layers:

- conjunctiva
- Bowman's membrane
- thick transparent fibrous layer
- Descemet's membrane
- endothelium.

The cornea must be continuously bathed in lacrimal fluid and aqueous humour, to provide nutrients and so on, as it does not have blood vessels. The level of hydration is critical for transparency of the eye.

The lens of the eye lies behind the iris and is held in place by ciliary muscles and the ciliary suspensory ligament. The ciliary muscles function to allow accommodation to enable the horse to focus the eye. The lens tissue is layered like an onion. The lens is derived from the ectoderm and consists of cuboidal epithelium; it has a softer cortex and firmer nucleus, which may get harder and sclerotic with age. It is avascular and has no nerves and must be supplied with nutrients from the aqueous humour. The vitreous humour in the posterior chamber of the eye is more jelly-like and contains water, hyaluronic acid and collagen. It helps prevent detachment of the retina by exerting pressure on it, holding it in place.

There are free nerve endings in the cornea which if stimulated cause reflex blinking, tear secretion and pain. The cornea must be transparent so that light can enter the eye.

Photoreceptors

Photoreceptors are highly specialised cells that respond to light, known as rods

Figure 11.7 Structure of rods and cones.

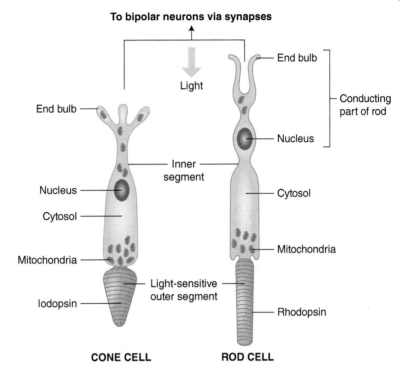

To bipolar neurons via synapses

Light

End bulb

Conducting part of rod

End bulb

Nucleus

Inner segment

Nucleus

Cytosol

Cytosol

Mitochondria

Mitochondria

Light-sensitive outer segment

Iodopsin

Rhodopsin

CONE CELL

ROD CELL

and cones which are found in the retina (Figures 11.7 and 11.8).

The retina has two layers – the neural layer and pigmented layer – and is found at the back of the eye, covering around 75% of its surface. The neural layer is an outgrowth from the brain and has several layers containing retinal neurons:

- photoreceptor layer
- bipolar cell layer
- ganglion cell layer.

These layers are separated by the inner and outer synaptic layers containing synapses. Light must pass through the ganglion layer, then the bipolar cell layer, and both the inner and outer synaptic layers before reaching the photoreceptor layer. The structure of the retina is shown in Figure 11.9. The pigmented layer consists of a layer of epithelial cells which contain melanin and is situated between the choroid and neural part of the retina. Melanin helps to absorb stray light rays which may obstruct images.

Both rods and cones contain pigments which undergo chemical changes in the presence of light. These are called photochemicals. Rods contain a pigment known as visual purple or rhodopsin, whereas cones contain iodopsin. Rhodopsin is formed from two chemicals: namely opsin, a protein, and retinal, a light-absorbing compound, the latter being derived from vitamin A. Rhodopsin decomposes and bleaches in the presence of light (similar to the effect of light on a negative in a camera), and splits it into its constituent parts, that is, opsin and retinal. This chemical decomposition starts a nerve impulse in the nerve fibre supplying the rod. Rhodopsin then regenerates in the dark. If, however, vitamin A is deficient, rhodopsin cannot regenerate because of the absence of retinal which is derived from vitamin A.

Cones do not function in dim light, they need bright light to see colour in detail. Cone cells contain the photosensitive pigment iodopsin, made up of photopsin, a protein that is different from the protein in rods and

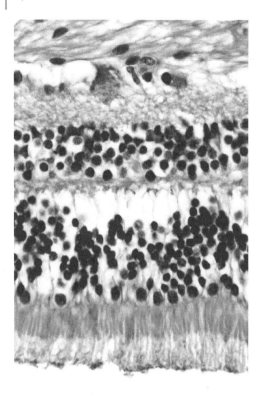

Figure 11.8 Retina under high magnification.
Source: Librepath, https://librepathology.org/wiki/
File:Retina_--_very_high_mag.jpg. CC BY 3.0.

retinal. There are two different types of cones in horses (three in humans) which respond to different wavelengths of light; one responds to blue light, the other to green. The third in humans responds to red. The colour seen by the horse's brain depends upon which cones are stimulated. The two types of cone produce the dichromatic colour horses see.

Transmission of Nerve Impulses to the Brain

The photoreceptor cells (rods and cones) are linked to bipolar cells in the retina. These link further with ganglion cells and the axons of these ganglion cells take information from the eye to the brain. Ganglion cells form a bundle and this becomes the optic nerve.

Specific neurons in the brain receive information on which part of the retina is stimulated. The brain then analyses this information and this is known as visual processing and is incredibly complex. Specific areas of the cerebral cortex are associated with different sensory functions and the visual cortex is located in the occipital lobes.

Accommodation (Focusing)

Horses have relatively poor 'accommodation'. This ability to change focus is achieved by changing the shape of the lens so as to sharply see objects near and far. Horses have weak ciliary muscles and so are not as efficient as humans in focusing. However, horses do not need to focus on objects very close to them. Recently, evidence has shown that a horse's head movements are linked to its use of its binocular field rather than to focus requirements.

Adaptation of the Horse's Eyes to Light

The eyes are capable of adapting to high levels of light intensity and low levels of illumination. Light adaptation occurs when the horse is exposed to bright light such as when coming out of a dark stable into bright sunlight. This causes photochemicals within the rods and cones to be altered in such a way that the amount of photochemical present is reduced. This decreases the sensitivity of the eye to light. At the same time, the pupil is constricted by a parasympathetic reflex constriction of the circular muscle of the iris.

On the other hand, when the horse moves from a light to a dark place or as the sun comes down there is a replenishment of photochemicals, enabling the eyes to detect very low levels of light intensity. Within 30 minutes of entering darkness, the sensitivity of the photoreceptors can increase by about 5000 times and 45 minutes later by 25,000 times. The pupil also dilates to allow more light to enter. Horse's eyes are adapted for bright light too in that structure within the eye called the granulae iridica or the corpora nigra, which appears to serve as a 'natural visor', helping improve the horse's limited depth perception.

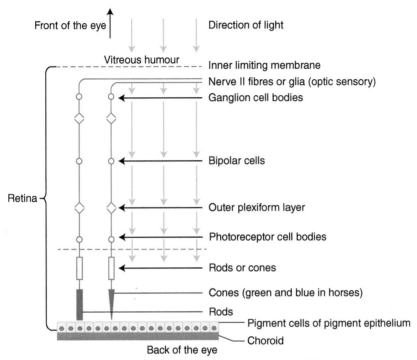

Front of the eye | Direction of light

Vitreous humour --- Inner limiting membrane
Nerve II fibres or glia (optic sensory)
Ganglion cell bodies

Bipolar cells

Retina {
Outer plexiform layer

Photoreceptor cell bodies

Rods or cones

Cones (green and blue in horses)

Rods

Pigment cells of pigment epithelium
Choroid
Back of the eye

The retina is comprised of pigmented epithelium, rods, cones, bipolar neurons and ganglion cells

Figure 11.9 Structure of the retina.

The time taken for the horse to adapt to sudden changes in light conditions – such as jumping into or out of a wood, jumping in an indoor arena and under floodlights or loading into a dark trailer – seems to be longer than in humans; this should be taken into account, giving the horse time for the eyes to adjust. For example, the horse may be walked into an indoor school and walked for as long as possible before the bell goes to begin the round. Also, when jumping the horse into or out of a wood, the horse should be slowed down to give the eyes time to adjust.

Eyelids
The horse has two eyelids and an inner one known as the third eyelid which is absent in humans. This third eyelid is pink in colour and consists of mucous membrane and cartilage. It assists in lubrication by spreading tears over the eye surface. The third eyelid is also known as the nictitating membrane and usually it can be seen only in the corner of the eye when the eye is open. One of the first signs of tetanus is the protrusion of the third eyelid partially across the eye. This becomes exaggerated if the horse is excited.

The eyelids consist of sheets of cartilage which are covered by skin on the outside and conjunctiva on the inside. The upper eyelid is the most mobile and closes over the eye. The eyelashes help to protect the eye and filter off dust particles.

Conjunctiva
The conjunctiva is a thin mucous membrane which is pink in colour and is found on the inside of the eyelids. From the inside of the eyelids, the conjunctiva folds back on itself to cover the front of the eye as a fine layer of transparent cells which form part of the cornea.

Lacrimal Apparatus

Tears are produced by the lacrimal glands which are situated beneath the supraorbital process. The tears are secreted on to the eye surface and collected in two tear ducts in the inner corner of the eye. These ducts then run down beneath the nasal bones and empty into the floor of the nostrils. The tears can be commonly seen as a clear fluid running from the nostrils. These openings can easily be seen if the nostril is pulled back slightly. If the tear ducts become blocked for any reason, tears will overflow the lower eyelid and run down the horse's face. This can be a problem, particularly in the summer when flies become attracted to this fluid. Some horses lose the hair on their face underneath the passage of tears and this can become sore.

Hearing and Balance

The sense of hearing is highly developed and acute in horses. They are able to hear sounds outside of the human range and can detect sounds from low to very high frequencies in the range of 14 Hz to 25 kHz, compared to the human range of 20 Hz to 20 kHz. They use hearing for three primary functions:

- to detect sounds
- to recognise sounds
- to locate the source of a sound.

A horse's ears can move 180° using ten different muscles, compared to only three muscles used by the human ear. This allows the horse to orient its head and neck toward the sound to determine what is making it (Figure 11.10). The sense of hearing deteriorates as the horse gets older.

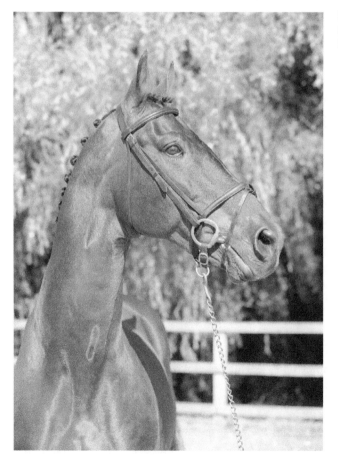

Figure 11.10 Horse listening to distant sounds. *Source*: Courtesy of Harthill Stud.

Sound travels by means of sound waves through air (or water or solids). Sound waves cause the eardrum to vibrate. These vibrations are converted into electrical impulses which are then sent to the brain for interpretation. Because the horse's sense of hearing is so acute, it can become distressed when placed in a noisy environment. It is a well-known fact that windy days can make horses more spooked, as sound waves are being carried by the wind and the horse has far greater difficulty in pinpointing the source.

Anatomy of the Ear

The ear consists of three parts: the outer, middle and inner ear (Figure 11.11).

- Outer ear – pinna, ear canal and tympanic membrane.
- Middle ear – maleus, incus and stapes (connects the middle ear to the eustachian tube).
- Inner ear – semi-circular canals and cochlear (detection of linear and angular movement, balance and hearing). The inner ear in particular is responsible for balance and informs the brain of the position of the head at all times.

Outer Ear

Most horse owners are familiar with the outer ear or pinna, which forms the visible part of the ear. This part consists of three cartilages. The conchal cartilage is the largest of the three. This cartilage funnels sound waves down into the ear canal towards the tympanic membrane (eardrum) and is funnel-shaped and lined with skin. The scutiform cartilage is a shield-shaped cartilage which acts as a lever for some of the ear muscles. It is located on the surface of the temporal muscle and attaches to the external ear muscles. The third cartilage is the annular cartilage which is shaped like a tube and connects the conchal cartilage with the external auditory canal.

Middle Ear

The tympanic membrane separates the outer from the middle ear and this is connected to three small bones – (from outside in) the malleus (hammer), incus (anvil) and stapes (stirrup) – which extend across the ear by means of ligaments. These tiny bones provide a mechanical link with the eardrum and form a bridge across the middle ear to a small opening in the skull covered by two membranous windows which lead to the inner ear. The stapes bone connects to one of

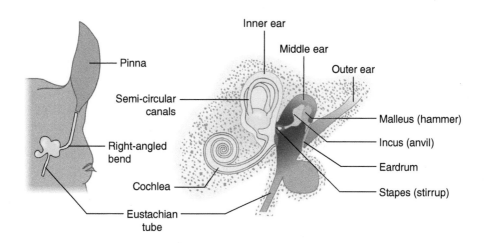

Figure 11.11 Anatomy of the horse's ear.

these two windows in the middle ear, known as the round window (fenestra rotunda) and the oval window (fenestra ovalis). The oscillations (vibrations) of the stapes hit the oval window and act like a miniature piston, setting the fluids of the inner ear and the cochlea into vibration. The middle ear also contains two muscles.

The middle ear is an air-filled cavity which connects to the pharynx (throat) by a tube known as the eustachian tube. This tube allows the adjustment of pressure between the middle ear and the outside. The opening into the pharynx from the eustachian tube is protected by a flap of cartilage which opens during swallowing.

The horse is unique in that it has two large sacs connected to each of the two eustachian tubes and these are known as the guttural pouches. They are situated between the pharynx and the skull and have a capacity of about 300 ml. The guttural pouches lie very close to important nerves and arteries, and there is a condition known as guttural pouch mycosis (caused by a fungus) which can be life-threatening if the vital nerves and blood vessels become affected.

Inner Ear

The inner ear is divided into the outer bony labyrinth and the inner membranous labyrinth, which consists of a series of membranous tubes filled with a fluid known as endolymph. The bony labyrinth is a series of cavities in the temporal bone which include the cochlea, vestibule and semi-circular canals and is bathed by a fluid known as perilymph, the whole structure being embedded deep in the skull (Figure 11.12).

The vestibule is the middle area of the bony labyrinth and is oval shaped. It contains the membranous labyrinth. This performs two functions: hearing, and balance and orientation. The membranous labyrinth in turn is made up of two sacs, namely the utricle and saccule.

Behind the vestibule sit three semi-circular canals:

- the horizontal semi-circular canal (lateral)
- the superior semi-circular canal (anterior)
- the posterior semi-circular canal (inferior).

The anterior and inferior canals are vertical, while the lateral canal is horizontal. The semi-circular canals all lie at right angles to each other and are continuous with the main membranous tubes of the inner ear, that is, they share its endolymph. When the horse moves its head from a resting position, the fluid or endolymph within the semi-circular canals is set in motion. According to the plane of movement (vertical, horizontal, etc.) the movement of endolymph is restricted to a particular canal in that plane. Thus if the horse is moving its head sideways, the fluid within the horizontal semi-circular canal will be moving the most. So, depending upon the angle of the head, the endolymph moves within the semi-circular canals and this results in impulses being sent to the brain. The brain can then interpret these signals and balance accordingly.

Cochlea The cochlea is a bony spinal canal structure which is wound spirally rather like a snail's shell. Transverse section through the cochlea shows it is made up of three channels:

- Cochlea duct – continues from the membranous labyrinth into the cochlea and is therefore filled with endolymph.
- Scala vestibuli – ends at the oval window.
- Scala tympani – ends at the round window.

The scala vestibuli and scala tympani are completely separated (except for an opening at the top of the cochlea), even though both are part of the bony labyrinth section of the cochlea and are therefore filled with perilymph.

There is a basilar membrane which lies between the cochlear duct and the scala tympani and resting on top of this is the organ of hearing known as the organ of Conti, consisting of supporting cells and hair cells. The hair cells are the receptors for sound or auditory sensation. A series of events follow sound waves entering the ear and causing movement of the small bones,

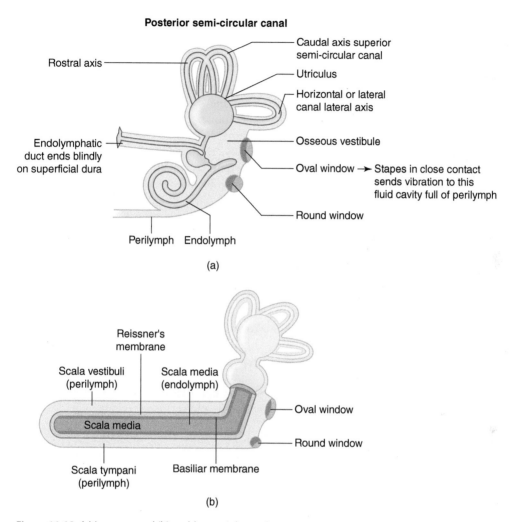

Posterior semi-circular canal

Rostral axis

Caudal axis superior semi-circular canal

Utriculus

Horizontal or lateral canal lateral axis

Endolymphatic duct ends blindly on superficial dura

Osseous vestibule

Oval window → Stapes in close contact sends vibration to this fluid cavity full of perilymph

Round window

Perilymph   Endolymph

(a)

Reissner's membrane

Scala vestibuli (perilymph)

Scala media (endolymph)

Scala media

Oval window

Round window

Scala tympani (perilymph)

Basiliar membrane

(b)

Figure 11.12 (a) Inner ear and (b) cochlea straightened out.

eventually resulting in pressure waves in the endolymph causing the basilar membrane to vibrate, moving the hair cells. Bending of the hair cells results in the sensory neurons generating nerve impulses, which are conducted along the vestibulocochlear nerve. The louder the sound, the higher the intensity of vibrations of the basilar membrane, leading to higher frequency of nerve impulses to the medulla oblongata of the brain. Each area of the basement membrane is able to detect different pitches. From the medulla oblongata, axons extend to the primary auditory area of the frontal lobe. The right and left areas each receive information from both the horse's ears.

Horses also use their ears to give visual signals to other horses and humans. The position of the ears provides signs as to the mood of the horse. Pricked ears are typical of horses that are alert, interested or startled. If the ears are pinned flat back, this is a threat signal. In the wild situation, the pinning back of the ears was a protective measure in the case of attack by a predator. If the ears are pinned back, they are less likely to be torn or damaged.

Taste and Smell

The senses of taste and smell are very closely linked in horses, so much so that they are often thought to be inseparable. Many horses are renowned for being fussy feeders. They seem readily to go off their feed and this may be partly to do with the fact that horses cannot vomit and they therefore have to be extremely careful in their choice of food. Unlike humans, who can be sick to get rid of an offending substance before it causes too much harm, it will have to pass right through a horse's digestive tract and this could cause quite serious health problems.

Taste sensations are produced from minute raised areas on the tongue called papillae on which the taste buds are situated (Figure 11.13). Taste buds are located on the tongue, soft palate and back of the throat, the highest concentration of taste receptors (nervous supply) being situated at the back of the tongue and these specialised receptors are enclosed in the membrane which covers the tongue. These nerve endings send messages to the brain. The taste buds consist of gustatory and support cells which are arranged in barrel-shaped groups with hair-like projections which protrude through a pore at the top (on the tongue surface). The taste buds of the horse are melon-shaped and slightly smaller than those found in cows and sheep. Although it is known that there are five specific tastes in man – sweet, salt, bitter, umami and sour (acid) – it is known that horses can at least distinguish salty and sweet. In fact, like people, horses are known to have a sweet tooth, appreciating such things as apples, carrots and honey. Horses are also known to tolerate substances (including medications) that people generally find very bitter. There are considerable differences between different species.

The sense of smell (olfaction) is commonly associated with seeking and selecting food and water, and is also a communication system within groups of horses. Horses, particularly those in the wild situation, need to be able to smell the presence of predators so they can make their escape. This highly developed sense of smell enables wild Equidae to detect blood from freshly killed animals up to 2 miles away. The sense of smell is also important in horses for reproductive patterns and social behaviour.

All horses have the ability to hold up their noses and curl the upper lip in a gesture known as Flehmen (see Figure 9.9). This is

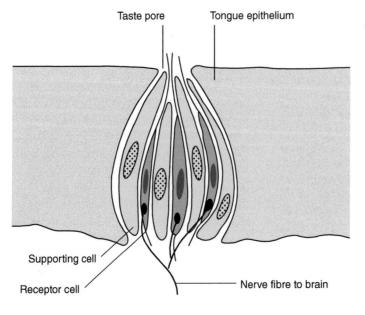

Taste pore   Tongue epithelium

Supporting cell

Receptor cell

Nerve fibre to brain

Figure 11.13 Structure of a taste bud.

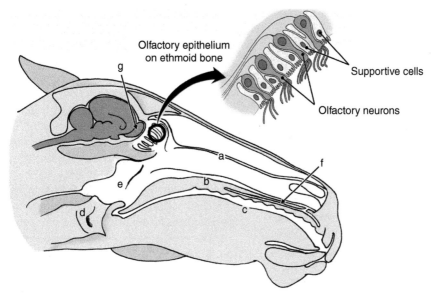

Figure 11.14 The olfactory system. The view is of the equine head in sagittal section. Inset shows a microscopic view of the olfactory epithelium, which covers the ethmoid bone within the caudodorsal nasal cavity. a, Nasal cavity; b, palate; c, oral cavity; d, larynx; e, pharynx; f, vomeronasal organ; g, olfactory bulb of the brain. *Source*: Frandson 2009. Reproduced with permission of John Wiley & Sons.

often seen when horses are presented with a strange or strong smell, but it is most often seen in stallions in their courtship activity with mares that are in oestrus. Horses also use their sense of smell to smell droppings on the pasture or a patch of grass which has been staled upon by another horse. Stallions or geldings showing stallion-like behaviour will then dung on top of these smells to mark the territory as their own.

The Olfactory System

The sense of smell is associated with the olfactory system (Figure 11.14). The horse's nasal passages contain two tightly rolled turbinate bones which increase the surface area of the nasal passages. The turbinates divide each nasal passage into three channels known as the dorsal meatus, medial meatus and ventral meatus, respectively. The dorsal meatus is closed at the back and it conducts air breathed into the olfactory region. Olfactory nerve cells are scattered among support cells throughout the mucous membranes within these areas of the nose.

Each olfactory cell bears a tuft of tiny hair-like projections which are the actual receptors for the sense of smell. Because the inside of the nose is moist, it follows that the material to be smelled must go into a solution before it can reach the sensory cells; however, some very fine particles may be smelled without actually dissolving first. There are several sinuses in each half of the skull, which fill partly with air during the breathing process, but they play no part in the sense of smell.

Jacobson's Organ

Otherwise known as the vomeronasal organ, Jacobson's organ is an elongated sac which opens into the nose. This organ is well developed in horses. Its lining contains olfactory cells and it is thought that these organs are particularly efficient at detecting scents from other horses. These are chemical signals known as pheromones. This enables groups of horses to recognise one another and individual herds in the wild have their own identification system. When new horses are introduced to a group, they will blow air into each other's nose as a process of recognition.

Summary Points

1) Horses use the central nervous system (CNS) and sensory receptors to give them the ability to see, hear, taste, smell, touch, feel pain, respond to changes in temperature and determine the position of their body.
2) Sensory receptors are specialised cells adapted for detection of changes to the internal and external environment. They are either neurons or connected to other neurons and may be enclosed in sense organs.
3) Both rods and cones contain pigments which undergo chemical changes in the presence of light. These are called photochemicals. Rods contain a pigment known as visual purple or rhodopsin, whereas cones contain iodopsin.
4) Horses are able to hear sounds outside of the human range and can detect sounds from low to very high frequencies, in the range of 14 Hz to 25 kHz, compared to the human range of 20 Hz to 20 kHz.
5) The organ of hearing is also known as the organ of Conti and consists of supporting cells and hair cells. The hair cells are the receptors for sound or auditory sensation.

Q + A

Q What is transduction?
A The changing of heat, pressure or light signals, for example, into electrical signals in neurons.

Q What are somatic receptors?
A These are receptors 'of the body' and so include receptors in the skin, such as mechanoreceptors, thermoreceptors and nociceptors, and those in muscles, joints, tendons ligaments and so on.

Q Name the two layers of the retina.
A The neural layer and pigmented layer.

Q How do horses see colour?
A By dichromatic vision – as a result of horses having two types of cones in their eyes: short-wavelength-sensitive cone (S), which is optimal at 428 nm, and mid- to long-wavelength-sensitive cone (M/L), which is optimal at 539 nm.

Q What is Jacobson's organ?
A Otherwise known as the vomeronasal organ, this is an elongated sac which opens into the nose. This organ is well developed in horses. Its lining contains olfactory cells and it is thought that these organs are particularly efficient at detecting scents from other horses. These are chemical signals known as pheromones.

12

Reproduction

Reproduction is a vital part of any mammalian life, the horse being no exception. Horses must reproduce in order to survive as a species. The survival of any species depends on the success of generations that follow. Genetic material (genes) is passed from one generation to another at the time of conception. Sexual reproduction involves the fusion of gametes from the mare and stallion. The mare's gametes are ova and the stallion's gametes are spermatozoa. Sexual reproduction also involves mixing of the genetic material of both parents to produce a foal that is genetically different from either – producing a genetically unique offspring.

All mares are naturally seasonal breeders, that is, they come into oestrus regularly during the season, which in their case is spring to autumn. In the breeding of Thoroughbred (TB) horses, extra demands are placed upon mares as an artificial breeding season is used to encourage mares to foal as near as possible to 1 January. All TB foals in the northern hemisphere are officially aged from this date irrespective of their actual date of birth. Those foals born nearer to 1 January will be bigger, stronger and faster when they are raced as 2 year olds than others born later in the year. As a result, the artificial breeding season for mares has been determined by the authorities as running from 15 February to 15 July (in the southern hemisphere, the TB breeding season runs from 12 August to 15 January). The natural breeding season of the mare would normally begin around mid-April until September,

with maximum ovarian activity occurring in mid-July. It is therefore quite obvious that a large number of TB mares will have difficulty conceiving when their fertility is not at its peak (Figure 12.1).

Reproductive Anatomy of the Mare

The reproductive system of the mare consists of two ovaries and the genital tract, which is composed of the vulva, vagina, cervix, uterus, cervix and fallopian tubes. All these are suspended within the body cavity by a sheet of strong connective tissue known as the broad ligament (Figure 12.2).

Vulva

The external genitalia of the mare are shown in Figure 12.3. The vulva protects the entrance to the vagina. This is the external opening of the mare's genital tract. The lips of the vulva are arranged vertically on either side of the vulval opening and are situated immediately below the anus. The vulval lips are covered by thin pigmented skin which contains sweat and sebaceous glands. Beneath the skin lie muscles which also fuse with the anal sphincter.

The lips of the vulva should meet evenly and have a good vulval seal to reduce entry from external potential pathogens and prevent air being sucked in, a condition known as pneumovagina. Previous births or vulvoplasty (Caslick's operation) where part of

Equine Science, Third Edition. Zoe Davies and Sarah Pilliner.
© 2018 Zoe Davies and Sarah Pilliner. Published 2018 by John Wiley & Sons Ltd.

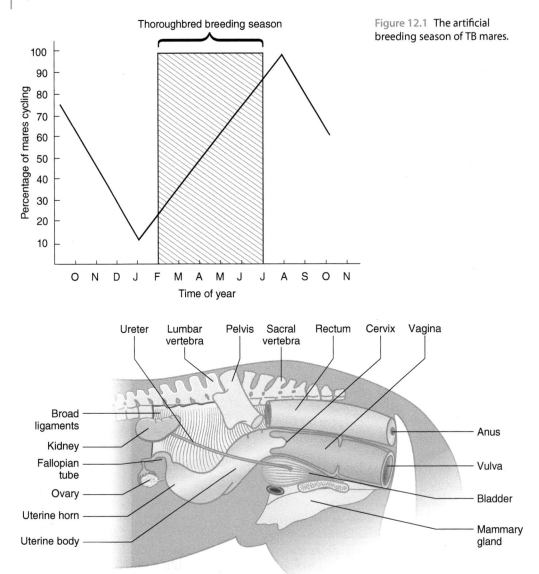

Figure 12.1 The artificial breeding season of TB mares.

Figure 12.2 The reproductive system of the mare.

the vulva is stitched following pregnancy confirmation may permanently alter the vulval seal, possibly allowing urine to collect inside or the vulva may have gaps which allow air to be sucked in, possibly carrying bacteria and other pathogenic organisms. The vulva elongates prior to parturition. The clitoris is located just inside the ventral commissure and has three sinuses associated with it. The central sinus is the largest. A swab is often taken from the clitoral fossa to test for contagious equine metritis (CEM), caused by *Taylorella equigenitalis*, a bacteria renowned for causing infertility. Mares must have a certificate showing they are free from this highly contagious disease before they will be accepted by a stud. Sinuses are the areas where mares may evert the clitoris during 'winking', which many mares do during oestrus.

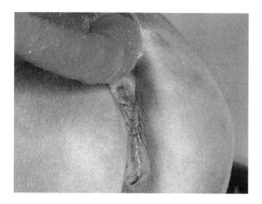

Figure 12.3 External genitalia of the mare. *Source*: Courtesy of Harthill Stud.

There are three seals within the genital tract:

- vulval seal
- vestibular seal
- cervix.

The vestibular seal is formed by the roof of the vagina and the floor of the pelvic girdle and hymen. The cervical seal opens during oestrus.

Vagina

Covered by peritoneum, the vagina is a muscular tube, lined by a mucous coat and is very elastic. The vagina secretes acid to kill bacteria, but this is also spermicidal and so stallions must ejaculate as close to or through the cervix as possible to avoid this. The vagina is approximately 20 cm (8 in) long and 12 cm (5 in) in diameter and extends from the cervix to the vulva. The terminal end of the vagina is known as the vestibule and this is separated from the main body of the vagina by a thin fold known as the hymen.

A vestibular seal is formed by the posterior vagina and by the pillars which support the hymen, and this helps to prevent the entry of dirt and bacteria into the uterus. Although the vagina plays this protective role, it is frequently liable to infections itself. On the floor of the vagina at the junction with the vestibule lies the urethral opening which allows urine to drain from the bladder. The vagina forms a channel for the entrance of the stallion's penis and for the birth of the foal. It follows therefore that it has to expand a great deal to allow a foal through and it is consequently composed of a thick muscular layer and an elastic mucous coat, which secretes mucus.

Cervix

The cervix is a tight, thick sphincter which lies at the opening of the uterus. When the mare is in dioestrus, that is, not in season, this is tightly closed. The cervix relaxes during oestrus. The lining of the cervix is highly folded and these folds slow the passage of spermatozoa following ejaculation, meaning that sperm may still be moving up the reproductive tract 24 hours after ejaculation. This increases the time period for successful ovulation and conception. The cervix plays a vital role in protecting both the foetus and the mare by being tightly closed when the mare is pregnant or not in season. This prevents the entrance of infection to the womb.

Uterus

The uterus is a muscular sac which consists of two horns, a body and a neck (cervix) (Figure 12.4). This is known as a bicornuate simplex uterus (previously termed bipartite) due to the large size of the horse's body compared to other mammals. Also there is no septum dividing the uterine body. Humans have a simplex uterus which consists of no horns, one body and one cervix.

In horses, the embryo will develop in the horn of the uterus, whereas in humans the embryo develops in the body. The horns of the equine uterus are about 25 cm (10 in) long and the body 18–20 cm (7–8 in) in length and 10 cm (4 in) in diameter. The uterus is a hollow muscular organ which joins the cervix at one end and the fallopian tubes at the other. It is attached by the broad ligaments, which are out-foldings of the peritoneum to the spine. Older mares that have had several foals tend to have larger uteruses.

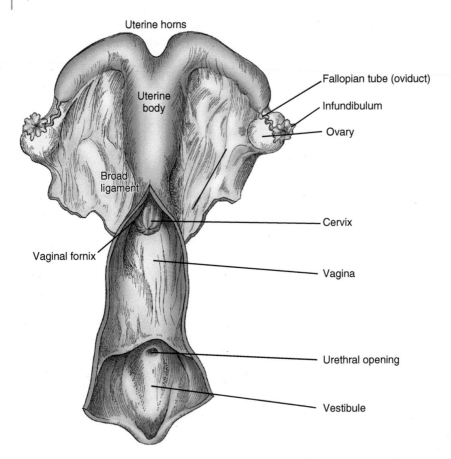

Figure 12.4 Anatomy of the equine uterus. *Source*: Frandson 2009. Reproduced with permission of John Wiley & Sons.

The wall of the uterus consists of three layers: an outer serous layer which is continuous with the broad ligament, a muscular layer called the myometrium which contains a layer of longitudinal muscle fibres, and an inner layer of circular muscle fibres and a mucous membrane which in the uterus is known as the endometrium. The endometrium comprises epithelial cells, connective tissue and glands.

Utero-tubular Junction

The utero-tubular junction separates the fallopian tubes from the uterine horns and is a narrowing. Fertilisation takes place just on the side of the fallopian tubes at the utero tubular junction. If fertilisation is successful the fertilised ova can then move into the uterine horn. It is thought that fertilised ova can actively control their own movement, probably via local secretions of hormones (oestrogens). Unfertilised ova remain in the fallopian tube and slowly degenerate.

Fallopian Tubes

Otherwise known as oviducts, fallopian tubes are continuous with the uterine horns and carry the ovulated mature egg to the horn. The horn end is known as the isthmus and the ampulla is the end near the ovaries. They are coiled and are approximately 25–30 cm (8–12 in) long and 2–3 mm (0.08–0.12 in) in diameter. Because they are continuous with the horns they have a similar structure. The ovarian end of the fallopian tube is funnel shaped and is known as the infundibulum.

This has irregular finger-like projections known as fimbriae which completely surround the part of the ovary where the egg is released, without being in direct contact. Here the fimbria attract and catch the released ova. The mucous membrane lining helps waft the ova towards the utero-tubular junction. The sperm, if present, will fertilise the egg in the fallopian tube before the resultant embryo passes into the uterus. The infundibulum is closely associated with the ova fossa, which is unique in mares and is the only site of ovulation.

Ovaries

The ovaries are a pair of bean-shaped glands of the mare and are the primary reproductive organs, containing many thousand eggs or ova. The ovaries are bean shaped due to the ovulation fossa – an indentation where ovulation takes place in mares. The ovaries also produce hormones (endocrine) and cells (cytogenic). Each mare is born with several hundred thousand immature eggs and no more will appear through her lifetime. There is little activity in the ovaries until puberty, which in the mare takes place between the first and second year. After puberty, mature eggs are released from the ovaries at regular intervals under hormonal control. Puberty begins at 10–24 months, with an average onset of about 18 months in mares.

The ovaries are situated between the last rib and the point of the hip, and they are also responsible for the secretion of the female hormone oestrogen. The ovaries vary in size and shape depending on the stage of the oestrus cycle. For example, the ovaries of maiden mares and those throughout the winter months are approximately 2–4 cm (1–1.75 in) long and 2–3 cm(1–1.5 in) wide, whereas in spring the ovaries may be double this size. The utero-ovarian artery and utero-ovarian nerve, respectively, provide the ovaries with a blood and nervous supply.

The ovaries are covered by a lining of smooth membrane known as the peritoneum, except at the attached border known as the hilus where nerves and blood vessels enter. The point of attachment of the hilus has a convex border. Another unique structure of the mare's ovary is the peripheral vascular area around an inner area of parenchyma which contains the developing and degenerating ovarian follicles, the corpus luteum and corpus albicans. The parenchyma surfaces at the ovulation fossa.

The ovaries are composed of:

- a central portion or medulla
- a dense outer section known as the stroma (or cortex).

The stroma and medulla are not separated by a distinct line but blend together at an indistinct corticomedullary border. The stroma is the region containing interstitial cells that provide support and the germinal cells which produce ova. The immature ova (known as oogonia) grow here and the development of follicles and the resultant formation of the corpus luteum take place here. The number of potential ova at birth is the final number, that is, no more are produced. Each ovum begins as a primordial germ cell and is surrounded by a gradually enlarging fluid-filled sac known as the Graafian follicle (Figure 12.5).

There are far more oogonia than the mare will need during her reproductive life. Oogonia have the full complement of chromosomes at 32 pairs (64) and are surrounded by a single layer of epithelial cells. These are known as primordial follicles. These develop prior to puberty into primary oocytes and then undergo the first stage of meiosis cell division. Following puberty, hormones from the anterior pituitary gland stimulate further development.

Following puberty, primary oocytes undertake later stages of meiosis, and not all will fully develop. Epithelial cells that surround the primary oocytes differentiate into follicular epithelial cells which secrete follicular fluid into the cavity around the oocyte. The primary oocyte then becomes larger and a thick outer jelly-like layer is produced around the outside known as the

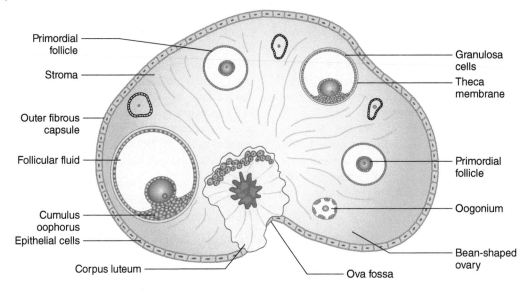

Figure 12.5 Section through an ovary.

zona pellucida. At this point it has half the number (or haploid number) of chromosomes, that is, 16 pairs (32), and is known as the secondary oocyte. It moves itself to the inner edge of the follicle, where it lies on follicular cells called cumulus oophorus. The theca membrane is then organised around the follicle by the storm. The follicle grows to around 3 cm and is known as the Graafian follicle.

At oestrus the mature Graafian follicle ruptures and the ova is expelled through the ovulation fossa into the dilated end of the fallopian tube. Follicles destined for ovulation are usually greater then 3cm and move towards the ovulation fossa in preparation. This process is known as ovulation. The ruptured follicle then undergoes three separate stages, known as the corpus haemorrhagicum (red body), corpus luteum (either of oestrus or pregnancy) and corpus albicans (non-functional). All follicle development and the corpus luteum development take place internally in the medulla of the ovary.

Immediately after the mature follicle has been released, the remaining follicle collapses and bleeding occurs into its centre, forming a clot called the corpus haemorrhagicum. Blood vessels and specialist cells known as fibroblasts enter the tissue to form the corpus luteum, which then begins to secrete the hormone progesterone. The corpus luteum does not project from the surface of the ovary, as in the cow and pig, but is embedded in the main body. Eventually the corpus luteum becomes non-functional if a pregnancy does not establish itself, and the active luteal cells are replaced by scar tissue.

In most mammals, from puberty onwards the primary oocytes develop and complete the final meiosis stages; however, in the mare, this first meiotic division occurs just after ovulation. This takes place at different rates, so that there is a regular supply of fully developed follicles for ovulation every 21 days during the breeding season. Normally one only will be ready for ovulation with each oestrus cycle.

The Oestrus Cycle

The oestrus cycle or sexual cycle describes alternating periods of sexual activity in the mare (Figures 12.6 and 12.7). It is controlled by hormones which are initially secreted by the pituitary gland. Mares begin oestrus cycles at puberty which is usually

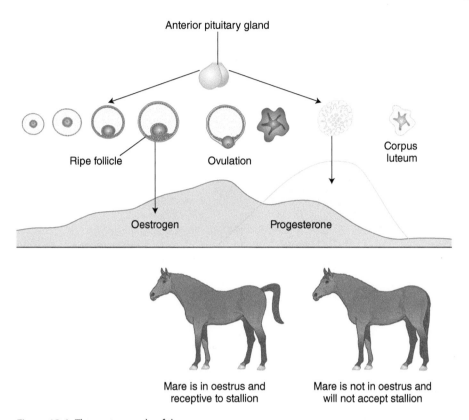

Anterior pituitary gland

Ripe follicle Ovulation

Corpus luteum

Oestrogen Progesterone

Mare is in oestrus and receptive to stallion

Mare is not in oestrus and will not accept stallion

Figure 12.6 The oestrus cycle of the mare.

around 1½ years of age. Mares are seasonally polyoestrus, which means that they come into oestrus many times during the breeding season and only during this time will they accept a stallion. In mares the season is spring through summer to autumn in the northern hemisphere. In the winter mares are in anoestrus which means there is no cyclical activity and the ovaries lie almost dormant. This is nature's way of ensuring foals will not be produced too early or late in the year when chances of survival in the wild would be less. Winter anoestrus is then followed by a period of change to regular cyclical activity or seasons. During this transitional phase the oestrus periods may be irregular or very long, up to a month or more. A mare's behaviour during this time is often not typical of a mare in season and therefore it may be difficult to assess accurately. During the first oestrus after the winter period, there is often a poor correlation between sexual behaviour and

ovarian activity. Sometimes these early heats do not show palpable follicles when the mare is investigated. However, once ovulation has occurred the mare will usually follow more regular oestrus cycles.

Oestrus may shorten from spring to summer. Early in the breeding season, through March and April, oestrus tends to be irregular and long, often with no ovulation. From May to July the periods become shorter and more regular, with ovulation as a normal part of the cycle. Ovulation usually occurs 1–2 days before the end of oestrus. Fertility increases during oestrus and is at a peak 2 days before rapidly falling off. Mares with longer oestrus periods should be bred on the third or fourth day and again 48–72 hours later. If oestrus is longer than 9 days, it is better to wait until the next oestrus cycle. Many mares with regular short oestrus periods throughout the year can be successfully bred at any time of the year.

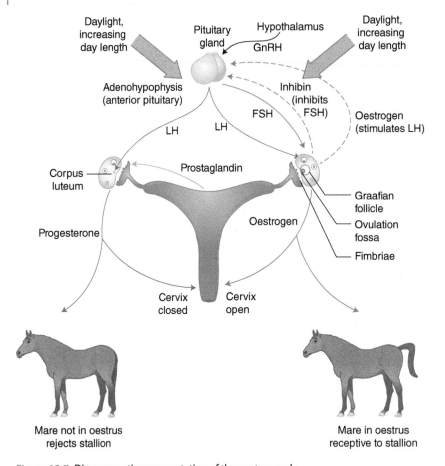

Figure 12.7 Diagrammatic representation of the oestrus cycle.

The oestrus cycle has two phases: oestrus ('heat', 'in season') when the mare is receptive to the stallion and ovulation takes place, and dioestrus (between oestrus periods) when the mare is unreceptive. The cycle typically lasts 21 days in the mare, oestrus lasting for approximately 5 days and dioestrus for 15–16 days. However, there is considerable individual variation in the length of oestrus cycles in mares. The oestrus cycle is a continuous pattern over the seasons of behavioural and endocrine changes. Mares will even come into season during lactation, unlike the ewe. This means mares can be pregnant and lactating at the same time, which is metabolically draining. The foal heat (first oestrus or heat period after foaling) occurs within 4–10 days following parturition, and usually only lasts for 2–4 days. Traditionally, mares have been covered on the ninth day post-foaling, but they often will not be very fertile at this time. The uterus usually has not had time to return to the normal 'non-pregnant' state and sometimes infection may be present after foaling. Some studs will therefore avoid this time for covering, but in TBs, where time is vital, the mares will often be covered.

Mares are termed polyseasonal spontaneous ovulators. Ovulation typically occurs on the last but one or last day of the oestrus cycle and this is fairly constant no matter what the length of oestrus is. A few hours before ovulation the tension in the follicle usually subsides. The presence of a large fluctuating follicle in the ovary is a sign of imminent ovulation.

Follicular Development or Oogenesis

The process of production of eggs and sperm is known as gametogenesis (Figure 12.8). Oogenesis is the name given to egg production and spermatogenesis to sperm production (see later). The end result of gametogenesis is to produce the eggs and sperm which have half the number of chromosomes of other body cells. This is required so that at fertilisation when the sperm fuses with the egg, the resultant embryo will have the full number of chromosomes (half from each parent). The process of gametogenesis involves a special type of cell division known as meiosis. Spermatogenesis and oogenesis vary slightly from each other in that during oogenesis only one egg and two polar bodies are formed. The polar bodies are simply by-products of the egg production process and, as far as we know, serve no useful function. Spermatogenesis, on the other hand, produces four sperms from one primary spermatocyte. There are, therefore, many more sperm produced than ova (see 'Spermatogenesis').

Ovarian Changes during the Oestrus Cycle

Just before the onset of oestrus, several follicles enlarge to approximately 1–3 cm (0.4–1.2 in) in size. By the first day of oestrus one of the follicles will be considerably larger than the others, having a diameter of approximately 2.5–3.5 cm (1–1.15 in). During oestrus this follicle matures and enlarges to about 3–7 cm (1.5–3.5 in). It contains follicular fluid. At this point ovulation takes place and the other follicles in the ovary begin to regress or reduce in size down to about 1 cm (0.4 in) in the following dioestrus period.

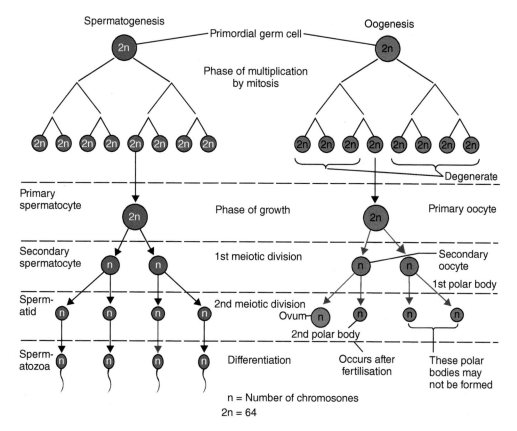

Figure 12.8 Gametogenesis – spermatogenesis and oogenesis.

The ovum is released and the remaining follicle then fills with blood, hence it is known as the corpus haemorrhagicum. The blood-filled follicle undergoes further changes over the next 3 days to become the corpus luteum, otherwise known as the yellow body. The corpus luteum is responsible for secreting the hormone progesterone. It reaches its maximum size approximately 4–5 days after ovulation and begins to regress at about 12 days after ovulation. As it regresses there is a corresponding fall in blood progesterone concentration.

Behavioural Signs of Oestrus in the Mare

As oestrus approaches, the mare will often become restless and irritable. She will frequently adopt the urinating posture known as micturition and eject urine while repeatedly exposing or 'winking' the clitoris (Figure 12.9).

Mares can often be seen 'showing' to geldings in neighbouring paddocks. When the stallion or teaser is introduced, the mare will tend to exaggerate these postures and she will raise her tail and lean her hindquarters towards the stallion. A clear mucus discharge may also be seen. The stallion will often exhibit 'Flehmen' where he rolls up his upper lip and stretches his neck outwards and upwards when the mare is in season. This is in response to pheromones present in the mare's urine. A mare that is not in oestrus will react violently towards the stallion's advances and will often kick out. This is the reason why a teaser is often used first, to prevent injury to a valuable stallion (Figure 12.10).

Summary of Mare Behaviour through the Cycle

- Oestrus – submissive, ears forward, legs straddled, tail held high, urinating, everting clitoris.
- Dioestrus – violent, ears back, squealing, tail clamped down.
- Transitional phase – ambivalent.
- Abnormal behaviour, idiosyncrasy.

Transitional mares are those in the phase between winter anoestrus (not cycling) and regular cyclic ovarian activity. The most common and easiest method to encourage early cycling is by simply leaving the lights on longer (see 'Light').

As oestrus approaches, some changes occur in the genitalia of the mare. The cervix becomes very relaxed and its protrusion can be felt lying on the floor of the vagina. The cervix also becomes a deep red colour and the vaginal walls glisten with clear mucus which lubricates the genital passages.

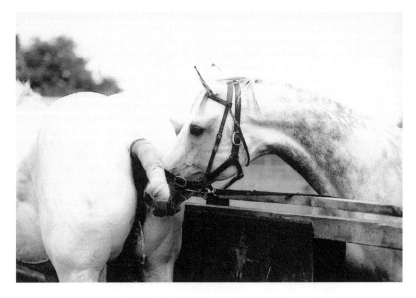

Figure 12.9 **Mare in season.**

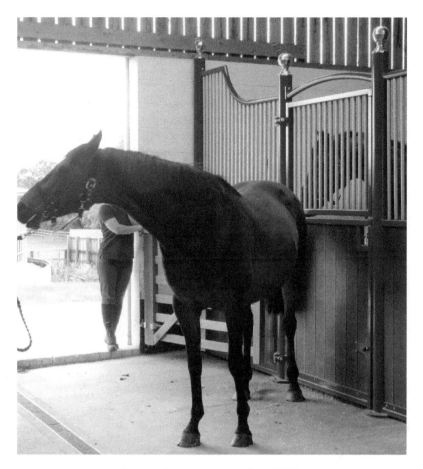

Figure 12.10 Teasing the mare. *Source*: Courtesy of Harthill Stud.

After ovulation, the cervix closes and the vagina becomes drier and paler in colour. The uterus also undergoes cyclical changes; as the corpus luteum grows and secretes progesterone, the uterus increases in tone and thickness, ready to accept an embryo if fertilisation occurs. During dioestrus and during the first few days of oestrus the uterus is flaccid.

Endocrine Changes during the Oestrus Cycle

The pituitary gland (hypophysis) is divided into two parts: the anterior pituitary (also called the adenohypophysis or pars anterior) and the posterior pituitary (or neurohypophysis). The anterior pituitary produces the gonadotropins luteinising hormone (LH) and follicle-stimulating hormone (FSH). The pituitary gland tends to be known as the 'master gland' because the hormones it produces regulate many other endocrine glands. Hormones involved in the oestrus cycle of mares are as follows:

- **Gonadotropin-releasing hormone (GnRH)** – a peptide hormone secreted by the hypothalamus in a pulsing manner which changes in amplitude through the ovarian cycle. It stimulates release of gonadotropins from the pituitary gland.
- **Gonadotropins** – glycoproteins, secreted by the anterior pituitary gland.
- **Luteinising hormone (LH)** – stimulates formation of the corpus luteum and with FSH stimulates oestrogen synthesis and ovulation.

- **Follicle stimulating hormone** (FSH) – stimulates ova production (growth and maturation of the follicle) and secretion of oestrogen (in the presence of LH).
- **Oestrogens** – steroid hormones, oestrogen is the generic term for an oestrogenic agent; the most potent oestrogen is oestradiol (estradiol), secreted by the ovary. Oestrogens stimulate the mare to be receptive to the stallion and cause changes in behaviour and the reproductive tract.
- **Inhibin** – a glycoprotein secreted by granulosa cells of developing follicles in the ovary. Inhibin has a negative feedback effect on FSH.
- **Activin** – a glycoprotein produced within granulosa cells in the ovaries. It is thought to play an almost directly opposite role to that of inhibin and is involved in many physiological functions, including stimulation of FSH synthesis in the pituitary gland; other roles include cell proliferation, cell differentiation, apoptosis and homeostasis. In mares activin has an effect on the anterior pituitary gland, resulting in increased FSH secretion.
- **Progesterone** – the most important progestogen and a steroid hormone, it maintains pregnancy and causes inhibition of sexual behaviour. Progestins are synthetic progestogens.
- **Prostaglandins** ($PGF_{2\alpha}$) – secreted by endometrial glands of the uterus and causes luteolysis of the corpus luteum.

The endocrine changes associated with the mare's oestrus cycle are as follows:

- Environmental factors such as increasing day length stimulate the hypothalamus to secrete the hormone GnRH, which in turn initiates the onset of oestrus activity in spring after the winter anoestrus period.
- GnRH causes the release of FSH from the pituitary gland which causes the development of follicles within the ovary. As these follicles develop they secrete oestrogen. These hormones are responsible for the changes in behaviour and physical changes in the genital tract as the mare comes into season and will accept the stallion.
- Rising levels of oestrogen then stimulate the pituitary gland to produce LH, and ovarian follicles secrete inhibin which reduces the amount of FSH being secreted. Ovulation occurs under the influence of LH and the ovum is released through the ovulation fossa into the fallopian tube ready for a possible fertilisation.
- The remaining follicle collapses and luteinises and oestrogen and inhibin secretions fall. A corpus luteum is formed in place of the burst follicle in the ovary. This corpus luteum, otherwise known as the yellow body, is responsible for the production of progesterone. This hormone has the opposite effect of oestrogen. Progesterone prepares the uterus to receive a fertilised egg and is essential for maintaining pregnancy.
- Rising progesterone from the corpus luteum and falling oestrogen is responsible for the changes in the mare's behaviour and genital tract which occur after ovulation. The mare then goes out of season (generally 24 hours post-ovulation).
- If conception takes place, maternal recognition of pregnancy occurs 14 days after ovulation. Recognition occurs because the blastocyst capsule secretes oestrogens preventing prostaglandin ($PGF_{2\alpha}$) secretion by the endometrial glands of the uterus. The corpus luteum continues to produce progesterone to maintain the pregnancy.
- If conception does not occur or there is a failure of recognition of a conceptus the uterus produces prostaglandins which results in luteolysis (which kills off the corpus luteum) in the ovary. As a result, progesterone secretion falls and this causes the anterior pituitary to secrete FSH and the cycle starts all over again.

Artificial Control of the Oestrus Cycle

In the management of horses there are times when some manipulation of the oestrus cycle is required. This is particularly likely in the breeding of TBs. Because of their artificial breeding season which begins on 15 February in the northern hemisphere, artificial means are often used to encourage the mare to come out of the winter anoestrus period and start coming into season early.

Light

The onset of cyclical activity in the mare is dependent upon the hours of daylight. The mare is stimulated into activity as the number of daylight hours increases due to the production of melatonin (see Chapter 9). If mares are stabled at the end of December and are subjected to artificial light, preferably of increasing duration, it is possible to advance the onset of normal cyclical activity so that there is oestrus and ovulation.

Melatonin affects the mare's reproductive system by inhibiting the secretion of LH and FSH from the anterior pituitary gland. This inhibitory effect is due to inhibition of GnRH from the hypothalamus, which is necessary for secretion of the anterior pituitary hormones.

Both tungsten and fluorescent lights have been used successfully, although the former seem to give better results. The provision of a minimum 100-watt bulb in each loose box is adequate. Day length should be increased from 1 October in a stepwise manner; that is, the light should be switched on at a later time each day, effectively increasing the day length by 30 minutes per week. A peak of 16 hours effective day length should be reached by 15 January and maintained for the rest of the winter. The lights do not have to be left on – it has been shown that a flash of light is all that is required to stimulate the pineal gland in the brain. More recently, a blue-light mask for mares kept out in the field for 24 hours a day has been developed; this follows research in humans which shows that release of melatonin is most strongly inhibited by blue light. Such a mask has been developed for field use (Figure 12.11). Scientists have evaluated a mobile blue-light mask's efficacy in suppressing mares' melatonin secretions, thereby inducing oestrus earlier in the year. The results found that exposing mares to as little as 10 lux via a

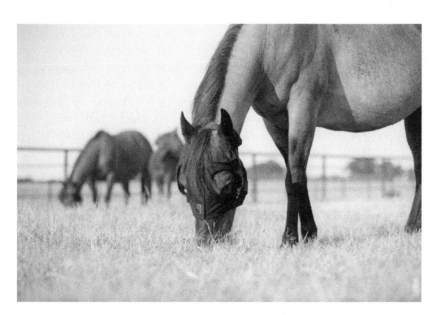

Figure 12.11 The Equilume™ Light Mask is an innovative method of providing light to horses to encourage the early onset of oestrus, following the winter anoestrus period. *Source*: Courtesy of Equilume Ltd.

blue-light mask effectively induced oestrus in healthy TBs.

Hormonal Methods

Many different hormones have been used to manipulate the oestrus cycle and there are a number of pharmaceutical options for inducing oestrus in transitional mares. The most common method is a progestin (synthetic progesterone) called altrenogest or (Regu-Mate™). Administering GnRH twice daily may also help hasten the breeding season; there are two GnRH analogues, namely deslorelin and buserelin. The administration of human chorionic gonadotropin (hCG) has also proven successful in inducing ovulation in mares within 48 hours of administration if the mare has a follicle measuring 3.5 cm before administration and she is in oestrus. Domperidone given orally stimulates prolactin production and therefore aids lactation in agalactic mares. It is also effective in bringing transitional mares into oestrus.

Once a mare has ovulated, oestrus and ovulation can be more easily manipulated. Altrenogest is mostly used for the following:

- synchronisation of oestrus for embryo transfer
- pregnancy maintenance, particularly high-risk pregnancies
- during transit abroad, as the stress of transportation may lower progesterone
- suppression of oestrus for problematical mares with dangerous behaviour when in season or when important competitions or races are affected.

Other more novel treatments are also used, including oxytocin injections during dioestrus, GnRH vaccines and intrauterine marbles. Marbles extend the corpus luteum function by tricking the mare into pregnancy. Researchers have also shown that infusing plant oil (such as corn or coconut oil) in the uterus might extend the corpus luteum function and suppress oestrus.

Postponing Ovulation

Breeders might wish to postpone ovulation – for example, if shipped semen has not arrived or the stallion of choice is not available for breeding. Altrenogest can be administered for 1 or 2 days when the follicle is 3.0–3.5 cm and this can delay ovulation, with fertility rates remaining the same.

Reproductive Anatomy of the Stallion

The male genitalia can be seen in Figure 12.12. The stallion's reproductive system consists of the following:

- two testes, each suspended by a spermatic cord and external cremaster muscle
- two epididymides
- two deferent ducts (vas deferens), each with an ampulla
- two seminal vesicles
- one prostate gland
- two bulbourethral glands
- urethra, penis and prepuce.

Function of the male reproductive system depends upon both endocrine and nervous stimulation. The reproductive tract is supported within the pelvic cavity by the genital fold externally by the scrotum and prepuce.

Scrotum

The testicles are carried in a sac known as the scrotum which is situated between the hind legs. The scrotum is a skin pouch composed of two scrotal sacs, one for each testis, separated by a septum. The sacs lie either side of and below the penis. Often one testis may be slightly larger than the other, leading to scrotal asymmetry. The scrotum has four layers consisting of:

- skin – contains sweat glands to keep the area cool
- tunica dartos – smooth muscle raises and lowers the testes
- fascia – allows mobility for vertical and lateral movement
- vaginal tunic – extends from the abdominal cavity through the inguinal canal to the

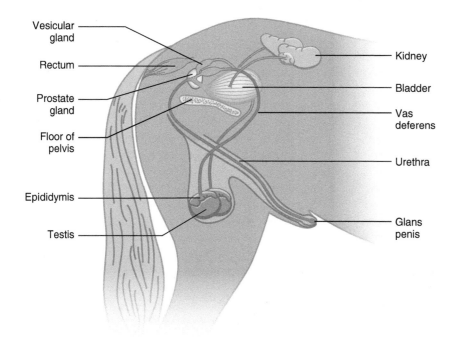

Vesicular gland
Rectum
Prostate gland
Floor of pelvis
Epididymis
Testis

Kidney
Bladder
Vas deferens
Urethra
Glans penis

Figure 12.12 Stallion genitalia. This figure was produced with kind permission of the copyright holder Wiley-Blackwell from Angus O. McKinnon, Edwards L. Squires, Wendy E. Vaala and Dickson D. Varner (2011) Equine Reproduction, Vols 1 & 2, 2nd edn. Oxford: Wiley-Blackwell.

bottom of the scrotum and contains watery fluid which aids movement of testes.

The scrotum is situated outside the body, as the temperature inside the body is too high for spermatozoa maturation and development. The temperature in the scrotum is approximately 4–7°C cooler than that in the body. The scrotum is designed to lose heat when the external temperature is warm. When it is cold, a muscle known as the cremaster muscle, retracts the testis against the body to reduce heat loss.

Testes (Testicles)

The stallion normally has two testes which are the male gonads that produce sperm and testosterone. They are egg-shaped and covered with a layer of heavy fibrous connective tissue known as the tunica albuginea. The mature testes are about 6–12 cm (2.4–5 in) long, 5 cm (2 in) wide and 4.7 cm (1.75–3.5 in) high (Figure 12.13).

In the foetus, the testes develop near the kidneys and well inside the body cavity. Approximately 1 month before birth, testes start to descend into the scrotum, although they are very small at this stage. They enter the inguinal canal before closure of the internal inguinal ring, during the first 2 weeks after birth, and descend into the scrotum. Hence newborn foals normally have both testes in the scrotum within 2 weeks of birth.

The testes are guided in their journey by a fibrous cord known as the gubernaculum which extends from the testis through the inguinal canal to the scrotum. This cord is quite thick to begin with, but becomes narrower once its function is complete. The testes have to descend through an opening in the abdominal wall before they reach the scrotum. This is known as the inguinal ring. The testes are held fairly close to the abdominal wall in the horse near to the inguinal ring. Sometimes one or both testes fail to descend and remain within the abdominal cavity; such

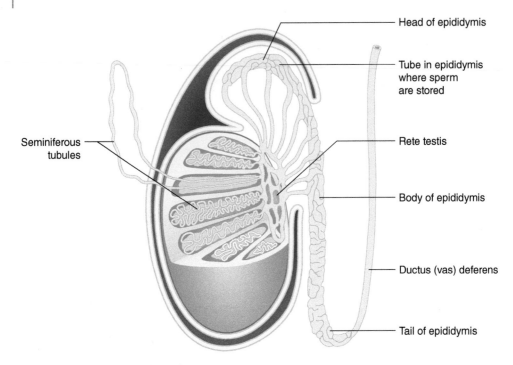

Figure 12.13 Cross-section through a testis.

horses are known as cryptorchids or rigs and often display stallion-like behaviour due to circulating testosterone. The condition is known as cryptorchidism.

By the time the horse is 2 years old, the testes have reached their full size. The growth of the testes is, however, controlled by hormones which also control sperm production. Once the testes are mature, the male hormone testosterone is produced. Age, season and sexual use will affect testis size and weight. Testicular function, semen constituents and circulating hormone levels also vary month to month. Leydig cells in the interstitial tissue of the testes produce steroid hormones, including testosterone. The pre-pubertal stage begins at approximately 6 months of age and few colts produce sufficient sperm for ejaculation before 14 months of age.

The testis consists of a mass of tiny tubes known as the seminiferous tubules surrounded by a heavy fibrous capsule called the tunica albuginea (see above). A number of fibrous divisions known as trabeculae divide the testis into sections called lobules which pass inward from the tunica albuginea to form a stroma (framework) to support the tubules. Within these small tubules are the cells that divide to form the spermatozoa or sperm (Figure 12.14). These cells also produce testosterone. The seminiferous tubules converge towards the front of the testis where they pass through the outer covering to merge into the epididymis.

Epididymis

The epididymis is a U-shaped, long, convoluted tube which collects the spermatozoa produced by the seminiferous tubules and connects with the vas deferens. The head of the epididymis attaches to the same end of the testes where blood vessels and nerves enter. The epididymis serves as a place for sperm to mature prior to ejaculation. Sperm are immature when they leave the testis and must undergo a period of maturation (usually 10–15 days) within the epididymis before they are capable of fertilising ova.

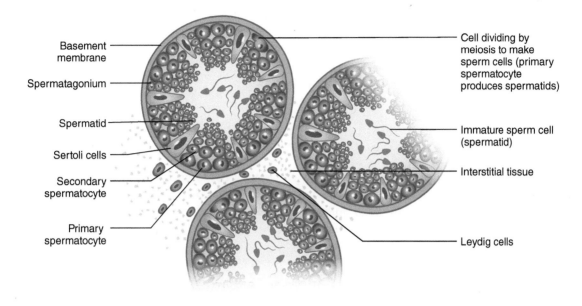

Basement membrane

Spermatagonium

Spermatid

Sertoli cells

Secondary spermatocyte

Primary spermatocyte

Cell dividing by meiosis to make sperm cells (primary spermatocyte produces spermatids)

Immature sperm cell (spermatid)

Interstitial tissue

Leydig cells

(a)

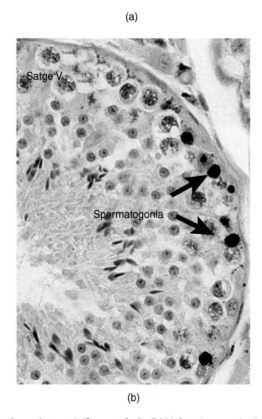

Satge V

Spermatogonia

(b)

Figure 12.14 (a) Section through a seminiferous tubule. (b) Light microscopic view of a cross-section of an equine seminiferous tubule, showing the nuclei of some spermatogonia. *Source*: McKinnon 2011. Reproduced with permission of John Wiley & Sons.

Vas Deferens

The vas deferens is a muscular tube which at the time of ejaculation propels the sperm and associated fluids from the epididymis to the urethra, a tube that carries urine from the bladder to the end of the penis. The vas deferens passes through the inguinal canal as part of the spermatic cord (which connects the testes with the rest of the body), and then it separates from the vascular and nervous parts of the cord and runs backward to enter the pelvic cavity. As the vas deferens approaches the bladder, the walls enlarge to form the ampulla (which is well developed in the stallion), after which it decreases in size to unite with the urethra.

Accessory Sex Glands

During ejaculation the accessory sex glands secrete approximately 60–90% of the total ejaculate volume. These glands produce a favourable medium for the carriage and nourishment of mature sperm. The accessory glands consist of the vesicular gland (seminal vesicles), the prostate and the bulbo-urethral (Cowper's) glands.

Vesicular Gland (Seminal Vesicles)

In the stallion the vesicular gland consists of a pair of hollow, pear-shaped sacs which lie either side of the bladder. The contraction of smooth muscles during ejaculation empties the secretions into the urethra. The excretory ducts of the vesicular glands open near the bifurcation where the ampullae merge with the urethra.

Several organic compounds found in secretion of the vesicular glands are unique in that they are not found in substantial quantities elsewhere in the body. Two of these compounds, fructose and sorbitol, are major sources of energy. Both phosphate and carbonate buffers are found in these secretions and are important in that they protect against shifts in the pH of semen. Such shifts in pH would be detrimental to spermatozoa.

Prostate Gland

The prostate gland is a bi-lobed discrete structure, shaped like a walnut. It is situated near the beginning of the urethra and releases a milky alkaline secretion into the urethra through a series of ducts.

Bulbo-Urethral Gland (Cowper's Gland)

In horses and other mammals, two glands – the bulbo-urethral glands – lie on either side of the urethra and release a clear fluid that flushes the urethra prior to ejaculation, although their true function seems unclear in stallions.

Penis

The penis is the male organ of copulation. It is composed of three general areas: the glans penis (free extremity, which is enlarged at the free end); the main portion (body); and two paired roots (crura) which attach to the ischial arch of the pelvis and together with the ischiocavernosus muscles are found in the shaft of the glans penis.

The penis is highly haemodynamic and musculocutaneous, containing many blood vessels and nerves. Erectile (or cavernous) tissue called the corpus cavernosum is contained within the tunica albuginea. When the stallion is sexually stimulated, the penis becomes engorged with blood – more blood enters through the arterial supply than leaves through the veins – causing the penis to double in length and thickness. The end of the glans penis is surrounded by a prominent margin or rose. This enlarges to three times its resting size after ejaculation. The end of the urethra projects through this rose. The free portion of the non-erect penis is covered by the sheath or prepuce which consists of a double fold of skin, so that two concentric layers surround the penis. This can be quite voluminous and may cause a sucking noise when the horse is trotting. Large glands in this area produce a fatty cheese-like substance called smegma. This can often become foul-smelling and irritating to the horse if allowed to accumulate.

Spermatogenesis

Spermatogenesis is the term for the formation of mature male gametes or sex cells from the most undifferentiated germ cells. It includes several mitotic cell divisions followed by two meiotic cell divisions, during which the chromosome number is reduced by half, that is, from diploid to haploid. This series of cell divisions is known as spermatocytogenesis.

Sperm are produced within the seminiferous tubules. The germinal epithelium which makes up the boundary of the seminiferous tubules contains the primary sex cells, otherwise known as germ cells. Seminiferous tubules are lined by germinal cells and Sertoli cells. Sertoli cells coordinate differentiation of germ cells and also form a testis–blood barrier. These cells are called spermatogonia and are attached to the wall of the tubule and nursed by the Sertoli cells. These cells are constantly dividing, and as new cells are formed they move gradually into the centre. Approximately 70,000 sperm are developed per second. They are dividing and maturing as follows on a 57-day cycle:

- spermatogonia
- primary spermatocytes
- secondary spermatocytes
- spherical spermatids
- elongated spermatids
- spermatozoa.

Once ready, spermatozoa are liberated from the seminiferous tubule, where they go into straight seminiferous tubules and an area known as the rete testis where fluid is added. The rete testis is a network of tubules which drains into the efferent ductules. The efferent ductules coalesce into a single epididymal duct. Sperm is then moved through efferent ducts into the proximal epididymis and fluid

is resorbed in the caput epididymis. Sperm must be matured in the corpus epididymis before being stored in the cauda epididymis and ampullae. Seminal plasma is added by the seminal vesicles and prostate gland and gel is also added by seminal vesicles ready for ejaculation.

This process of multiplication and development of the spermatogonia to form spermatozoa is known as spermatogenesis (see Figure 12.8).

The sex cells undergo several changes:

- Spermatogonia – these increase in number by multiplying through a process called mitosis. The resultant cells all have the same number of chromosomes as the cell from which they derived and these are known as primary spermatocytes.
- Primary spermatocytes – these travel inwards and undergo a type of cell division known as meiosis, where the chromosome number of the resultant cells is reduced by half. One primary spermatocyte produces two secondary spermatocytes each with half the number of chromosomes. The two secondary spermatocytes produced then divide again by mitosis (so they still retain the same chromosome number) to form four spermatids.
- Spermatids – each spermatid undergoes a series of changes from a non-moving cell to a cell capable of movement by the development of a tail (flagellum). This is now known as a spermatozoon. The spermatozoon becomes active after a maturation process which takes place in the epididymis. These spermatozoa become capable of fertilising the egg in the mare after they undergo a further process called capacitation in the mare's genital tract (see 'Fertilisation').

Of the four sperm cells produced from each primary spermatocyte, two cells will contain the X or female sex chromosome and two will contain the Y or male sex chromosome. The whole cycle of sperm

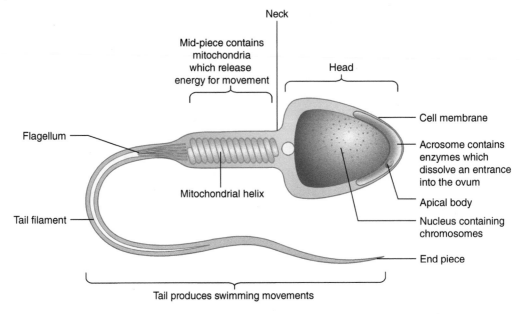

Figure 12.15 A spermatozoon.

development takes approximately 57 days in the stallion. The mean daily production of sperm is in the order of 7×10^9. The more a stallion is used, that is, the higher the frequency of ejaculation, the faster sperm are produced. Each spermatozoon consists of a head, mid-piece and tail (Figure 12.15). The head contains the nucleus and is capped by a structure known as the acrosome. This structure plays an important part in fertilisation.

Acrosome Reaction

Acrosomes are membranous sacs containing hydrolytic enzymes which include acrosin and hyaluronidase. These are released from the acrosome to allow cells to penetrate the zona pellucida and fuse with the oocyte plasma membrane. The acrosome reaction during normal fertilisation is highly complex and dependent upon the extracellular environment and calcium (Ca^{2+}) and sodium (Na^+) ions. All of these complex steps provide a delivery method for depositing the spermatozoon's genetic information in the oocyte cytoplasm and at the same time activate the oocyte's metabolism. These events are crucial to normal development.

During spermatogenesis, the cytoplasm of the cell is pushed down the tail length, leaving the head, mainly composed of the nucleus, containing half the number of other body cells. The mid-piece, or neck, contains a large number of mitochondria which are responsible for producing energy to move the tail quickly from side to side. Researchers have now found that stallion sperm use oxidative phosphorylation (a metabolic pathway by which cells use enzymes to oxidise nutrients) to produce energy for movement, rather than anaerobic glycolysis. The tail itself consists of muscle fibrils.

Semen – the ejaculate – is made up of sperm and seminal fluid produced by the accessory sex glands. The seminal fluid nourishes the sperm on their journey to the egg. In experimental conditions, sperm taken from the epididymis (i.e. in the absence of seminal fluid), when mixed with artificial medium, were still capable of producing fertilisation.

Endocrine Pathways in the Male

The hypothalamus regulates sexual behaviour, with GnRHs secreted in short pulsatile bursts in response to nervous sensory stimulation from the hypothalamus. The adenohypophysis (anterior pituitary) also produces the gonadotropins LH and FSH. LH acts upon the Leydig cells in testicular tissue to secrete androgens including testosterone. Leydig cells, also known as interstitial cells of Leydig, are found next to the seminiferous tubules in the testicle. They produce testosterone in the presence of LH. Testosterone stimulates spermatogenesis and sexual behaviour in stallions.

Sertoli cells (also known as nurse cells) nourish developing spermatogonia and are activated by FSH secreted by the adeno-hypophysis and have FSH-receptor on the membranes. They are specifically located in the seminiferous tubules (since this is the only place in the testes where the spermatozoa are produced). Sertoli cells also release inhibin and activin following puberty, which help regulate spermatogenesis. Episodic pulsing bursts of LH control testosterone production.

Fertilisation

The egg enters the fallopian tube down the funnel-shaped fimbriae in the mare. It then travels to a small enlargement called the isthmus. Here, if the mare has been covered by a fertile stallion, it will be met by millions of sperm. The viability and survival times of spermatozoa in the mare's reproductive tract are different between fertile and sub-fertile stallions and between fertile and infertile mares. It is also different for fresh and frozen/thawed semen. Possible explanations for this include a selective phagocytosis of damaged or dead spermatozoa. It may also be due to problems with myometrial activity in some sub-fertile mares or physiological changes in spermatozoa during the cryopreservation process.

As previously mentioned, the spermatogonia must undergo a change after they have been deposited in the mare's genital tract, so as to enable them to actually penetrate the egg to fertilise it. This process is known as capacitation. This enables the acrosome in the head of the sperm to form small holes through which an enzyme called acrosin can be released. This enzyme is capable of breaking into the zona pellucida region of the egg.

Once the sperm has penetrated the ovum, it injects its own genetic material into it. Following penetration of the zone pellucida the cell membrane of the single spermatozoon fuses with the vitelline membrane of the ovum, thereby initiating the second meiotic division by the ovum (see Figure 12.8), resulting in formation of the second polar body.

Once fertilisation has occurred, the ovum will not allow any more sperm to enter it. It immediately undergoes divisions (Figure 12.16). Up to the blastula stage, the dividing cells are still enclosed in the zone pellucida of the fertilised ovum. The zona is shed (a process called hatching) before the embryo can attach to the wall of the uterus for placentation. Foetal membranes are formed from the outer layer of the blastula called the trophoblast.

Pregnancy Diagnosis

Pregnancy diagnosis is mostly done by transrectal ultrasound, where an ultrasound probe is inserted into the rectum to view the underlying uterus. The first ultrasound examination is accurate at 14–16 days post ovulation, and breeding should take place 14–16 days after the last date of covering or artificial insemination. At this stage the embryonic vesicle is not fixed in the uterus and is still mobile. It is an ideal time for identification of twin pregnancies, and transrectal ultrasound is the best method for twin detection. Figure 12.17

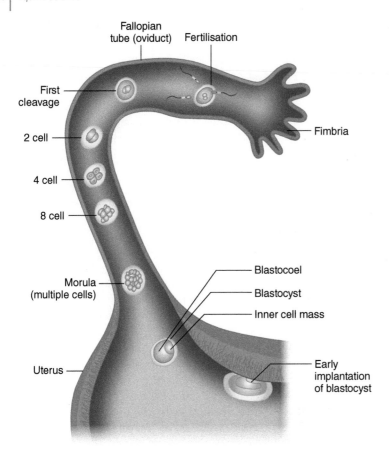

Figure 12.16 Events immediately following fertilisation.

shows the presence of a viable embryo at 14 days.

If only one pregnancy scan is to be carried out due to costs, then a scan between 21 and 34 days of pregnancy is advised, although if twins are identified at this stage it is much more difficult to treat and much more likely to result in the loss of both embryos. Later scans can be carried out, but after day 90 the pregnancy begins to drop down in the abdomen and transrectal ultrasound is much less useful. For Miniatures where rectal ultrasound may not be appropriate, a blood or urine test should be carried out instead.

Blood tests and urine tests include eCG before 120 days gestation or oestrone sulphate or conjugated oestrogens after 100 days gestation. Conjugated oestrogens are blended equine oestrogens, which may include oestrone sulphate, equilin sulphate and equilenin sulphate. Non-invasive pregnancy diagnosis for difficult mares or Miniatures should be done as above, between days 45 and 95 of gestation or oestrogen after day 100 of gestation (mare's serum) or 150 days (mare's urine).

Foetal Sexing

Transrectal ultrasound scans can accurately reveal the sex of the unborn foetus in utero. Vets have been able to successfully sex foetuses with around 90% accuracy from days 55 to 70 gestation. Researchers in Brazil have also found that a simple blood test from the mare can be used, although the method is not yet

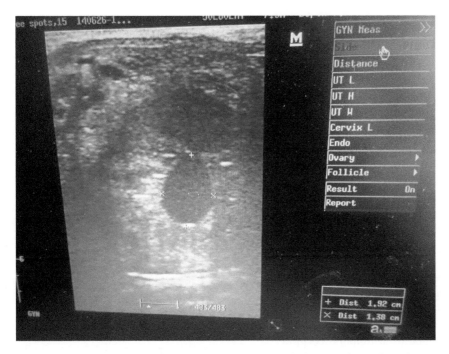

Figure 12.17 Day 14 sonogram of an equine embryo. *Source*: Courtesy of Harthill Stud.

commercially available; genetic material from the foal (known as circulating cell-free foetal DNA) detected in the mare's blood is analysed for the presence of the male gene or sex-determining-region Y gene. Biopsies from embryos recovered from mares for embryo transfer or reimplantation can also be sexed and checked for possible genetic conditions. In future, vets will be able to request genetic screening of the mare and foetus.

Twins

During oestrus a single ovum is released from the ovary during ovulation. In the mare there is a slight increase in ovulations from the left ovary and so the chance of multiple pregnancy is higher. The uterus of the mare can only generally accommodate one foal and one placenta. Most twin pregnancies are lost in mid to late gestation. TB mares are more susceptible and approximately 10–13% of all pregnancies in TBs and Standardbreds

are twin conceptuses. This is of particular concern to the TB industry because of economic implications. Sometimes, one twin may undergo mummification in the uterus and will appear at birth with the surviving twin. However, the mummified twin will still have taken up space from the maternal placenta and the chances are that the other twin will not grow to its full potential size.

If twins are detected early on in pregnancy by ultrasound scan, an attempt is usually made to 'pinch' one embryo out. If this is not successful an injection of prostaglandin may be given to abort both embryos. The mare will then be left to come back into season before a further covering takes place.

Endocrine Maintenance of Gestation

Maternal recognition of gestation occurs at 14 days. The blastocyst capsule secretes oestrogens which act locally to prevent the secretion of prostaglandins. A second wave of ovarian follicles ovulates and supplements progesterone secretion via secondary corpora lutea.

Equine Chorionic Gonadotropin

The chorionic girdle forms endometrial cups which secrete eCG (previously referred to as pregnant mare's serum gonadotropin (PMSG)), a glycoprotein, at 35–100 days (a pregnancy test for eCG is carried out at 45–95 days). eCG is really equine LH and is encoded by the same gene for pituitary LH. In contrast to LH from most other animals, equine LH (eCG) acts in a similar way to FSH. High blood levels of eCG stimulate development of ovarian follicles which then ovulate or luteinise, resulting in development of secondary corpora lutea. These work with the primary corpus luteum to secrete progesterone to maintain pregnancy until placental progesterone synthesis takes over. eCG is widely used for super-ovulation in other animals for embryo transfer.

Progesterone

In pregnant mares not only are there different sources for progesterone secretion but also a variety of progestogens and oestrogens are secreted. (The term 'progestogen' refers to any of a group of naturally occurring or synthetically derived steroids similar to progesterone, which bind to progesterone receptors and have progesterone-like effects.)

From ovulation until approximately day 40 of pregnancy, progestogens and oestrogens are solely secreted from the primary corpus luteum. Besides progesterone, the equine placenta synthesises progesterone or large amounts of progestogens (e.g. 5-alpha-pregnane), which serve the same function as progesterone, that is, maintenance of pregnancy. Sufficient progesterone is required to maintain the pregnancy

until about day 100. Low or inadequate progesterone levels are thought to be a major cause of early embryonic death. Toward the end of gestation, blood levels of progestogens are typically 100 times the maximal level of progesterone.

Pregnant mares that suffer from colic or laminitis may benefit from supplementation with progesterone and a non-steroidal anti-inflammatory for pain relief.

Oestrogens

Mare's urine contains high concentrations of oestrogens during the second and third trimesters of pregnancy and has been harvested to produce Premarin^{TM} for hormone replacement therapy in humans. Oestrogens are synthesised in the placenta from androgens that are produced by the foetal gonads. Foetal gonads secrete oestrone sulphate from 100 days to full term (pregnancy test for oestrone sulphate is carried out at 120–300 days). The gonads of the foetus secrete large quantities of the androgen dehydroepiandrosterone (DHA) into the umbilical blood system. Within the placenta, DHA is metabolised into different oestrogens, most prominently oestrone, equilin and equilenin. Both equilin and equilenin are oestrogens that are apparently unique to pregnant horses.

Relaxin

Relaxin is a protein hormone produced by the foeto-placental unit, rather than as previously thought the corpus luteum. It is detected in mare's serum starting at about day 80 of pregnancy, and remains at high levels until term. It is thought to act with progesterone to promote loosening of pelvic ligaments in preparation for parturition. Gradual increases in relaxin during late gestation also help the mammary glands to develop and prepare for lactation.

Gestation

The gestation period or pregnancy extends from fertilisation of the ovum to parturition. The gestation period includes:

- fertilisation
- early embryonic development
- implantation of the embryo in the wall of the uterine
- placentation
- development of foetal membranes
- growth of the embryo/foetus to term.

The average gestation period of the mare is 333–336 days (11 calendar months from the date of last service). There is a range in TBs of 310–384 days. In other breeds a range of 322–345 days has been suggested. Donkeys have a gestation period of 13 months. The foetus determines its own gestational life as it approaches full term. The genetic make-up and environmental factors, such as nutrition of the foetus, all have a bearing on the length of gestation.

The embryo is surrounded by fluids which cushion and protect against the effects of movement and gravity (Figure 12.18). The wall of the uterus also allows protection and the embryo cannot lose fluids or heat except through its immediate surroundings. The mare is therefore responsible for controlling heat and water balance. The uterus is a highly muscular organ, which allows the foetus to expand as it grows in size. First pregnancies often result in smaller foals than expected, because the uterus is being stretched for the first time. In subsequent pregnancies, the uterus is able to expand more easily. The uterus is also kept very effectively closed by the cervix. This prevents the entrance into the uterus of micro-organisms which may harm the developing foetus.

Implantation and Placentation

The function of the placenta is to allow exchange between the mother and the foetus. The placenta is attached to the wall of the uterus and is connected to the foetus by the umbilical cord. This cord contains the blood vessels that allow the circulation of blood between the foetus and the dam. It is important to note that

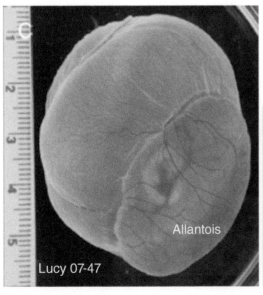
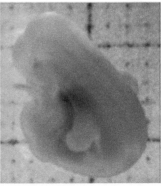

Day 27.5:
Diameter ~4 cm

Allantois

Lucy 07-47

Figure 12.18 A 27.5-day-old embryo. *Source*: McKinnon 2011. Reproduced with permission of John Wiley & Sons.

the foetal and maternal blood never mix, but instead come into close contact. There are six layers of cells between the maternal and foetal blood supplies. Implantation is the term for the attachment and penetration of the blastula to the epithelium of the uterus, whereas placentation is the development of extra embryonic membranes.

Early in gestation, between days 12 and 15, the embryo moves freely throughout the lumen of both uterine horns in response to contractions of the uterus. This movement and contact between embryo and endometrium of the dam is thought to be an important part of maternal recognition of pregnancy in horses. At approximately day 16 of gestation, a combination of an enlarged embryo and increased uterine tone leads to the embryo becoming fixed in one spot within the uterus and this is called fixation. The equine conceptus then develops extra-embryonic membranes. For the first 3–4 weeks of gestation, however, the yolk sac of the embryo is quite large, maintaining nutritional support of the embryo.

The chorion is the outermost membrane and is in contact with the endometrium of the uterus. The next layer (moving from outermost inward) is the allantois, a continuous layer that encloses a sac called the allantoic cavity. The chorion and the outer layer of the allantois fuse to form the chorioallantois. The inner of these foetal membranes, the amnion, encloses the amniotic cavity containing the amniotic fluid and the foetus in the amniotic sac or 'bag'. On the outer side, the amniotic sac is connected to the yolk sac, to the allantois and, through the umbilical cord, to the placenta.

At this early stage, a large part of the surface of the embryo is composed of a choriovitelline layer. The allantois can first be seen at about day 20, after which it expands rapidly and soon provides the dominant blood supply to the fused chorioallantois. Through day 35 there is no discernible attachment of foetal membranes to the endometrium. By day 40, attachment occurs.

These invading foetal cells form structures called endometrial cups which are unique to the horse family. At about day 90, the endometrial cups begin to degenerate and eventually they slough off.

Between day 40 and 150 of gestation, the placenta develops to full maturity. Early in pregnancy, the placental surface is smooth, but by day 70 it develops minute finger-like projections called microvilli. The equine placenta is classified as diffuse, that is, it includes the entire surface of the chorioallantois except for a small area adjacent to the cervix called the cervical star where attachment cannot occur.

Bundles of microvilli invade into receiving depressions in the uterine endothelium. These bundles of microvilli are known as microcotyledons. They increase the surface area of the placenta which increases the area for passage of nutrients, oxygen and waste products both to and from the foetus. Within each microcotyledon, the foetal and maternal blood supply come into very close contact to allow efficient exchange.

By day 150, a strong attachment is formed between the mother and the foetus. This consists of six layers of cells; three of these are on the maternal side (the epithelium, endometrium and wall of the blood vessel) and three on the foetal side (endoderm, mesoderm and ectoderm).

Embryology

Embryology is the study of pre-natal development. After fertilisation has taken place in the oviduct and the head of the spermatozoon has fused with the ovum a single cell is formed, which, as mentioned previously, now contains 32 chromosomes from the stallion and 32 from the mare to make the full complement of 64. This new cell is known as the zygote. Once the zygote is formed, it becomes resistant to the entry of further sperm.

A zygote carries information in the form of the genetic code for the growth of a new horse. This requires cell division, migration, differentiation and growth. During this process the zygote becomes a morula, blastula, gastrula and embryo. This is a highly intricate process following conception. Approximately 15 days after conception, all cells are identical but then they begin to transform into approximately 400 different cell types making up every part of the horse's body. Any errors at this most critical time may have devastating consequences.

Early on, the zygote divides repeatedly into blastomeres (daughter cells) moving down the oviduct towards the uterus. This increase in cell number is called cleavage. Although the number of cells increases, the volume remains the same, so it appears like a cluster of very small cells, known as the morula. This takes about 72 hours and consists of about 60 cells

As the morula reaches the uterus, a cavity called the blastocoel forms within it, transforming the morula into a hollow ball called a blastula (known as the blastocyst in mammals). This blastula or blastocyst stage is collected for embryo transfer. The blastocyst comprises a layer of cells, the trophoblast, surrounding the blastocoel, into which a collection of cells, the inner cell mass, protrudes. The inner cell mass eventually forms the body of the embryo. The trophoblast will develop into the outer embryonic tissues, including the placenta.

The area of the inner cell mass closest to the trophoblast is called the epiblast, while the area adjacent to the blastocele is called the hypoblast. As the inner cell mass develops, a cavity forms dorsal to the epiblast known as the amniotic cavity. The epiblast begins to thicken with proliferating cells on the longitudinal axis of the embryo. This thickening is called the primitive streak, and here the epiblast cells migrate into the interior of the embryo, taking up residence deep to the outer layer of cells (now called ectoderm) and displacing the hypoblast to create a deep layer, the endoderm. Between the ectoderm and endoderm the third and

Table 12.1 Main derivatives of embryonic germ layers.

Germ layer	Main derivatives
Ectoderm	Epidermis, coat, mane and tail hair, skin glands, brain and spinal cord, neural crest, sensory nerve cells, parts of the skeleton, blood vessels, head and neck
Mesoderm	Trunk and limb muscles, nucleus of intervertebral discs, vertebrae, ribs, kidneys, gonads, connective tissues of limbs, walls of digestive and respiratory tracts, heart blood vessels
Endoderm	Epithelial lining and glands of digestive and respiratory tracts

final germ cell layer, the mesoderm, is established. This migration of cells is known as gastrulation; with it the embryo establishes the three primary cell lines that will give rise to all of the tissues in the adult body.

These three primary germ layers are the ectoderm, mesoderm and endoderm (Table 12.1). Ectoderm and endoderm are epithelial tissue forming sheets. Mesoderm is a mesenchyme tissue containing mesenchyme cells that are star-shaped and do not attach, migrating freely. The mesoderm begins to differentiate into three regions: the somites (40 pairs of body segments repeating units or building blocks), intermediate mesoderm at the side of the somites, and the lateral plate which splits to form the coelom or cavity plate. The embryo is still a flat disc before folding then begins.

Phases of Equine Embryo Development and Migration

- Phase 1 – oocyte and early cleavage embryos: days 0–6.
- Phase 2 – blastocyst before completion of yolk sac: days 6–8.
- Phase 3 – rapid expansion of the conceptus and yolk sac completion: days 8–17.
- Phase 4 – conceptus fixture: days 16–17.
- Phase 5 – capsule loss: after day 20.

- Phase 6 – cell to cell communication with endometrium: days 21–28.

Phase 1

The transport of embryos through the oviduct requires energy use by the embryo using adenosine triphosphate (ATP). Cell differentiation and division also requires energy and so embryos are highly metabolically active. Total nuclear DNA increases 100 times as the zygote develops into a blastocyst. There are important interactions or epigenetic processes (see Chapter 2) between the embryo's inherent genotype and the environment within the oviduct, which may have important outcomes for the short- and long-term viability of the embryo and foetus or even the neonate or adult horse. This is an area of new research which may impact on mare management in the future.

The oocyte and early embryo have polarity and must also transit through the oviduct, passing unfertilised oocytes that remain there.

Phase 2

The embryo passes into the uterus at roughly 6 days post ovulation. It is still surrounded by the zona pellucida which has not expanded yet and it is between the stages of the morula and blastocyst. Many morphological and physiological changes occur at this point both inside and outside the differentiated trophoblast cells (see 'Embryology').

Inside, the blastocyst cavity enlarges and becomes more defined and the lining of endoderm cells becomes demarcated. Outside the blastocyst, the capsule (a glycoprotein layer) is laid down between the trophoblast and inner surface of the zona pellucida, which is then shed during the first day in the uterus. The embryo is now encapsulated. The capsule is very strong and essential if the pregnancy is to continue. The blastocyst is highly mobile from the time it enters the uterus. It appears to be 50–100 times more active than the bovine blastocyst.

Phase 3

The conceptus migrates through the uterine horns up to around day 15. There is rapid growth between days 11 and 16 as the conceptus communicates with the mare by moving throughout the uterus. The capsule continues to develop and it is thought that selective proteins bind to the capsule, allowing the delivery of 'messages' or substances to the embryo and endometrium as a form of communication. The production and metabolism of steroids, for example oestrogens, is also important for the maintenance of the pregnancy. At days 16–17 the conceptus becomes 'fixed' and is no longer mobile.

Phase 4

Phase 4 seems to be a mechanical process as the conceptus travels to the narrow flexure at the base of a uterine horn. Following fixation, amniotic folds arise around the embryo and then meet and fuse to complete the amnion. This process is completed while the capsule is still present.

Phase 5

Some time after day 20 the capsule is lost and its fragments can be seen around this time.

Phase 6

Following loss of the capsule the embryo has a completed amnion, developing circulatory system and an emerging allantois and looks like a small foal's body shape, with a diameter of approximately 4 cm. The allantois has become much more prominent.

Timeline of Embryonic Development

- Day 1 – 2 cell.
- Day 2 – 4 cell.
- Day 3 – 8 cell.
- Day 3/4 – 8 to16 cell, activation of embryonic genome.

- Day 6 – morula/blastocyst enters the uterus.
- Day 7 – endoderm appears.
- Day 8 – capsule appears.
- Day 10 – sex of the foetus can be determined using ultrasound, by establishing direction of migration of the pedicle that will become either the penis or clitoris. Upward migration towards the anus of course indicates a female.
- Day 11 – mesoderm appears.
- Day 14 – conceptus can be viewed by ultrasound (regular circular shape).
- Day 23 – heart beat, limb buds appear.
- Day 25 – allantochorionic placenta developing.
- Day 33 – developing allantois (outgrowth of the embryo's hindgut which forms the bladder, carries blood vessels in the umbilical cord and later combines with the chorion to form the placenta) is visible, and the yolk sac is regressing.
- Day 34 – forelimb and hindlimb buds protruding and the embryo is now known as a foetus (Figure 12.19).
- Day 50 – the embryo becomes a foetus, the legs, head, tail and eye are all clearly defined externally. Internally organs and skeletal structures are in place. The overall size is approximately 1 inch in length.

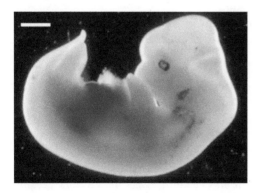

Figure 12.19 A 34-day-old equine foetus – forelimb and hindlimb buds protruding. *Source*: McKinnon 2011. Reproduced with permission of John Wiley & Sons.

The Foetal Endocrine System

The foal has an active endocrine system early in foetal life. Together with the placenta, the equine foetus synthesises precursors for the major hormones of pregnancy, namely progestogens and oestrogens, which maintain the pregnancy up to parturition. Once delivered and independent from the homeostatic mechanisms of the mare and the placenta, the foal has to respond dynamically to the extrauterine environment in order to survive. The transition from life as a foetus in utero to a free-living foal ex utero is reflected in a series of endocrine changes that can be measured within minutes or hours of birth.

The early embryo must communicate with the mare prior to implantation in the early stages of pregnancy. Likewise, in late pregnancy, oestrogens from placental metabolism of precursors in the mare's placenta have been found to be derived from foetal gonads. The foetus is now thought to have an active and developed endocrine system which plays an active role in gestation.

Preparation for Parturition (Birth)

The foal needs to be mature enough before it is born. Development takes place throughout the pregnancy in preparation for the drastic change in the foal's environment which takes place at birth. The foal grows a good coat of hair while in the uterus, and the lungs and nervous system should be fully developed by the end of the gestational period. The heart and circulation are already working while the foal is in the uterus, although after birth they will need to work harder. All the body systems including those of the glands, hormones, digestive and liver enzymes must be in place before birth and most of the organs are working (although not necessarily fully developed). Foals that are premature will be underdeveloped and face an uphill struggle to survive.

A normal pregnancy should last for more than 320 days. Any foal born before this will be classed as premature. Foals born between 320 and 355 days are considered to be 'full-term'. Any foals born after 355 days are post-mature and some problem may have occurred in the uterus while the foetus was growing. Birth should take place only when the foal is mature enough and ready to enter its new environment. It is commonly thought that the foal begins the birth process by sending some kind of signal (probably hormonal) to the mare that it is mature. However, although the foal determines the length of pregnancy, the mare is able to determine the exact time of foaling. Most mares foal at night because in the wild situation it would be more difficult for predators to see them.

It is known that prostaglandins play a critical role in parturition in the mare. In particular, $PGF_{2\alpha}$ appears to be instrumental in eliciting the uterine contractions and is involved in all three stages of foaling. The exact pattern of endocrine events leading to birth in the mare – for example, how prostaglandins and other hormones such as relaxin contribute to cervical relaxation and uterine contraction in the mare – have yet to be fully explained. Oxytocin acts directly on uterine smooth muscle to enhance uterine contractions during parturition.

One of the most common tests used to determine readiness for birth is milk electrolytes, usually calcium. If the mare is more than 310 days gestation and calcium is greater than 400 parts per million this indicates foaling is likely in the next 24 hours.

The Three Stages of Parturition

Stage 1

Uterine contractions gradually move the unborn foal and water bag (chorioallantois) to the cervix. Stage 1 is characterised by signs of abdominal discomfort and restlessness due to uterine contractions. Patches of sweat on the flank and behind the elbows usually appear a few hours before foaling. Increasing pressure in the uterus causes the chorioallantois to protrude through the internal os of the cervix. The chorioallantois usually ruptures at the cervical star, and the release of allantoic fluid marks the end of the first stage of parturition. The duration of this stage lasts 1–4 hours in the mare.

Stage 2

Delivery of the foal takes place, with passage of the foal through the cervix into the vagina. This results in the Ferguson reflex and stimulates the mare to have abdominal contractions. The combination of uterine contraction and abdominal contraction forces the foal through the birth canal and the foal is delivered. The presence of the foal in the birth canal also initiates oxytocin release from the neurohypophysis. Oxytocin acts directly on uterine smooth muscle to enhance uterine contractions and thereby assists delivery of the foal. The amnion appears at the vulvar lips as a whitish, fluid-filled membrane (Figure 12.20). In mares, plasma levels of oxytocin gradually rise during the latter stages of gestation and then increase greatly as parturition begins. Second stage labor usually lasts 15–30 minutes.

Stage 3

Stage 3 involves delivery of the placenta up to 3 hours after the foal is born.

Induction

Induction is sometimes used for mares with a history of poor neonatal outcomes for their foals or other health problems. The criteria for induction are more than 330 days gestation and calcium levels in the milk greater than 400 ppm. Problems associated with induction include higher risks of red bag delivery (premature separation of the placenta prior to or during a mare's foaling) and retained placenta. Fortunately red bag delivery is an infrequent occurrence in healthy

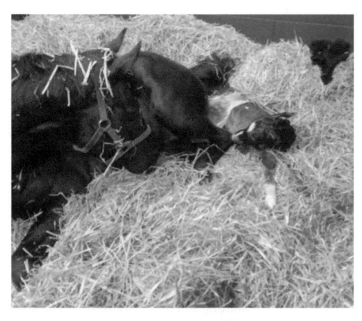

Figure 12.20 Mare giving birth: presentation of the forefeet. In a normal presentation the first visible sign is a transparent bluish-white amnion which surrounds the foal, then come the forefeet with one slightly extended in front of the other for easier passage of the shoulders. *Source*: Courtesy of Elkington Stud.

foaling mares. However, if it occurs, prompt action is required to prevent a stillborn or weak foal.

Lactation

In the weeks leading up to foaling, the mare's udder (mammary glands) develops and enlarges. The mammary glands are modified sweat glands and the mare has four, in two pairs. Each pair of glands exit through a central teat, that is, there are two teats supplying the four glands. The mare's mammary glands are situated between the hind legs. Each of the four mammary glands is completely separate from the other – there is no mixture of milk between the four quarters. They are supported by the medial and lateral suspensory ligaments.

The tissues of the mammary glands are made up of millions of alveoli with connecting ducts or branches, rather like a bunch of grapes. Milk is formed in the epithelial cells of the single alveolus. The alveoli are grouped together in units known as lobules. These lobules are, in turn, grouped together in larger units known as lobes. The alveoli are surrounded by myoepithelial cells (muscle cells) which are capable of contraction. These muscle cells are also found in the smaller ducts and they contract as part of the milk ejection or 'let down' reflex. During the gestational period, progesterone stimulates lobular and alveolar development, leading to an increase in size of the udder, particularly in the last 3 months of pregnancy. It is only in the 2–4 weeks before foaling that milk is produced. This is known as lactogenesis.

Lactogenesis

The milk is made from components either directly or indirectly from the blood. Milk contains much more sugar, fat (lipid), calcium, phosphorus and potassium, but less protein, sodium and chlorine than blood. The protein in milk is primarily casein with small amounts of albumins and globulins. These

Table 12.2 Composition (%) of milk from various species.

Species	Fat	Protein	Lactose	Ash
Horse	1.9	2.5	6.1	0.5
Donkey	1.3	1.8	6.2	0.4
Zebra	4.8	3.0	5.3	0.7
Dog	9.5	9.3	3.1	1.2
Whale	33.2	12.2	1.4	1.4
Jersey cow	5.5	3.9	4.9	0.7

albumins and globulins are the principal proteins of blood; most of the milk fat is in the form of triglycerides, whereas phospholipids and cholesterol are the blood fats. Table 12.2 gives the average composition of milk for some species.

The composition of milk reflects the needs of the young of the species. Colostrum, which is known as the first milk, contains a high concentration of immunoglobulins which confer immunity to the foal. The high level of these proteins in the colostrum falls drastically after about 12 hours and the foal also loses the ability to absorb them 'whole', that is, without digesting them first, after about 1 or 2 days. Many of the vitamins are present in substantially higher levels in colostrum compared with normal milk. The transfer of vitamin A across the placenta to the foetus is known to be poor in many mammals and consequently the newborn will have very low levels. The high levels in colostrum are therefore extremely important.

Some species, for example humans and rabbits, can transfer antibodies across the placenta before birth, but this is not the case in horses. The newborn foal is therefore dependent upon the colostrum as a vital source of antibodies or passive immunity until it is able to build its own immunity.

Lactation Curve

The amount of milk produced by individual mares varies considerably. In general however, the milk yield increases during the first 3 months of lactation (Figure 12.21). The actual amount of milk produced depends upon the requirement by the foal, so smaller pony breeds will produce less milk than TB's.

TB's produce approximately 4–8 litres per day in the first 2 weeks and this increases to 10–18 litres per day at 3 months. After 3 months, the foal's demands start to decrease as it is beginning to graze with the mother. Consequently, the milk yield starts to drop and continues to fall until the mare stops producing milk after about a year. In the natural state the mare will dry up a few weeks before she is due to foal the following year. Human intervention leads to the weaning of foals at about 6 months of age, and consequently the foal will not be receiving as much nutrition from the mother. Foals weaned later at 10–11 months of age will derive more nutrients from the mare and will be less likely to suffer setbacks at weaning, as the mare is naturally weaning the foal herself.

Applied Reproductive Technologies

Applied reproductive technologies (ART) refers to different technologies used to achieve pregnancy in mares and includes procedures such as artificial insemination (AI), in vitro laboratory fertilisation, gamete intrafallopian transfer (GIFT), oocyte transfer and intracytoplasmic sperm injection (ICSI). Cloning is also now used, although this is still very costly.

Artificial Insemination

The first references to AI in horses date back to Arabic texts in the 1300s, but it was not until the technique of semen conservation in liquid nitrogen was developed in the 1960s that AI became an established technique. Although semen preserving techniques have improved tremendously, many owners still prefer to use chilled rather than frozen semen on their mares.

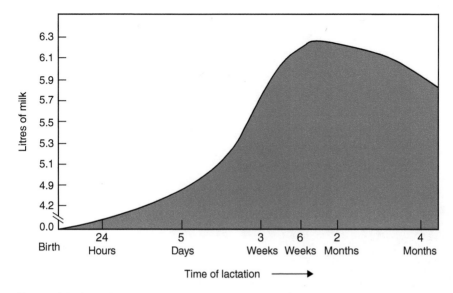

Figure 12.21 Lactation curve.

AI is used widely and with great success in the breeding of sports horses. However, TB horses produced by AI are not eligible for entry in the General Stud Book and thus are unable to race. For TB foals to be registered with the Jockey Club, they must have been conceived by live cover and had a natural gestation. Foals must have been delivered by the same mare at covering. However, other breed societies regularly use AI and other techniques.

Advantages

- Efficient stallion use – a single ejaculate can be divided and used to inseminate a number of mares.
- Regular evaluation of semen quality.
- The use of chilled and frozen semen means that semen is available to mares worldwide.
- No risk of injury to the mare or stallion through natural covering.
- Lower risk of the spread of venereal diseases.
- Mares and foals do not have to travel to stud.

Disadvantages

- Skill and knowledge are required for the technique to be successful.

- Additional veterinary and associated costs.
- Lack of recognition by some stud books.
- Risk of overuse of some popular stallions.
- Semen from some stallions will not tolerate chilling, freezing or thawing.

Collection of Semen

Semen is collected using an artificial vagina (AV). The AV is a rigid container lined with two rubber liners. Warm water is introduced between the two liners at a temperature above 45°C. This high temperature allows for cooling. The water also controls the pressure within the AV so that when the stallion's penis enters the AV it represents the mare's reproductive tract as closely as possible. The amount of water placed in the jacket and the temperature of the inner liner can be adjusted to suit the individual stallion's preferences. The temperature usually lies between 43 and 45°C. The inside of the AV is lubricated with obstetric gel. A pre-warmed collection bottle is attached to the end of the AV. The stallion's semen is collected using either an in-season mare or a phantom or dummy mare (Figure 12.22). As the stallion mounts, his penis is deflected into the AV. After ejaculation the stallion is allowed to dismount and the AV is removed.

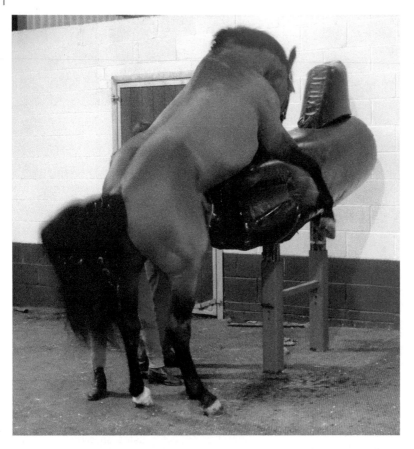

Figure 12.22 The stallion is encouraged to mount a phantom or dummy mare. *Source*: Courtesy of Harthill Stud.

Semen Preservation

Semen is filtered to remove the gel fraction and diluted with an appropriate pre-warmed extender. The volume, concentration, colour and motility of the ejaculate are evaluated under the microscope to determine its quality. Depending on the requirements of the stud and location of the mare, AI can be carried out using fresh, chilled or frozen semen.

Fresh Semen

Fresh semen is used by some studs to replace natural covering with their own or visiting mares. Semen is collected in the normal way and in-season mares are inseminated immediately. The semen may be diluted if several mares are ready to be inseminated.

Chilled Semen

AI using chilled semen involves the collection, evaluation, dilution and chilling of semen from the stallion which is then inseminated into the mare.

- Evaluation – the motility of the sample is checked using a microscope with a warming table at 37°C.
- Dilution – the semen is filtered to remove the gel-fraction and diluted with an extender at 37°C.
- Chilling – the semen is cooled to 5–8°C over a 2- to 3-hour period.

Throughout these processes it is vital to avoid cold shock to the sperm. Cold shock severely compromises the ability of the sperm to fertilise the egg due to cellular and motility changes. The rate of cooling from room temperature is critical and a specialised container is used that lowers the temperature of the semen steadily until the storage temperature is reached. The semen can be stored for up to 3 days in the container, allowing it to be transported worldwide.

In order for the use of chilled semen to be successful, the following factors must be considered:

- Semen is of sufficient quality.
- The storage ability of semen will vary between stallions.
- Appropriate cooling, storage and handling of the semen.
- The correct timing of insemination relative to ovulation.
- Correct insemination technique.
- Appropriate post-insemination examination and treatment.

Frozen Semen

Semen is collected in the usual manner and the gel-free fraction diluted with a transport medium. The semen is centrifuged to concentrate the sperm into a lower volume of seminal plasma. The resulting sperm are diluted with nutrient-rich freezing extender. The semen is then packed into plastic straws and frozen in liquid nitrogen down to a temperature of −196°C. At this temperature the sperm will remain viable indefinitely and may be used to inseminate mares years after collection.

The use of frozen semen and the thawing process have previously resulted in lower conception rates, but recent research has shown that mares inseminated once with 800 million sperm had a 48% per cycle conception rate, whereas mares inseminated twice with 800 million sperm each time had a 57% per cycle conception rate; that is, there is a significant improvement when using the latter technique.

Frozen semen is thawed in warm water before insemination into the mare. Timing of insemination is crucial and ideally is carried out within 6 hours either side of ovulation. Stallion semen is very sensitive to freezing and many do not have semen that will freeze. Problems normally occur in the rewarming phase, when motility may fall by 75%. However, the process of freezing semen does enable the blood lines of stallions to be continued long after their death.

Timing of Insemination

Semen should be inseminated into the mare 24 hours before ovulation. The semen does not require warming beforehand. The vet will confirm that the mare is ready for insemination through rectal palpation of the ovaries to determine the size and consistency of the follicles. After insemination, injection of the mare with human chorionic gonadotropin may be used to stimulate ovulation within the next 24–48 hours.

Insemination Technique

The mare is suitably restrained, usually in stocks, her tail bandaged and the vulva and perineal region thoroughly cleaned and dried. The semen is loaded into a sterile syringe which is then attached to an insemination pipette. The catheter is gently inserted into the vulva and through the cervix so that the semen is inseminated into the mid-uterine body. The vet should check that the mare has ovulated within 24 hours. If the time of ovulation has been miscalculated, it may be necessary to repeat the procedure. The mare is then treated as any other pregnant mare, using ultrasound scanning at 14 days to confirm pregnancy.

Under ideal circumstances the success for chilled semen is comparable with that of fresh semen. However, if the semen is not properly handled or inseminated at the wrong time, the conception rate falls dramatically.

Embryo Transfer

Embryo transfer is being increasingly used in the breeding of sports horses that, for a number of reasons, are unable to breed themselves. In simple terms, it involves removing a 6- to 8-day-old embryo from a donor mare and transferring it to a recipient mare that then carries the foal to term.

Advantages

- Mares can breed foals while still competing.
- It allows more extensive use of the mare's genetic potential.
- It enables a mare that cannot carry a foal to term to breed.
- It allows sub-fertile mares to breed.
- It allows a filly that is too young to carry a foal herself to breed.

Disadvantages

- The procedure is expensive.
- A suitable recipient mare is needed.
- The technique requires highly skilled vets and technicians.
- The success rate is low.
- Stud books may limit the number of foals that can be registered to one mare in a season. The TB industry will not recognise any foal born through embryo transfer.

Donor and Recipient Mares

The donor mare will have a thorough examination of the ovaries, uterus and cervix, along with the usual swabs to ensure that she is free from disease or infection. Ideally she should show a normal oestrus pattern. The recipient mare should be in good physical condition and a reasonably 'roomy' type, able to carry a foal without compromising its growth and development. Careful veterinary examination should be made to ensure that she is free from disease and has regular ovarian activity. Ideally she should have previously bred a foal herself and proved herself a good mother, able to supply sufficient milk for the foal. The mare should have a good temperament and be free from stable vices, as these may be learned by the foal.

The Synchronisation Process

The first step is to synchronise the oestrus cycles of the donor and recipient mares. Ideally they should ovulate within 24 hours of each other so that their reproductive tracts are in a similar physiological state, enabling the recipient to receive the embryo and take over and maintain the pregnancy. Synchronisation is accomplished by the use of prostaglandin to advance the onset of oestrus, followed by the use of LH to bring about ovulation. Thorough and regular teasing of both mares to establish whether or not they are in season plus rectal palpation of the ovaries to determine the size of the follicles are essential. Blood tests will also be taken. These will continue to be taken into the first weeks of the recipient's pregnancy to monitor the progesterone levels. Progesterone is essential for the maintenance of pregnancy and if the levels are not correct progesterone therapy will be necessary. This is discontinued once the uterus has taken over progesterone production from the corpora lutea.

Collection of the Embryo

The donor mare is covered or inseminated as normal and 7 days later the embryo is removed from the uterus and transferred to the recipient mare. This may be done surgically, but more commonly a non-surgical technique is used that involves flushing the embryo from the uterus. The donor mare is secured in stocks, her tail bandaged and the perineal area thoroughly cleaned. A catheter is placed into the uterus through the cervix and held in place on the uterine side by an inflatable cuff. About 2 litres of nutrient solution kept at body temperature is then passed into the uterus through the catheter. The vet palpates the uterus per rectum while the fluid is drawn off.

The fluid is allowed to settle in the laboratory and examined under a low-powered microscope. The embryo, if present, is transferred within 2 hours into the recipient mare. Embryos can be cooled to 5°C and kept for up to 24 hours if it is not possible to transfer the embryo immediately.

Transfer of the Embryo

Transfer can be performed either non-surgically or surgically. In non-surgical transfer the mare is placed in stocks and the embryo is placed in the uterus using a special inseminator. There is a higher risk of damage to the embryo and the possibility of infection; however, the procedure poses less risk to the mare and is less costly. Antibiotics are administered after the transfer has taken place.

In surgical transfer a small incision is made, under general anaesthetic, just in front of the udder. One horn of the uterus is brought out, a small hole made and the embryo injected into the uterine horn. Alternatively, the procedure can be carried out under local anaesthetic with the mare in stocks and sedated.

After transfer, as previously mentioned, the recipient mare's progesterone levels should be monitored and she should be scanned for pregnancy approximately 14 days after the transfer. She should then be treated like any other in-foal mare.

Gamete Intrafallopian Transfer

In GIFT the mare's ovum and the stallion's sperm are deposited in the fallopian tube of a surrogate mare. This technique is useful for sub-fertile stallions such as a stallion with a low sperm count.

Oocyte Transfer

Oocyte transfer is sometimes used for mares with physical problems, such as an obstructed fallopian tube. An oocyte is removed from the mare's follicle and transferred into the fallopian tube of a recipient mare, which is then covered.

Intracytoplasmic Sperm Injection (ICSI)

The technique of ICSI involves the injection of a single sperm into the egg in the laboratory. The resultant fertilised egg is then grown in a culture to form the embryo, which is then transferred to a recipient mare. This procedure may benefit mares with uterine adhesions, recurrent anovulatory follicles or infections.

Summary Points

1) The ovaries are bean shaped due to the ovulation fossa – an indentation where ovulation takes place in mares.

2) In gestation, between days 12 and 15, the equine embryo moves freely throughout the lumen of both uterine horns in response to contractions of the uterus. This movement and contact between embryo and endometrium of the dam is thought to be an important part of maternal recognition of pregnancy in horses. At approximately day 16 of gestation, a combination of an enlarged embryo and increased uterine tone leads to the embryo becoming fixed in one spot within the uterus and this is called fixation.

3) Pregnancy diagnosis is mostly done by transrectal ultrasound, where an ultrasound probe is inserted into the rectum to view the underlying uterus. The first ultrasound examination is accurate at 14–16 days post ovulation and breeding and should take place at 14–16 days after the last date of covering or artificial insemination.

4) Some species, for example humans and rabbits, can transfer antibodies across the placenta before birth, but this is not the case in horses. The newborn foal is therefore dependent upon the colostrum as a vital source of antibodies or passive immunity until it is able to build its own immunity.

5) Mares may be induced artificially to start the birth process. This is sometimes used for mares with a history of poor neonatal outcomes for their foals or other health problems. The criteria for induction are more than 330 days gestation and calcium levels in the milk greater than 400 ppm.

Q + A

Q When is the artificially imposed breeding season of TBs for international racing?

A For mares this has been determined by the authorities as running from 15 February to 15 July (in the southern hemisphere, the TB breeding season runs from 12 August to 15 January).

Q What is the corpus haemorrhagicum?

A Immediately after the mature follicle has been released, the remaining follicle collapses and bleeding occurs into its centre, forming a clot called the corpus haemorrhagicum.

Q What is the acrosome reaction?

A The membranous sac at the head of the acrosome contains hydrolytic enzymes which include acrosin and hyaluronidase. These are released from the acrosome to allow cells to penetrate the zona pellucida and fuse with the oocyte plasma membrane.

Q What is spermatogenesis?

A This is the term for the formation of mature male gametes or sex cells from the most undifferentiated germ cells. It includes several mitotic cell divisions followed by two meiotic cell divisions, during which the chromosome number is reduced by half, that is, from diploid to haploid.

Q When would high transrectal ultrasound be inappropriate for use?

A For Miniature breeds.

Q Is artificial insemination allowed to be used in TB's bred for racing?

A AI is used widely and with great success in the breeding of sports horses. However, TB horses produced by AI are not eligible for entry in the General Stud Book and thus are unable to race.

13

Genetics

The purpose of genetics is to understand inheritance and genetic diseases of horses. A few model organisms were developed to study genetics, such as yeast, *Drosophila*, *Arabidopsis* and mice. These organisms have a well-established genetic background, a relatively short life cycle, a relatively large number of offspring from a single mating and genetic variations. Equine genetic research now includes epigenomics and nutrigenomics, with widespread health, fitness and performance benefits for equine athletes.

The Genetic Code or Genome

The complete genetic code is called the genome. In November 2009, the first genome sequence of the domestic horse (*Equus caballus*) was published in the international journal *Science*. This major achievement was the result of a concerted effort by the worldwide equine research community. DNA from a single Thoroughbred mare called Twilight (Figure 13.1) was used to construct the genome sequence. This information is now being used to assist genetic research in horses all over the world.

The genome represents the genetic material or the core instructions for an animal. In the horse (as in all mammals) the genetic material or DNA is found mostly in the chromosomes within the nucleus of the cell. The genes of the horse are similar to other mammals. However, researchers now know that there is also a fractional but functionally vital amount of DNA present in mitochondria

within the cytoplasm. Although most DNA is found within chromosomes in the nucleus, it is thought that mitochondrial DNA, though much smaller in quantity, has a significant role to play. Even the horse's life span is written into its DNA.

Chromosomes

Chromosomes of the horse have been studied for over 100 years. A chicken has 78 chromosomes, which is more than a horse at 64, but it is important to understand that it is the quality of the chromosomes that counts. All organisms have the same DNA; it is simply what the genes or DNA code for and the translation process that make the real difference.

In horses, every nucleated body cell (i.e. each body cell with a nucleus) has 64 chromosomes (2n=64), arranged in 32 pairs. One pair determines the gender of the horse. Females have a matched homologous pair of X chromosomes. Males have an unmatched heterologous pair – one X and one Y chromosome. Homologous means 'the same'; heterologous means 'different'. The remaining 31 pairs of chromosomes are known as autosomes. The word 'autosome' may be defined as the chromosomes that determine physical/body characteristics, that is, the phenotype of the horse (excluding the sex). The X chromosome is almost identical in terms of the order of genes between horses and human. Horse chromosome 11 matches human 17.

Equine Science, Third Edition. Zoe Davies and Sarah Pilliner.
© 2018 Zoe Davies and Sarah Pilliner. Published 2018 by John Wiley & Sons Ltd.

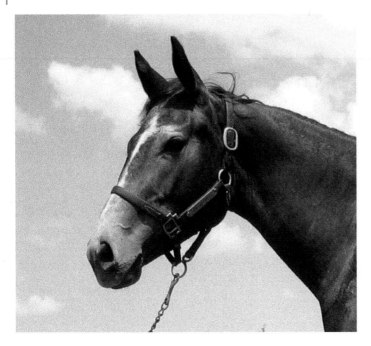

Figure 13.1 Thoroughbred mare 'Twilight' – the DNA donor for the sequencing project. *Source*: Chowdhary 2013. Reproduced with permission of John Wiley & Sons.

The horse genome also seems to include vast regions of DNA that do not code for genes, as does the human genome, but they are now thought to have some function. A karyotype is the term used for the complete set of chromosomes in a species or an individual organism (Figure 13.2).

It is thought that most chromosomal abnormalities in horses involve the X or sex chromosome, many of which will have an effect on fertility. There are also numerical abnormalities such as a complete lack of an X chromosome and this is known as monosomy. Sex reversal has been described in horses where the karyotype does not agree with the phenotype. This is where an XY karyotype that should be a male horse shows the phenotype or characteristics of a female or mare (i.e. XX).

Gene Expression

DNA has two main functions: (1) to act as a memory bank for all the genetic information in the cell, which can then be replicated at cell division, producing exact copies of the cell after division; and (2) to serve as a template for the synthesis of mainly proteins. This second function is very loosely described as gene expression.

So what makes a heart cell, for example, different from a nerve cell or skin cell? The answer is the proteins produced by the cell. DNA carries the instructions or codes for all these proteins and is found in every living thing on earth. DNA instructs every cell in the horse's body what it is to become and when and where. All equine cells, whether in the heart, skin or muscle, contain exactly the same DNA; they must do because they have developed from the fusion of one egg and one sperm, and all daughter cells from cell division (mitosis) contain exact copies of the parent cells. Cells therefore can differentiate into different types even though all the cells contain the same DNA. This is because genes in individual cells can be switched on or off. They can make a protein if switched on or not

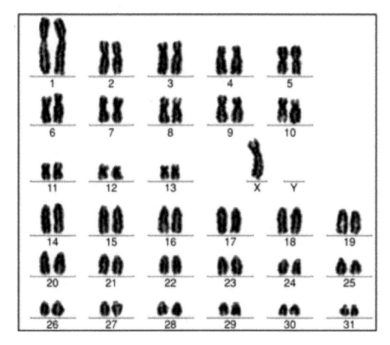

Figure 13.2 A karyotype of a mare with 63XO (Turners Syndrome) resulting in infertility. *Source*: Chowdhary 2013. Reproduced with permission of John Wiley & Sons.

if switched off. For example, although all the cells of the horse's body contain an albumin gene, only the liver cells make albumin to secrete into the bloodstream. This is because the genes are highly regulated, some are active and some are silent.

The heart cell proteins will be switched off in liver cells, for example, but on in heart cells; that is, the gene is expressed in heart cells but not in liver cells. This is called gene expression, or more accurately tissue-specific gene expression. This is controlled by regulatory proteins which bind to DNA switching the gene on. Genes do not produce their proteins continuously. Researchers in France discovered gene regulation in bacteria, using *Escherichia coli* (*E. coli*). They found that when lactose was available the bacteria were able to turn on a group of genes to metabolise the sugar. Lactose removed an inhibitor from the DNA and this resulted in the necessary genes being switched on. The gene producing the inhibitor is known as a regulatory gene. Cells therefore have not only a genetic

programme for proteins but also a regulatory programme for expression of those genes.

Also the expression of genes can vary with different stimuli. For example, when blood glucose levels fall in the horse, the alpha cells of the pancreas secrete the hormone glucagon. This will circulate in the blood until it reaches the liver, where it causes a 15-fold increase in expression of a gene involved in gluconeogenesis which then restores blood glucose.

Mitochondrial DNA

Mitochondria are cell organelles that act as the power house of the cell. The mitochondria are thought to have originally existed as free-living alphaproteobacteria and adapted to a symbiotic relationship within all eukaryotic cells approximately 1.5 billion years ago. These mitochondria are exclusively passed down the maternal line directly from the dam to her offspring. This is due to the structure of the male sperm, which contains the stallion's mitochondria in the mid-section, rather than in the head section. The mid-section does not permeate the egg during fertilisation and therefore the male mitochondria are lost and only the dam's egg mitochondria are passed on to the offspring. This unique hereditary trait allows the maternal line to be investigated without influence from any paternal factors.

All aerobic respiration occurs within the mitochondria. The mitochondria genome is approximately 16,660 base pairs in length compared to 2.7 million base pairs in nuclear DNA. Mitochondrial DNA contains genes, all of which are essential for normal mitochondrial function. Some of these genes provide instructions for making enzymes involved in oxidative phosphorylation including NADH1, NADH2 and NADH3 as part of the electron transport chain. The remaining genes provide instructions for making molecules called transfer RNA's (tRNA's) and ribosomal RNA's (rRNA's). These types of RNA help assemble protein building blocks (amino acids) into functioning proteins.

Mitochondria make up about 70% of the cytoplasm and are replicated clonally within the cell, that is, they make exact mitochondrial copies. This mitochondrial DNA has proved very useful in determining the history and evolution of horses.

The Y Chromosome

The Y chromosome is quite distinct from the X chromosome, but around 300 million years ago they were structurally similar, that is, homologues. Now the Y chromosome is relatively small and male specific and contains much fewer genes than the X chromosome, with most of the functional genes being lost. It was therefore largely ignored by researchers for many years. However, studies in other mammals including the mouse, cat and chimpanzee have shown this is not the case and that the Y

chromosome contains important functional genes that play an important role in sperm production and fertility. Typically the Y chromosome was not used in whole genome sequencing but studied separately due to requirements for different, more complicated techniques in studying it. Therefore the whole genome draft sequence of the horse did not include the Y chromosome. Recently, though, researchers have closely studied the horse's Y chromosome. Some of the male-specific genes present only in the Y chromosome play a vital role in fertility.

Alleles

An allele is a form of the gene. Alleles are found at the same loci on homologous chromosomes and are separated during meiosis (see Chapter 2). Genes carried on pairs of homologous chromosomes are also paired and instruction sequences run down each homologous chromosome in the same order. Paired genes therefore control the same characteristic and may give identical instructions; however, they may also give slightly different instructions from each other. The two different genes for the same traits are known as alleles or allelomorphs. Figure 13.3 shows terms used to describe genes and chromosomes.

Dominance

One gene may be dominant to the other, which is therefore termed recessive. A dominant gene will mask the effect of the recessive gene. Sometimes two alleles may be equally dominant and this is known as incomplete dominance or blending. For example, a lack of dominance between a gene for red colour and one for white may result in a mixture or a roan colour in horses.

Co-dominance occurs when a pair of genes controlling the same characteristic gives different instructions but neither is dominant. Both are represented in the

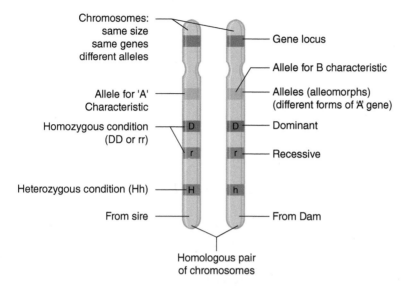

Figure 13.3 Terms used to describe genes and chromosomes.

result. An example of this is blood group in humans. The blood group AB results from co-dominance of the gene for A group and the gene for B group.

Sex Cells

Sexual reproduction in all animals involves the fusion of one egg and a sperm that is, the process of fertilisation. These sex cells are also known as gametes. Gametes are produced by meiosis to ensure that eggs and sperm have half the number of chromosomes (haploid = n). The diploid number of chromosomes is often referred to as 2n. Each equine species has a distinct chromosome number:

- Horse (*Equus caballus*) 2n = 64
- Donkey (*Equus asinus*) 2n = 62
- Grévy's zebra (*Equus grevyi*) (Figure 13.4) 2n = 46
- Plains zebra (*Equus burchelli*) 2n = 44
- Mountain zebra (*Equus zebra*) 2n = 32

Hybrids

Hybrids or interspecies crosses between equine family members are usually viable because their genes (housed on chromosomes that appear to have undergone major physical rearrangement during the adaptive radiation of *Equus* species) are largely homologous. However, because the chromosomes have changed so much during evolution, some chromosomes cannot pair properly during meiosis to allow crossing over and successful segregation of homologues into new daughter cells. Hence, the hybrids are almost always sterile, as they cannot produce viable gametes.

The horse and donkey (ass) belong to separate species, which differ quite markedly in size and phenotype. They do not share a common gene pool although they can mate with each other and produce offspring. A jack donkey and a mare will produce a mule, whereas a stallion and a jenny donkey will produce a hinny; both mules and hinnies are sterile.

Heredity

Horses vary even within the same breeds, to a great extent. There are differences in, for example, size, colour, bone, weight, condition, temperament, even thickness of skin.

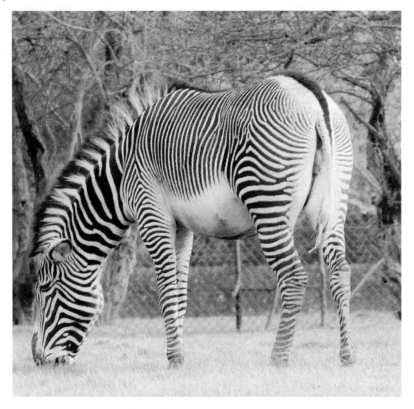

Figure 13.4 Grévy's zebra. *Source*: Courtesy of Rebecca Eastment.

These differences are known as variation. Variation may be:

- genetic (inherited)
- environmental.

Genes provide the horse or pony with a range of heights and weights into which the animal should fit, but environmental factors such as feeding will determine the position in the range. Reproduction leads to variation when the egg and sperm (gametes) join together. Half the genetic information is provided by each of the two parents, the sire and dam.

As already mentioned, the sire and dam each have 64 chromosomes or 32 pairs in most of their cells and this is known as the diploid number (see 'Meiosis', Chapter 2). The gametes (egg and sperm) have half this number, i.e. 32 chromosomes. This is known as the haploid number. At fertilisation the egg and sperm join, resulting in cells with 64 chromosomes (32 pairs) again. Thus half the genes come from the sire and half from the dam. This results in a huge number of possible gene combinations, producing variation in the resulting foals.

Sex Determination

The sex chromosomes carry the gene that determines the sex of the horse. A foal's sex is actually determined by the genetic information it receives from the sire at fertilisation. All eggs have one X sex chromosome, whereas the sperm are either X or Y in a 50:50 ratio. At fertilisation, therefore, the sperm has a 50% chance of being X or Y. If the egg is fertilised by a Y-containing sperm, the offspring will be a colt, whereas if it is fertilised by an X-containing sperm, it will result in a filly. To summarise:

- colts inherit an X from the dam and a Y from the sire
- fillies inherit an X from the dam and an X from the sire.

Of the resulting offspring, 50% are male and 50% are female.

Genotype and Phenotype

Genotype refers to the genetic makeup of the animal, whereas phenotype refers to the appearance. Phenotype is often therefore a result of both genotype and environment.

Polygenic or Multiple Gene Traits

Most traits are influenced by more than one gene working together; where the exact loci are and the genetic mechanisms involved are as yet unknown. An example of a polygenic trait is blue eye colour and white markings in horses and also conformation traits.

Multiple Alleles

There are occasions when more than two alleles control a particular characteristic, as only two alleles may occupy a locus on a pair of homologous chromosomes. An example of multiple alleles is the ABO blood group in humans, which is controlled by three alleles:

- I_A – antigen A produced on the erythrocyte
- I_B – antigen B produced on the erythrocyte
- I_O – no antigens are produced on the erythrocyte.

The alleles I_A and I_B show equal dominance, but both are dominant to I_O. Possible combinations are therefore:

- $I_A I_A$
- $I_A I_O$
- $I_A I_B$
- $I_B I_B$
- $I_B I_O$
- $I_O I_O$.

Sex Linkage

Some traits are sex linked. The X and Y chromosomes have been named from their shapes. The Y chromosome is actually shorter and therefore contains less genetic information than the X chromosome. This sometimes results in the X chromosome having no match on the Y chromosome. This allele on the X chromosome will therefore express itself in the male. Alleles found on only the X of the sex chromosomes are known as sex-linked traits.

Lethal Genes

Genes may cause a lethal condition and these are therefore known as lethal genes. There are several lethal genes in horses, including:

- lethal white foal syndrome (LWFS)
- foal immunodeficiency syndrome (FIS)
- lavender foal syndrome (LFS)
- severe combined immunodeficiency (SCID) in Arabian foals.

Most lethal alleles only have the lethal effect when the horse is homozygous for the gene. The heterozygotes are therefore known as carriers for the lethal condition.

Lethal White Foal Syndrome (LWFS)

LWFS-affected foals are born white or mostly white and may be deaf and/or have blue eyes with a condition termed atresia coli. This is an incomplete development of the large colon and the foal cannot defecate. There is no treatment.

Foal Immunodeficiency Syndrome (FIS)

Previously known as fell pony syndrome, FIS was responsible for many fell pony deaths. The carrier rate in the UK and Netherlands is thought to be estimated at 4–60%. FIS was first reported in 1996 in purebred fell ponies, but was also then seen in Dales ponies and some coloureds. Foals are born normally but soon deteriorate and become lethargic and anaemic and highly susceptible to infections. Many of the affected foals die within 3 months. A genetic cause was suspected and researchers developed a DNA test to identify carriers. Two carrier parents can produce a foal with FIS and the DNA test allows parents to be chosen that are not carriers or where only one is a carrier, and this removes the FIS possibility in foals.

Lavender Foal Syndrome (LFS)

Foals with LFS have a characteristic dilute coat colour that is described as lavender, pale grey, pewter or light chestnut. These foals suffer from multiple neurologic abnormalities, preventing them from standing and nursing. The condition is most commonly reported in Egyptian Arabians, where it has an autosomal recessive mode of inheritance.

Severe Combined Immunodeficiency (SCID)

SCID-affected foals are purebred or part-bred Arabs and they always die within the first 6 months of life, regardless of the level of veterinary care administered. SCID is a deficiency of the immune system which predisposes the newborn foal to infection. The immune system has two major defence systems: the B lymphocytes, which produce antibodies, and the T lymphocytes, which are responsible for cell-mediated immunity. The SCID mutation results in an inability to produce either B or T lymphocytes, so the affected foal effectively has no immune system, leaving it susceptible to infective pathogens.

There is a new DNA test for SCID which requires a small blood sample. A molecular biology technique known as the polymerase chain reaction (PCR) is used to specifically amplify only the tiny region of the DNA that is affected by SCID. The samples are then run on a diagnostic apparatus which determines the length of the DNA fragments generated during PCR. If the horse is normal the length will be 163, if the horse is affected the length will be 158, and if the horse is a carrier both of these lengths will be present. There are many different DNA tests available for horses, which are shown in Table 13.1.

Congenital Curly Coat Syndrome

A non-lethal genetic syndrome is curly coat syndrome. A congenital 'curly coat' syndrome is also recognised in some horses including Quarter-horses, Percherons, Arabs, Appaloosas and Morgans. This is viewed as a desirable feature by some breeders. Curly coat patterns may be acquired in other horses from time to time, although most such cases only manifest later in life and may be a result of Cushing's syndrome.

A prominent curly, dense coat is present from birth and develops into a dense, wavy coat quality (Figure 13.5). This condition may be restricted to the mane and tail (wavy mane syndrome) but may also affect the whole body. Some hair loss, including the tail and mane, is also often present. The coat is often less curly in summer.

Epigenetics

Epigenetics refers to heritable changes in gene expression that do not involve changes to the underlying DNA sequence, that is, a change in phenotype of horses without a change in genotype. Epigenetics is a new area of research and there is some debate as to its accuracy at present. It is currently thought that epigenetic change is a regular and natural occurrence, but it can also be influenced by several factors including age, exercise, pharmaceuticals, diet, environment and disease state. Epigenetic modifications may manifest in the same way that cells terminally differentiate to end up as skin

Table 13.1 Genetic disease and allelic variants identified by DNA testing.

Disease[a]	Gene	Alleles	Breeds[b]	Mutation description	References
GBED	*GBE1*	*N, G*	QH and related	ECA26 (see ref.)	Ward et al. (2004)
HERDA	*PEIB*	*N, HRD*	QH and related	ECA1g.128056148G>A	Tryon et al. (2007)
HYPP	*SCN4A*	*N, H*	QH and related	ECA11g.15500439C>G	Rudolph et al. (1992)
LWO	*EDNRB3*	*N, O*	Several[c]	ECA17g.50624681-50624682TC>AG	Metallinos et al. (1998), Santschi et al. (1998), Yang et al. (1998)
JEB	*LAMC2*	*N, J*	BE and related	ECA5g.20256789-20256790insC	Spirito et al. (2002)
JEB	*LAMA3*	*N, Js*	AS	ECA8g.3724_10312del6589	Graves et al. (2009)
LFS	*MYO5A*	*N, L*	AR and related	ECA1g.138235715del	Brooks et al. (2010)
MH	*RyR1*	*N, MH*	QH, PT	ECA10g.9554699C>G	Aleman et al. (2004)
PSSM	*GYS1*	*N, P*	Several[d]	ECA10g.18940346G>A	McCue et al. (2008)
SCID	*PRKDC*	*N, S*	AR and related	ECA9g.35528429-35528433del	Shin et al. (1997)

Source: This figure was produced with kind permission of the copyright holder Wiley-Blackwell from Bhanu Chowdhary (2013) Equine Genomics. Oxford: Wiley-Blackwell.
a) GBED, Glycogen branching enzyme deficiency; HERDA, hereditary equine regional dermal asthenia; HYPP, equine hyperkalemic periodic paralysis disease; LWO, lethal white overo; JEB, junctional epidermolysis bullosa (hairless foal syndrome – JEB 1 and 2); LFS, lavender foal syndrome; MH, malignant hyperthermia; PSSM, polysaccharide storage myopathy; SCID, equine severe combined immune deficiency.
b) QH, Quarter-horse; BE, Belgian Draft; AS, American Saddlebred; AR, Arabian; PT, American Paint Horse.
c) Breeds with overo white spotting.
d) Widespread including QH and related, Warmbloods and Draft breeds.

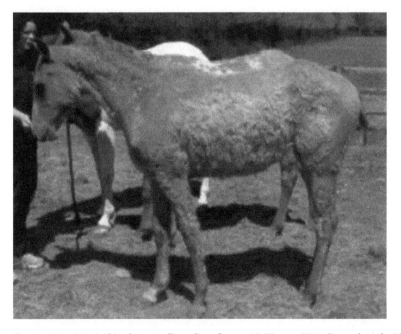

Figure 13.5 A typical 'curly coated' yearling. *Source*: McKinnon 2011. Reproduced with permission of John Wiley & Sons.

cells, liver cells, brain cells and so on. Epigenetic changes may also have more damaging effects that may result in ill health.

At least three systems – DNA methylation, histone modification and non-coding RNA (ncRNA)-associated gene silencing – are currently considered to begin and sustain epigenetic change. New and ongoing research is continuously uncovering the role of epigenetics in a variety of equine disorders. In cells, DNA is wrapped around coin-shaped proteins called histones for compaction and gene regulation. The attachment of small molecules to the DNA strand or histones modifies or regulates the genes, affecting the ability of transcription factors to reach their target genes. For example, adding a methyl group (CH_3) to DNA generally makes adjacent genes less accessible and therefore less active, whereas attaching an acetyl group ($COCH_3$) to histones 'relaxes' that part of the DNA strand, making it more accessible to transcription, that is, the genes are more accessible.

Epigenetic factors may cause changes to mitochondria via exercise. Proteins are used to make mitochondria within muscle cells. A key regulator of these proteins is a molecule known as **PGC**-1α in skeletal muscle fibres which may affect endurance. Changes during exercise stimulate production of this protein and, aided by specialised transcription actors, produce components for building mitochondria. It appears that a variant of **PGC**-1α is not present at all before exercise, but high levels can be found after only 1 hour of aerobic work. This suggests certain genes may be turned on by exercise.

Muscle Disorders

Several heritable diseases affect energy metabolism and muscle contraction and seriously affect athletic performance. These include:

- exertion rhabdomyolysis (ER)
- recurrent exertional rhabdomyolysis (RER)
- hyperkalemic periodic paralysis (HYPP)

- malignant hyperthermia (MH)
- glycogen branching enzyme deficiency (GBED)
- polysaccharide storage myopathy type 1 (PSSM 1)
- polysaccharide storage myopathy type 2 (PSSM 2).

Nuclear Transfer (Cloning)

The first cloned equids were born in 2003. To date, more than 20 cloned horses have been produced, and some have in turn reproduced, giving birth to healthy offspring. Cloning involves taking the nucleus of a cell from the donor horse and transferring it into the cytoplasm of an oocyte; the oocyte is then signalled to develop into an embryo. The cells from the donor horse are typically grown from a tissue biopsy sample, such as from under the mane on the horse's neck. Oocytes used for cloning must be mature (in metaphase II) (see Chapter 2). The mature oocyte is enucleated by removing the metaphase plate and polar body using a small-diameter pipette. The equine donor cell is then combined with the enucleated oocyte, either by electrofusion or by directly injecting the cell into the cytoplasm of the oocyte. The recombined oocyte is activated to stimulate embryonic development. Once the recombined oocyte has been activated, it may be transferred surgically to the oviduct of a recipient mare, or may be cultured in vitro to the blastocyst stage for transfer directly to the uterus of a recipient mare, as for normal embryo transfer.

The main problems noted in live cloned foals appear to be crooked front legs, umbilical problems and neonatal maladjustment syndrome. Fifty percent plus of cloned foals showed these signs to some extent, although these conditions mostly responded well to treatment.

Parental Similarity of Clones

Clones may not be completely identical to the donor. This is because epigenetic changes (see above) may cause the way a gene is used in a cloned foal to differ from that of the donor. This may affect phenotype. More importantly, epigenetic changes may cause placental insufficiency in cloned pregnancies, potentially resulting in maladjustment syndrome in the foal or a small foal.

Mitochondria have their own small DNA molecule coding for about 13 proteins and some functional nucleic acids. As discussed previously, mitochondrial DNA is passed through the generations via the oocyte only, not through sperm. The embryo is formed by division of the oocyte cytoplasm, thus the mitochondria of the host oocyte used for cloning become the mitochondria of the offspring. The result of cloning of a mare is therefore that the mitochondrial genotype of the cloned foal will differ from that of the donor animal. It is not known whether this may affect phenotype.

To summarise, the offspring of a cloned mare will have different mitochondrial DNA compared to that of the donor, but a cloned stallion will have the same mitochondrial DNA as the donor. Top-class competition horses have now been cloned, such as the eventer Tamarillo (offspring Tomatillo) and Cruising (offspring Cruising Encore and Cruising Arish). In 2012 the Fédération Equestre Internationale (FEI) changed its rules to allow clones to compete. The reason for cloning in most cases is to maintain the superior horse's genome for future generations.

Mutation

Mutation is a spontaneous change in the DNA structure or quantity which results in a change to the organism. Only mutations that arise in the formation of the sex cells or gametes are inherited. The rate of mutation is slow, but external factors may increase the rate of mutation. These external factors, such as radiation and chemicals, are known as mutagenic factors.

Mutations tend to be random. Darwin's theory of evolution is based on mutations that result in a beneficial trait in the animal,

helping it to survive and giving it an advantage over other animals in the group. Other mutations may be lethal and as such cannot be passed on to future generations. There are two types of mutation:

- gene mutation
- chromosome mutation.

Both of these may occur in somatic (body cells) and germ cells (sex cells), but somatic cell mutations are not passed to the next generation. In general, these occur as the horse gets older and this is thought to be a cause of cancer. However, when a mutation occurs in a germ cell which then goes on to fertilisation and become a zygote, the mutation is passed on to the new foal. Germ cell mutations therefore result in changes to the genome of the foal.

Gene Mutation

Gene mutation occurs due to a change in the base sequence of DNA. This change can render the whole gene useless and may even be lethal. The change in a single base is known as point mutation. The change to one base therefore can be catastrophic. This is because this minute change will alter a codon, resulting in it now coding for a totally different amino acid which itself may result in a different polypeptide chain and resultant protein. An example of gene mutation is sickle cell anaemia in humans. There are several types of gene mutation:

- Substitution – nucleotides are replaced with others with different bases.
- Addition – more nucleotides are added to the DNA.
- Deletion – nucleotides are lost from the DNA.
- Duplication – a portion of nucleotide within DNA is repeated.
- Inversion – a nucleotide sequence is reversed within DNA.

Mutation → different base sequence →

different amino acid → different polypeptide

→ different protein or protein shape →

protein now does not function in the horse.

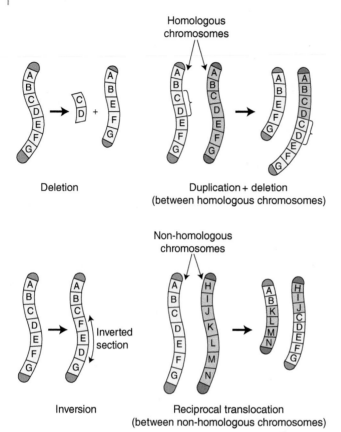

Homologous
chromosomes

Non-homologous
chromosomes

Deletion

Duplication + deletion
(between homologous chromosomes)

Inverted
section

Inversion

Reciprocal translocation
(between non-homologous chromosomes)

Figure 13.6 The four basic types of chromosome mutation.

The least damaging gene mutations are inversions and substitutions because they alter only one amino acid. Deletions and additions are potentially more damaging because they result in frame shifts; that is, the loss or addition of one base causes the whole sequence to shift along the DNA strand, altering all the codes.

The rate of gene mutations depends on many factors, such as species of animal and genes at different loci. The rate, however, can be greatly increased by environmental factors known as mutagens, for example X-rays, chemicals and smoke.

Chromosome Mutation

During mitosis, chromosomes are copied, condensed and pulled apart on the spindle, before separating into the daughter cells, and sometimes faults occur during this process so that the structure of the new chromosome in one or both of the daughter cells is altered. Chromosome mutation generally affects whole blocks of genes within the chromosome, as opposed to one gene as found in gene mutation. There are four basic types of chromosome mutation (Figure 13.6):

- deletion
- duplication and deletion
- inversion
- reciprocal translocation.

Non-Disjunction

Non-disjunction occurs when pairs of chromosomes fail to separate during anaphase I in meiosis. One of the gametes now has an additional chromosome and the other lacks one. At fertilisation the result will be either 2n+1 or 2n−1.

Polyploidy

Sometimes chromosomes fail to separate properly during meiosis and this results in the gamete having the diploid number (2n) of chromosomes instead of the necessary haploid number (n). If this gamete fuses with another normal haploid sex cell, then the resultant embryo will be triploid in number, that is 3n. This is known as polyploidy.

Single Nucleotide Polymorphisms

A single nucleotide polymorphism (SNP, pronounced snip) is a DNA sequence variation occurring when a single nucleotide – A, T, C or G – in the genome (or other shared sequence) differs between members of the equine species or between paired chromosomes in an individual horse. They are sometimes referred to as genetic markers. SNPs are now used routinely in equine genetic research, enabling thousands of genes to be tested at the same time.

The horse Twilight was selected for whole genome sequencing by the National Human Genome Research Institute (NHGRI) as a representative of the order Perissodactyla. Her genome was sequenced at the Broad Institute of Harvard and MIT. This project has produced the EquCab 2.0 assembly. From this dataset researchers were able to manufacture an equine whole genome SNP array known as the EquineSNP50 BeadChip, which contains 54,000 SNP assays per sample for use in research.

The Myostatin Gene and Performance

The equine gene encoding myostatin (the MSTN gene) has been found to have a highly significant association with racing performance in Thoroughbreds. Myostatin is a growth and differentiation factor that functions as a negative regulator of skeletal muscle mass development.

The research into myostatin and performance was a genome-wide SNP-association study for optimum racing distance and was performed using the EquineSNP50 Bead-Chip genotyping array in a cohort of 118 elite Thoroughbred racehorses divergent for race distance aptitude. The most significant SNP was located on chromosome 18 close to MSTN. The results complement a recent investigation of functional responses to exercise training in Thoroughbred skeletal muscle, which identified MSTN mRNA transcripts as the most significantly altered following a 10-month period of training. Research provides clear evidence that the previously reported polymorphism in equine MSTN at locus g.66493737C>T is the most powerful genome-wide predictor of optimum racing distance, that is, sprint, middle distance or long distance in Thoroughbred horses. A genetic test is now available to horse breeders and trainers for this polymorphism. The Equinome Speed Gene Test may be used to make a prediction about the type of horse an individual is most likely to be and may be used to improve decision-making in selection, breeding and training.

Recent research has also found a key gene in horse height known as LCORL which limits growth and size in horses. The stronger LCOR is expressed, the smaller the horse.

Coat Colour and Genetics

For most alleles of horse coat colours it is impossible to tell by looking at the horse whether it is homozygous or heterozygous for any coat colour gene. As previously mentioned, each somatic cell contains a duplicate set of genes. Each set is derived from the single genes inherited at conception by both the dam and the sire. The genes code for similar but not necessarily identical genetic information. The alternative forms of each gene are called alleles. If both alleles are identical copies, the animal is said to be homozygous, for example EE or ee, but if the alleles are different for the same trait, the animal is said to be heterozygous for that gene, that is, Ee. This is important for coat colour. The expressed version of the gene is known as dominant (denoted by uppercase letter) and the unexpressed one is known as recessive (denoted by lower case). A horse homozygous for a certain allele will always pass it on to its offspring, while a horse that is heterozygous carries two different alleles and can pass on either one.

Coat colour alleles affect the pigment melanin which gives skin and coat colour. There are two chemically distinct types of melanin:

- phaeomelanin – perceived as red to yellow colour
- eumelanin – perceived as brown to black.

All colour genes in horses affect either the production or distribution of phaeomelanin and eumelanin. Alleles affecting melanocytes (pigment cells) do not alter the pigment chemicals themselves, but rather by acting on the placement of pigment cells produce distinct patterns of unpigmented pink skin and corresponding white hair. Horses have three basic coat colours:

- red (chestnut)
- bay
- black.

All the above are controlled by the action of the following two genes:

- the extension (E) locus gene on gene MC1R (alleles E or e)
- the agouti (A) locus gene on gene ASIP (alleles A or a).

In the 1990s, scientists in Sweden demonstrated that genetic differences in the MC1R gene are responsible for the red base coat colour in horses. Red is a recessive trait, so all chestnuts must be homozygous for that colour (i.e. ee). If the E allele is dominant (i.e. E), black pigment will be expressed, so all bay and black horses must have either EE or Ee genotypes. Table 13.2 shows common coat colours and dilutions with their genetic formulae. Genes G and W both have alleles that effectively block the actions of other coat colour genes.

Table 13.2 Common coat colours and dilutions with their genetic formulae.

Colour	Genetic formula
Grey	G
White	W
Red	ee,aa,CC,dd,gg,ww,toto
Bay	E,A,CC,dd,gg,ww,toto
Black	E,aa,CC,dd,gg,ww,toto
Palomino	ee,CCcr,dd,gg,ww,toto
Mouse dun	E,aa,CC,D,gg,ww,toto
Cremello	CcrCcr
Bay tobiano	E,A,CC.dd,gg,ww,TO

Bay/Black

In horses that have EE or Ee it is the A gene that determines black or bay colour. Bay is the dominant phenotype of the two (A) and so the genotype of a bay horse is expressed as:

- E/Aa – bay
- E/AA – bay
- E/aa – black (the recessive colour and always homozygous recessive for the agouti gene).

When black pigment is present, the agouti gene (A locus) determines whether or not the pigment is expressed over the whole body or only the points, that is, the legs, tail and mane. The gene for expression at these points is always dominant. All other equine coat colours stem from red, bay or black.

White (Albino) (WW or Ww)

If a horse has the dominant W allele at birth, which is relatively rare, the foal will lack any pigment in the coat hair and skin; this is known as albino, with pink or blue eyes and white hair, and sometimes is referred to as white (Ww). All horses that are not white will therefore be ww, that is, double recessive for that gene. The homozygous WW foals are not viable.

Grey (GG or Gg)

The grey coat colour gene is named STX17. Horses with the dominant G allele will be

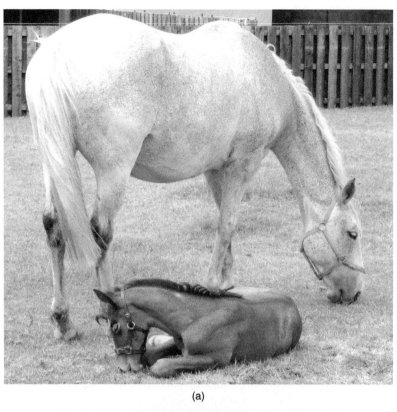

(a)

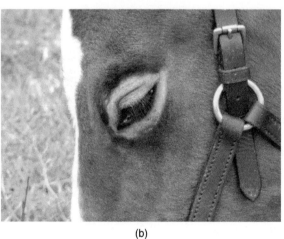

(b)

Figure 13.7 (a) Grey mare with 'bay' foal with grey around the eyes (b). *Source*: Courtesy of Harthill Stud.

born any colour (usually dark) but grey, and this will change with age as they eventually lose their colour pigment in the hair and become more white or white with added flecks of red or black colour. Earliest

signs of grey will be seen around the eyes (Figure 13.7).

However, grey horses have pigmented skin all the time before any colour change. Grey is produced by a dominant gene (i.e. G), so a grey horse's genotype will be GG or Gg and one of the parents must be grey. All non-grey horses must therefore be gg.

Roan

Roan colours often look very similar to greys, particularly when greys are changing their coat colour. Roans do not whiten over time but retain the mixture of white and other colour over the body with darker heads and legs. The mutation of this gene is not known yet, but it is thought to be linked to the MC1R and KIT genes that appear to play a role in the pinto (black and white patches) genetics. The KIT gene in horses is responsible for many different white patterns. It has four known white pattern alleles: roan, tobiano, sabino and dominant white.

Spotting Patterns

Most of these genes produce horses with a base colour with a variety of white patches or spots.

Sabino (SB1)

Sabino is another painted coat colour pattern and is a subclass of the overo coat pattern. These horses are generally a solid colour with white facial markings, white legs and belly spots. The KIT gene is also involved with creating this colour pattern.

This pattern is common in many breeds of horse and is also prized by breeders. Sabino1 is the gene responsible and is dominant in that a single copy of the gene causes the distinctive white patterns. However, two copies of the gene result in a horse that is born almost entirely white. This gene occurs in many horse breeds. There are similar sabino patterns that are not a result of this gene. For example, Clydesdale horses are famous for their sabino markings but appear to have a different gene for sabino. Clearly, there are probably several different genes that may cause sabino patterns. A molecular DNA test is available for sabino1.

Foals with a homozygous genotype can be born all white and healthy (unlike some other white foals that are affected by the deadly overo lethal white syndrome (OLWS)). Therefore white foals suspected of having OLWS should be tested for OLWS first, before euthanasia.

Tobiano (TO or to)

The tobiano gene is responsible for the white patches that occur on the bodies of horses, almost always crossing the midline of the back. Tobianos normally have dark-coloured heads with white legs and white patches. The pattern is popular and found among a large number of horses registered in the Paint Horse Registry. This colour occurs due to chromosomal inversion (i.e. part of the chromosome appears flipped upside down) of the KIT gene. Tobiano is dominant and so horses with this gene will always produce spotted offspring. Recently, scientists in Kentucky identified the probably genetic basis for tobiano patterns and a molecular test has been developed.

Overo (O)

Similar to tobiano, overo causes extensive white markings and is well represented among horses in the Paint Horse Registry (Figure 13.8). However, unlike tobiano, overo patterns almost never cross the midline of the back and often look as if they are growing up from the belly. Overo white patterns are caused by a dominant gene. However, horses with two copies of the gene are born completely white but with multiple developmental defects, resulting in death soon after birth, that is, this can be a lethal gene. Horses with one copy of the gene are, however, normal and highly sought after by breeders because of their attractive patterns. A molecular test has been developed to identify the gene.

Appaloosa (LP)

The Lakota or Nez Pierce Native Americans bred horses with distinctive white colour

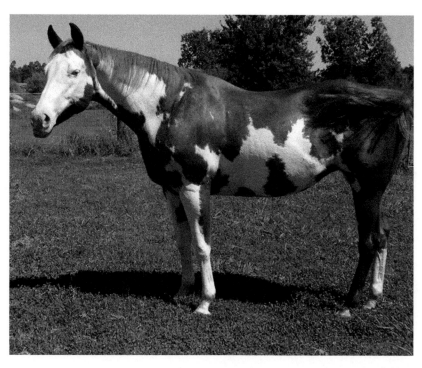

Figure 13.8 Deaf American Paint Horse with frame splashed with white overo phenotype. *Source*: Chowdhary 2013. Reproduced with permission of John Wiley & Sons.

patterns in the American Northwest Territory during the 1800s. The patterns included white hips with dark spots, white body with dark spots throughout, partial or full roaning and more. The spotting patterns include leopard, blanket, snowflake and roan. Permanent identification of Appaloosas can be difficult, since the white patterns may not be stable from birth. In addition, Appaloosa horses possess characteristics defined as striped hooves, mottled muzzles and white sclera around the eye. Observations suggested that a single gene determined whether or not the horse had the appaloosa characteristics and a colour pattern, while other factors, possibly genes, determined the precise colour pattern. Researchers have determined that the gene for appaloosa is on horse chromosome 1, but they do not know which gene. Horses homozygous for the appaloosa mutation are also affected by a complete loss of night vision, named congenital stationary night blindness.

Cream (C or Ccr)

The cream dilution gene causes a loss of pigment or dilution in cells expressing brown or red pigment. It is an allele of a C gene known as CCcr and is thought to be a mutation on gene MATP. A chestnut horse with the dilution gene becomes a palomino as the dilution gene dilutes red pigment to yellow (Figure 13.9).

- A palomino is a chestnut that is heterozygous for the cream dilution gene (ww,gg,ee,CCcr).
- A cremello is a chestnut homozygous to the cream dilution gene (CcrCcr). It has cream-coloured hair, pink skin and blue eyes.
- A buckskin is a bay horse heterozygous for the cream dilution gene (ww,gg,A,E,CCcr) (Figure 13.10).
- A perlino is a bay horse homozygous for the cream dilution gene.

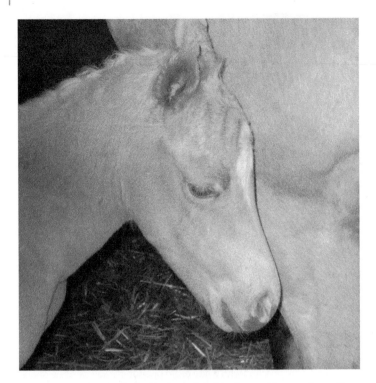

Figure 13.9 Palomino foal with deep pink skin. *Source*: Coetzee, https://commons.wikimedia.org/wiki/File: Palominofoal-pinkskin.png. CC0 1.0.

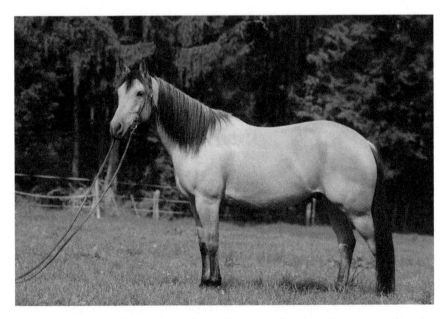

Figure 13.10 Buckskin Quarter-horse. *Source*: Tierpfotografien, https://commons.wikimedia.org/wiki/File: Quarter_Horse_Buckskin.JPG. CC BY-SA 3.0..

Two copies will cause greater dilution and horses appear almost white. A bay horse with the dilution gene becomes a buckskin where the red pigment is diluted to yellow. Perlino and cremello also occur from this dilution gene. The gene is dominant and only one copy is necessary for its effect on the phenotypic colour.

Silver (Z)

The silver dilution gene dilutes eumelanin to a chocolate or silver colour. It is often known as silver dapple and the effect on black pigmented hair is caused by a mutation on gene PMEL17. Horses with the dominant silver gene show a dilution to grey for any black hairs. This dilution produces a chocolate body colour with flaxen mane and tail.

Champagne

Champagne is caused by a mutation to gene SLC36A1 and is dominant. This gene acts on the base coat colour, lightening it. Champagne-coloured horses are born with blue eyes which change to amber with age.

Pearl

Pearl dilutions are caused by a mutation on gene MATP. Two copies of the mutation will produce a diluted base colour, while one may produce golden undertones to the coat colour.

Dun (D or d)

The mutation behind the dun coat colour is unknown. It is a dominant trait affecting all the horse's primary base colours. The D allele dilutes both eumelanin and phaeomelanin on the body but not on the points. A horse with a chestnut base would be red dun in colour, while a horse with a bay base would be yellow dun. All dun horses have dorsal stripes, and some may also have zebra stripes on their legs, although this is rarer. The dun gene is only found in a few breeds.

White Markings

White markings are socks or stockings on the limbs and a blaze, star or snip on the head. Although multiple genes and a complex mode of inheritance are thought to play a role, there appears to be an association for a locus of major effect near the KIT gene. The KIT gene in horses is responsible for many different white patterns.

Melanomas in Grey Horses

Many grey horses have a high incidence of skin melanomas that generally take the form of firm, black nodules under the tail base and in anal, perianal and genital regions, as well as the perineum, lips and eyelids. Although some melanomas are benign, others can metastasise to internal organs. Melanomas are reported in 70–80% of grey horses older than 15 years of age. A high level of expression of STX17 was seen in melanomas from grey horses.

Exercise-Induced Pulmonary Haemorrhage (EIPH) or Epistaxis

Researchers investigated 117,000 horses that suffered from EIPH. The most severe forms are now thought to be caused by a combination of genes and external factors. Horses affected by EIPH are known as 'bleeders' as they haemorrhage from their lungs.

EIPH has been detected in three-day eventers, steeplechasers and polo ponies, among others. The common denominator is strenuous exercise. It may even result in death in racehorses after extreme effort, for example following the end of a race.

EIPH is influenced by multiple genes that each contribute a little to the problem. Exposure to certain environmental risk factors may lead to expression of these genes. The next step will be to identify the genes and risk factors, allowing for better treatment.

Summary Points

1) In November 2009, the first genome sequence of the domestic horse (*Equus caballus*) was published in the international journal *Science*.
2) Although most DNA is found within chromosomes in the nucleus, it is now known that mitochondrial DNA, though much smaller in quantity, has a significant role to play, particularly in mares.
3) In horses, each nucleated body cell has 64 chromosomes, arranged in 32 pairs.

Of those 32 pairs, one pair (the sex chromosomes) determines the gender of the horse.

4) Most lethal alleles only have the lethal effect when the horse is homozygous for the gene. The heterozygotes are therefore known as carriers for the lethal condition.
5) There are two chemically distinct types of melanin: phaeomelanin, perceived as red to yellow colour, and eumelanin, perceived as brown to black.

Q+A

Q When was the first genome sequence of the domestic horse (*Equus caballus*) published?
A November 2009.

Q What are two different genes for the same traits known as?
A Alleles or allelomorphs.

Q Name four examples of lethal genes in horses.
A Lethal white foal syndrome (LWFS), foal immunodeficiency syndrome (FIS), lavender foal syndrome (LFS) and severe combined immunodeficiency (SCID) in Arabian foals.

Q In which horses is a congenital 'curly coat' syndrome recognised?
A Quarter-horses, Percherons, Arabs, Appaloosas and Morgans.

Q What are the three basic coat colours of horses?
A Red (chestnut), bay and black.

Q What is the Equinome Speed Gene Test?
A This test may be used to make a prediction about the type of athletic horse an individual is most likely to be and may be used to improve decision-making in the selection, breeding and training of horses for racing.

14

The Urinary System

The urinary system is primarily involved in the extraction and removal of waste products from the blood. It filters the blood. In particular it is responsible for the removal of nitrogenous waste, and together with the digestive system it removes most of the waste products produced in the body, except gaseous carbon dioxide which is removed via the lungs. While removing these waste products, the urinary system is closely involved with the water balance, acid–base balance and salt balance. These processes are highly complicated and involve the influence of hormones. The products of excretion of the horse are shown in Figure 14.1.

The urinary system is composed of two kidneys, two ureters, one bladder and the urethra (Figures 14.2 and 14.3). Each day approximately 1000–2000 litres of fluid are delivered to the kidneys of the horse. Since only approximately 5–15 litres of urine are excreted daily, the kidneys must remove most of the substances present in them. If the kidneys did not reabsorb fluid entering them, horses would lose their entire water and salt content in less than half a day.

Kidneys

The kidneys are a pair of reddish-brown organs and in the horse lie on either side of the body, approximately midway between the withers and the croup underneath the spine. The left kidney lies farther back towards the last rib, whereas the right kidney lies under the last three ribs. In this position they are well protected from external injury. The kidneys are situated outside the abdominal cavity but are bound to the upper wall of the abdomen by a layer of peritoneum which prevents the kidneys moving about as the horse moves. There are often large collections of fatty tissue around the kidneys which also helps to protect them.

The kidneys play a crucial role in homeostasis, regulating plasma salts, and have a hormonal role. They filter plasma from the blood through the glomerulus. In other words, they are highly efficient sieves, which allow the passage of smaller particles such as plasma salts through, but not the larger blood cells. On the whole, the filtrate is reabsorbed further along the nephron and all that remains is substances the horse's body no longer requires. The kidneys also play a vital role in the water balance of the horse. The horse's entire circulatory volume is effectively filtered and reabsorbed every half an hour. The functions of the kidney are to:

- regulate water balance and ion levels (solute reabsorption)
- maintain volume and contents of extracellular fluid such as plasma
- regulate pH, that is, acid–base regulation;
- maintain osmotic balance
- excrete waste products, such as urea, toxins and electrolytes.

From the substances that are filtered through, the kidneys selectively reabsorb water and other useful constituents to prevent their depletion in plasma, while other

Equine Science, Third Edition. Zoe Davies and Sarah Pilliner.
© 2018 Zoe Davies and Sarah Pilliner. Published 2018 by John Wiley & Sons Ltd.

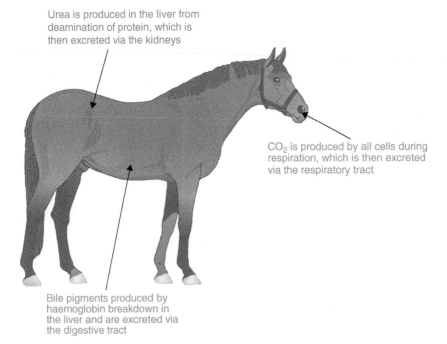

Urea is produced in the liver from deamination of protein, which is then excreted via the kidneys

CO_2 is produced by all cells during respiration, which is then excreted via the respiratory tract

Bile pigments produced by haemoglobin breakdown in the liver and are excreted via the digestive tract

Figure 14.1 Excretory products of the horse.

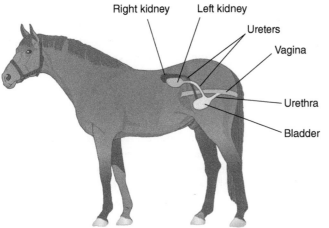

Right kidney   Left kidney

Ureters

Vagina

Urethra

Bladder

Figure 14.2 Position of the urinary organs.

waste products are allowed through the system to be evacuated. Most domestic animals have bean-shaped kidneys similar to humans, but the horse has two different-shaped kidneys: the left is bean-shaped and the right is heart-shaped. In the adult horse each kidney weighs approximately 700g and measures 15–18 cm in length.

The indented portion of the kidney is known as the hilus. This is where the blood vessels and nerves enter and the thin muscular tube known as the ureter and lymphatic vessels leave. If the kidneys are cut open, two main regions known as the cortex and the medulla are evident (Figure 14.4). The cortex is the outer light-red region and the

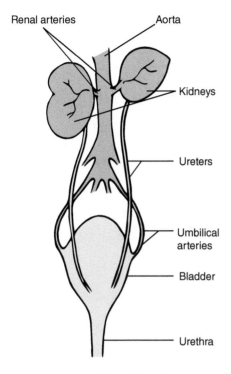

Renal arteries   Aorta

Kidneys

Ureters

Umbilical
arteries

Bladder

Urethra

Figure 14.3 Dorsal view of the urinary system.

degree of fusion occurs, resulting in fusion into the renal crest; however, the function of the kidney remains the same. Thus in horses the renal cortex lacks the divisions in to individual lobes as seen in the human kidney (Figure 14.5). This applies also to goats and sheep. In all these animals, the renal papillae are actually fused to make the longitudinal renal crest (which projects into the renal pelvis). Urine discharged from the collecting tubules of the renal crest is collected in the renal pelvis.

The renal pelvis is a funnel-shaped cavity and is the origin of the ureter, which then takes urine to the bladder. The water and solutes dissolved in the urine that enter the renal pelvis stay in the urine for evacuation or excretion; that is, there are no further changes. The cortex or outer part of the kidney is situated between the medulla and the thin connective tissue capsule which surrounds the whole kidney itself. The cortex is velvety and granular. The granular appearance comes from the large number of filtering capsules otherwise known as glomeruli. The outer part of the kidney is a tough fibrous capsule which prevents the kidney expanding as it fills.

The kidney has a wide variety of cell types. For the most part, renal tubules and/or ducts comprise most of the renal parenchyma and are lined by specialised epithelial cells. Renal interstitial tissue is sparse in the cortex and gradually increases toward the papillae. The distribution of the renal blood system supplies more blood to the cortex.

Nephrons

Apart from blood vessels and a small amount of connective tissue, the kidney consists of a mass of tubules known as nephrons (Figure 14.6). The horse has approximately 2.5 million nephrons, each being a hollow tube which starts in the cortex as a blind-ended thin-walled sac (Bowman's capsule) into which a knot of blood vessels passes

medulla is darker and within it can be seen cone-shaped pyramids known as the renal pyramids; urine drains from the tips of these pyramids into the renal pelvis and then into the ureter. The medulla can be spilt into two areas – the outer and inner medulla – and different parts of the nephron reside in these two areas. Each kidney has a system of tubules which each end in the ureter, a single larger tube which takes fluid into the bladder before it is eventually expelled via the urethra outside the horse's body. The medulla appears striated or lined because of these radially placed collecting vessels or tubules (part of the nephron). Renal columns are extensions of the renal cortex and fill space between the renal pyramids. The hilus marks the boundary of an area known as the renal pelvis.

During development, the horse begins with a multi-lobed structure, but a varying

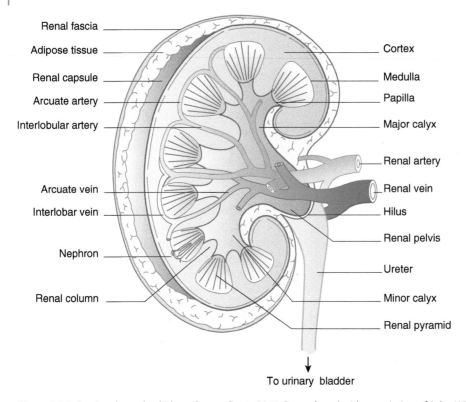

Figure 14.4 Section through a kidney. *Source*: Peate 2011. Reproduced with permission of John Wiley & Sons.

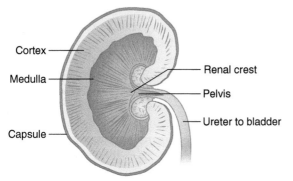

Figure 14.5 Renal papillae fused into the renal crest.

(the glomerulus). Each unit of a Bowman's capsule together with its own glomerulus is known as a Malpighian corpuscle (also known as a Malpighian body) (Figure 14.7). The number of nephrons remains the same from birth of the foal and new ones cannot be made to replace injured or diseased ones.

Following on from the Bowman's capsule, the next part of the nephron becomes coiled into a series of loops, which again are situated in the renal cortex and this part is known as the proximal convoluted tubule. Then the nephron loops down into the medulla as a thin-walled tube known as the loop of Henle, which returns to the cortex again to end in another series of coils known as the distal convoluted tubule. This empties into a series of collecting ducts which eventually

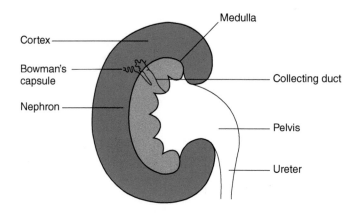

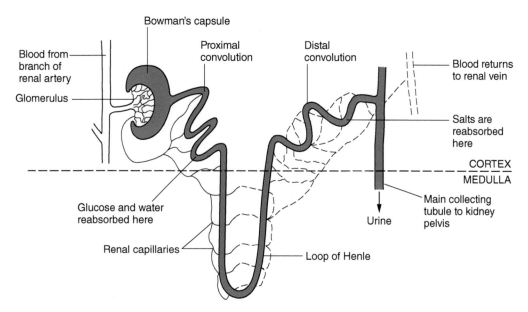

Figure 14.6 Structure of a nephron.

discharge into the renal pelvis. The blood supply to the nephron is such that most of the blood passes into the glomeruli for filtration before reaching the rest of the kidney. There are two capillary beds (one after the other) – one that surrounds the Bowman's capsule and the other that intermingles with the tubular parts of the nephron. This renal microcirculation is a unique anatomical anomaly in that the glomerular capillaries are between two arterioles rather than an arteriole and a venule (see Figure 14.6). The afferent arterioles go into the glomerulus and the efferent arterioles leave it. Ultrafiltration requires blood being filtered under high pressure, and this is achieved by:

- blood arriving from the first branch of the aorta (i.e. under pressure)
- the afferent arteriole being shorter and having a larger diameter than the efferent arteriole.

This produces hydrostatic pressure that forces blood against a filter consisting of

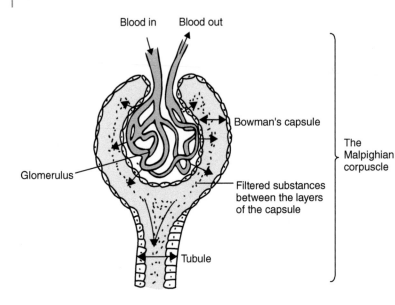

Blood in   Blood out

Bowman's capsule

The Malpighian corpuscle

Glomerulus

Filtered substances between the layers of the capsule

Tubule

Figure 14.7 Malpighian corpuscle showing blood passing from glomerular capillaries to the tubules.

three layers. The layers that separate the plasma in the glomerular capillaries from the cavity of the Bowman's capsule are:

- the lining of the endothelium of the glomerular capillaries
- the basement membrane on which the capillary wall rests
- cells of the renal capsule.

Of the three layers that act as the barrier through which filtration takes place, only the basement membrane acts as a barrier to the free movement of substances. Together the glomerular endothelium and the podocytes act as a filtration membrane. The walls of the capillaries in the renal capsule are more permeable than normal and the cells have small slits or fenestrations through which plasma contents can pass. Figure 14.8 shows a glomerulus of a mouse kidney, showing the very small filtration slits.

The renal capsule is also lined with unique cells called podocytes, which again do not fit tightly together, forming a network of more slits that fit over the capillary. This effectively results in two coarse filters, one either side of the continuous basement membrane, which is a finer filter preventing the passage of all larger molecules, such as proteins, and these stay in the blood.

Because blood in the glomeruli is under such high pressure, there is no tendency for fluid to enter back into the glomeruli blood vessels. The hydrostatic pressure of blood going into the glomerulus is opposed by two other pressures, namely:

- glomerular capsule pressure – fluid already in the capsule and renal tubule
- blood colloid osmotic pressure.

If either of these pressures increases, glomerular filtration rate will fall. If blood pressure increases or decreases slightly, then small changes in the diameter of the afferent and efferent arterioles can maintain net filtration rate at a steady rate. If the efferent arteriole is constricted slightly, blood flowing out will increase net filtration pressure.

Blood cells and larger substances such as proteins are retained within capillaries in the glomeruli and only water and smaller substances such as mineral salts, glucose, amino acids and urea are filtered out. The glomerular filtrate therefore contains water, salts, glucose, amino acids and excretory products such as urea. If there is a fall in blood pressure, for example if the horse is haemorrhaging (bleeding), the filtration process may stop and no urine will be formed. Urea is the main nitrogenous waste product

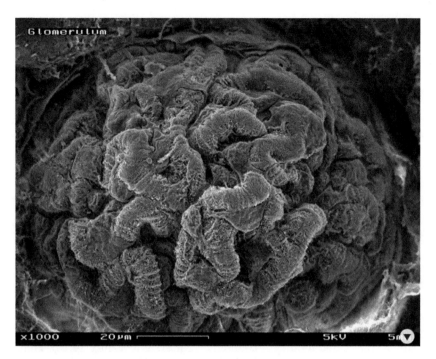

Figure 14.8 Glomerulum of mouse kidney under a scanning electron microscope, magnification 1000×. *Source*: SecrectDisc, https://commons.wikimedia.org/wiki/File:Glomerulum_of_mouse_kidney_in_Scanning_Electron_Microscope,_magnification_1,000x.GIF. CC BY-SA 3.0.

found in mammals. It is soluble in water and fairly toxic. Urea is manufactured in the liver in a cyclical chemical reaction, known as the ornithine cycle, from ammonia (Figure 14.9).

To summarise the functions of the nephron, ultrafiltration of the blood takes place, where fluid is forced through the glomerulus capillaries, forming a filtrate similar to blood but lacking proteins and blood cells. The filtrate is then modified by absorption and secretion to add and remove ions, before urine is formed.

Role of Tubules in Formation of Urine and in Homeostasis

The main role of tubules is to resorb large volumes of fluids and most of the substances dissolved in that fluid. The mechanisms of resorption and secretion in the kidney tubules use both active and passive transport. Water moves passively through the walls of the renal tubules down an osmotic gradient. Substances dissolved in the filtrate fluid, however, move passively in and out of the tubular fluid down chemical and electrical gradients. However, some compounds have to be actively transported against chemical and electrical gradients, and this requires the use of energy.

If a substance is removed from tubular fluid to the blood, it is said to be reabsorbed, whereas if it is moved from the blood to the tubules it is said to be secreted. The tubules may add more of the substance to the tubular fluid (tubular secretion) or may remove some or all of the substance from the tubular fluid (reabsorption) or may do both – a highly complicated process.

Proximal Convoluted Tubule

The proximal convoluted tubule is also known as the first convoluted tubule. This is the portion of the duct system of the nephron of the kidney that leads from the Bowman's capsule to the loop of Henle. In the proximal

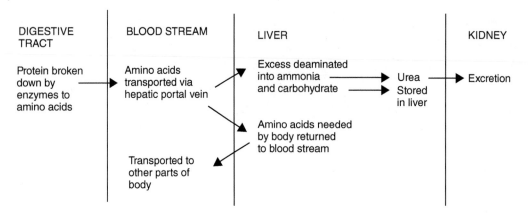

Figure 14.9 Control of water balance.

convoluted tubule, many solutes are totally resorbed by active transport, including amino acids and glucose. Normally all blood glucose is reabsorbed, unless levels in the blood are much higher than normal, such as in diabetes. The proximal convoluted tubule is also very close to blood vessels known as peritubular capillaries carrying blood away from the glomerulus. In the renal system, peritubular capillaries are tiny blood vessels that travel alongside nephrons, allowing reabsorption and secretion between blood and the inner lumen of the nephron.

The plasma in these vessels contains plasma proteins which were not filtered and so result in a high solute potential and relatively low hydrostatic pressure, allowing the blood to resorb a large portion of filtered water by osmosis. The cells that line the first convoluted tubule are adapted for active transport, with a large surface area created by microvilli and many mitochondria providing energy for active transport in the form of adenosine triphosphate (ATP).

Loop of Henle

The loop of Henle is a long U-shaped part of the tubule. It extends deep into the medulla and then turns to loop back up to the cortex. The loop creates a region of high solute concentration in the medulla. As the collecting ducts pass through this area, the osmotic gradient between the outside of the collecting duct and the inside results in water being drawn out of the collecting ducts by osmosis. This makes the urine more and more concentrated as water is removed as it passes down the duct. The loop of Henle works by a countercurrent system (Figure 14.10). Fluid in the two limbs of the loop of Henle flows in opposite directions, hence it is known as a countercurrent system.

The loop of Henle works as follows:

- The ascending limb of the loop of Henle actively pumps chloride ions (Cl^-) out of the filtrate, and the counter ion sodium (Na^+) follows. This part of the loop in impermeable to water and so water cannot follow by osmosis.
- This sodium chloride is pumped out of the ascending limb into the surrounding tissue fluid. Now water that is in the descending limb moves out under osmosis, leaving the descending limb with increased solute concentration, creating a region of high solute concentration in the medulla.
- Fluid passing down the collecting duct must pass through the region of high solute concentration When the horse is dehydrated and needs to conserve water, antidiuretic hormone (ADH) makes the collecting duct more permeable so more water is lost by osmosis into the tissues; that is, water is conserved as it does not go into the urine. The regulation

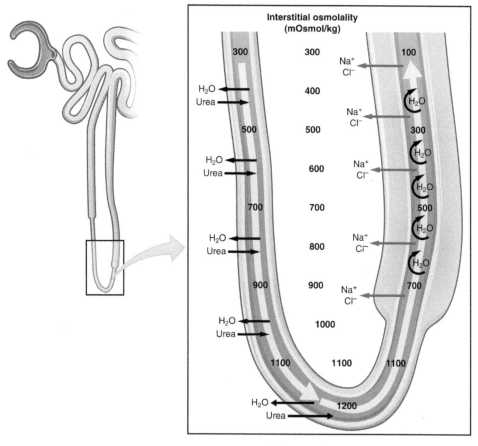

Figure 14.10 The loop of Henle countercurrent multiplier system. *Source*: OpenStax, https://commons
.wikimedia.org/wiki/File:2621_Loop_of_Henle_Countercurrent_Multiplier_System.jpg. CC BY 3.0.

of permeability in the distal convoluted tubules and the collecting ducts and therefore the control of urine concentration is controlled by ADH.

- Water lost from the urine is collected by vessels of the blood system. They are peritubular capillaries and surround the proximal and distal tubules, but around the loop of Henle in the medulla the blood capillaries are straight and are known as the vasa recta renis or arteriolae rectae renis. The vasa recta renis form long descending and ascending loops and are important for the countercurrent exchange system which produces concentrated urine when required.

Distal Convoluted Tubule

Also known as the second convoluted tubule, the distal tubule effectively acts to fine tune the remaining fluid according to the needs of the horse's body at the time. The distal convoluted tubule is important in the regulation of water, it is partly responsible for the regulation of salt balance (potassium and sodium) and regulates pH. It is also the primary site for the kidneys' hormone-based regulation of calcium.

The distal convoluted tubule regulates pH by absorbing bicarbonate and secreting hydrogen ions (H^+) into the filtrate, or by absorbing hydrogen ions and secreting bicarbonate into the filtrate. Sodium and potassium levels are controlled by secreting K^+ and absorbing Na^+. Sodium absorption by the distal tubule is mediated by the hormone aldosterone. Aldosterone increases sodium reabsorption. Sodium and chloride (salt) reabsorption is also mediated by a group of four kinases called WNK kinases. Calcium regulation also occurs by reabsorbing calcium ions in response to parathyroid hormone. Arginine vasopressin receptor 2 is also expressed here.

Regulation of Water

The kidneys play a vital role in the control of body water, by altering the amount excreted when there are large variations in water intake. When horses are deprived of water, the quantity of urine produced is low and the concentration of urine is high. Of water that enters the tubule, about 85% is reabsorbed in the proximal part and the remaining 15% is passed on to the further parts of the tubule. It is this fraction of the filtered water that is modified by the kidney according to the state of the body's water balance (hydration). If the horse's body is dehydrated, most of the water in the distal end of the tubule will be reabsorbed, whereas if the body is overhydrated almost all of this water will be excreted in the urine. This is the way the horse's body maintains water balance (Figure 14.10).

Regulation of Permeability of the Collecting Ducts by ADH

The permeability of the distal parts of the nephron to water is controlled by the ADH, which is secreted by the posterior lobe of the pituitary gland. ADH acts by negative feedback. When the concentration of water in blood decreases by as little as 1%, the osmoreceptors (that are sensitive to solute concentration in the blood) in the hypothalamus stimulate production of ADH in the posterior pituitary, which is then secreted into the blood. ADH production will also

be stimulated by massive loss of blood volume following severe dehydration. The hypothalamus responds in two ways:

- it stimulates production of ADH from the posterior pituitary gland;
- it stimulates the thirst centre in the brain.

The term diuresis refers to the condition when large volumes of dilute urine are produced. Antidiuresis means the opposite and applies when water is reabsorbed and smaller amounts of a more concentrated urine are produced. The name of antidiuretic hormone therefore describes its effect on nephrons in the kidney. The release of ADH from the pituitary gland increases permeability of the distal convoluted tubules and collecting ducts to water, allowing more water to diffuse out into the tissue fluid and making a reduced volume of urine which is more concentrated. In the absence of ADH, the collecting tubules remain impermeable to water and no concentration of urine occurs. ADH makes the tubules more permeable to water by inserting proteins that act as channels for water into their plasma membranes. ADH is a peptide hormone which fits into receptor sites (proteins) on the cells' surface membranes of the distal convoluted tubules. Once in situ, they stimulate cyclic adenosine monophosphate (AMP) which activates protein molecules known as aquaporins, which then move to the cell surface to act as water channels or aqua pores, making the membrane more permeable to water.

As water permeability of the cells increases, water moves from the tubular fluid into the cells and then into blood. As water increases in the blood, ADH production by the hypothalamus decreases and water permeability is reduced and more dilute urine is produced.

In the condition known as diabetes insipidus, which rarely occurs in horses, the posterior pituitary gland either does not secrete ADH or secretes insufficient amounts of the hormone. This means that the urine is not concentrated and affected horses will pass large quantities of pale, thin, dilute urine. These horses will also need to drink more to replace these losses in the urine and therefore may show excessive thirst as one of the symptoms of the condition. Other signs include weight loss, weakness and exercise intolerance. Frequently, this condition in horses is the result of a tumour in the pituitary gland. It can be treated, but this is often not practical.

Aldosterone

In addition to regulating body water, kidneys are responsible for regulating the plasma concentration of body salts (electrolytes) such as sodium and potassium. The majority of sodium and potassium in the glomerular filtrate is reabsorbed by the proximal convoluted tubule and the loop of Henle. However, the collecting duct is also capable of sodium and potassium transport, and it is here that adjustments are made when regulating sodium and potassium balance. Aldosterone is a steroid hormone from the adrenal cortex and functions as a major regulator of sodium and potassium transport in the collecting duct.

Regulation of aldosterone secretion from the adrenal cortex relative to sodium balance is via the renin–angiotensin system. The renin–angiotensin–aldosterone pathway has three functions:

- maintenance of blood pressure
- maintenance of sodium concentration in the blood
- maintenance of water levels in the blood.

The pathway works as follows:

- Low blood pressure/blood flow is sensed by the juxtaglomerular apparatus in the kidney (which are cells next to the glomerulus). This is because a decrease in sodium ions reduces the amount of water in the blood, and thus the blood will have a lower pressure.
- The glomerulus releases the hormone renin into the blood stream.

- Renin moves to the liver, where it converts an inactive peptide (protein) angiotensinogen to active angiotensin I.
- Angiotensin I goes to the lungs, where an enzyme known as the angiotensin converting enzyme (ACE) converts angiotensin I to angiotensin II. Angiotensin II has the ability to constrict blood vessels, thus increasing blood pressure. It also stimulates the adrenal glands to produce the hormone aldosterone.
- Aldosterone stimulates the reabsorption of sodium ions in the distal convoluted tubules. Increasing sodium reabsorption means that water and chloride ions will follow, thereby increasing blood volume.
- The increase in blood volume may also trigger the release of a hormone known as atrial natriuretic hormone, which inhibits the release of aldosterone, keeping the body's water and sodium levels at the homeostatic levels. This is termed negative feedback.

If a horse's diet is deficient in salt (i.e. sodium), aldosterone will be secreted to conserve sodium in the distal convoluted tubule. The horse is able to self-limit its salt intake, and if it needs extra salt, a salt lick should be available at all times, so that it can help itself. Those horses that overuse a salt lick may have salt added to the concentrate feed instead.

Acid–Base Balance

Large amounts of chemical reactions take place in the body and acids are being continuously produced by cells as a result of metabolism. Also, a large number of these potential acids may come from the horse's diet. However, in spite of all this acid production, the pH of the blood plasma and other body fluids must remain constant. The normal average pH of arterial blood is 7.4, whereas the venous blood is 7.35 due to the extra carbon dioxide being carried back to the lungs. The pH within cells in the body varies from 4.5 (very acid) to 8.0 (alkaline) depending upon the type of cell. The kidneys have an important role to play in the acid–base balance by controlling the excretion of bicarbonate in the urine, thereby making it more or less acidic and compensating for alkalosis or acidosis in the body. There are three ways the horse's body functions to prevent the development of an abnormal pH:

- extracellular and intracellular chemical buffers
- ventilatory control of plasma carbon dioxide as required
- urinary excretion of bicarbonate or an acid urine as required.

Extracellular and Intracellular Chemical Buffers

Keeping the hydrogen ions level (pH) is of critical importance, as the three-dimensional shape of all body proteins is very sensitive to changes in pH. This will lead to a failure in enzymic reactions as all enzymes are proteins. With high-protein diets, cellular metabolism produces more acids than bases and therefore such diets tend to produce more acidic blood.

Buffers are substances that quickly bind to hydrogen ions, removing the highly reactive H^+ from solution. Buffers therefore help prevent rapid changes in the pH of the horse's body by converting strong acids and bases into weak acids and bases. There are three major mechanisms for maintenance of the acid–base balance:

- protein buffer system
- carbonic acid–bicarbonate buffer system
- phosphate buffer system.

Protein Buffer System
The protein buffer system is the main buffer system. Many proteins act as buffers, and proteins in the body fluids, that is, intracellular fluid and plasma, act as buffers. Haemoglobin is a particularly effective buffer within erythrocytes. Albumin is also an effective buffer in plasma. The carboxyl

group ($-COOH$) and amino group ($-NH_2$) of amino acids in proteins are the functional components of the protein buffer system. When pH rises the carboxyl group releases H^+. This H^+ can then react with any OH^- in the solution to form water. Conversely, when pH falls the amino group combines with H^+, forming an $-NH_3^+$ group. Proteins can therefore act as a buffer to both acids and bases.

Carbonic Acid–Bicarbonate Buffer System
The carbonic acid–bicarbonate buffer system is based upon bicarbonate ions (HCO_3^-) which act as a weak base and carbonic acid (H_2CO_3) which acts as a weak acid. Bicarbonate ions are significant anions in intracellular and extracellular fluid. Kidneys resorb filtered bicarbonate ions so this important buffer is not lost in the urine. If pH falls and there is an excess of hydrogen ions (H^+), bicarbonate HCO_3^- can function as a weak base and remove the excess acid. Conversely, if there is a shortage of H^+, carbonic acid H_2CO_3 can function as a weak acid and provide H^+ ions.

$$H^+ + HCO_3^- \rightarrow H_2CO_3$$

Hydrogen ion   Bicarbonate ion   Carbonic acid (weak acid)

$$H_2CO_3 \longrightarrow H^+ + HCO_3^-$$

Carbonic acid   Hydrogen ion   Bicarbonate ion (weak base)

Phosphate Buffer System
The phosphate buffer system acts in a similar way to the carbonic acid–bicarbonate system. The components in this case are dihydrogen phosphate ($H_2PO_4^-$) and monohydrogen phosphate (HPO_4^{2-}). Phosphates are major anions (negative ions) in the intracellular fluid and minor ones in extracellular fluids. Dihydrogen phosphate acts as a weak acid and is able to buffer strong bases such as hydroxide ions (OH^-). Conversely, monohydrogen phosphate ions act as weak bases and can therefore buffer H^+ released by strong acids such as hydrochloric acid HCl. The concentration of phosphates is highest in the intracellular fluid and therefore the

phosphate buffer system is very important for regulating pH within the cells' cytosol. It also acts as a buffer in urine.

Carbon Dioxide Exhalation

Breathing plays an important role in the maintenance of pH in body fluids. An increase in carbon dioxide in body fluids lowers pH by increasing hydrogen ion concentration, that is, it makes body fluids more acidic. Conversely, a decrease in carbon dioxide in body fluids results in a rise in pH, that is, body fluids become more alkaline.

$$CO_2 + H_2O \longleftrightarrow H_2CO_3 \longleftrightarrow H^+ + HCO_3^-$$
carbon dioxide+   carbonic   hydrogen ion+
water   acid   Bicarbonate ion

Changes in rate and depth of breathing can alter the pH of body fluids very quickly. With increased respiratory rates, more CO_2 is exhaled, concentration falls and blood pH rises. If respiratory rates slow down, less CO_2 is exhaled and blood pH falls.

Excretion of Hydrogen Ions

The excretion of hydrogen ions is the only method of actually removing acids from the horse's body, but it is slow. Cells of the renal tubules secrete hydrogen ions which are then excreted into the urine. Kidneys also make new HCO_3^- and reabsorb filtered HCO_3^- which conserves this very important buffer.

Acid–Base Imbalances

Alkalosis is the condition in which the pH of the horse's body fluids (including blood) is abnormally high (pH above 7.45) and acidosis is a condition in which the pH is abnormally low (pH below 7.35). Acidosis or alkalosis may be either metabolic or respiratory, to indicate the cause of the pH imbalance.

- **Metabolic acidosis** – refers to when the body produces too much acid or the kidneys are not removing enough acid from the body.
- **Respiratory acidosis** – refers to acid–base imbalances that come about as a result of primary or initial changes in carbon dioxide levels.

An acid–base imbalance occurs when the normal buffering mechanisms are overwhelmed. If pH falls below 7 the horse may die. Alkalosis can cause overexcitability of the CNS (Central Nervous System) and peripheral nerves, causing muscle spasms, nervousness and eventually convulsions. Changes in blood pH that lead to alkalosis or acidosis can be countered by 'compensation' – the body's physiological response which aims to normalise pH. These are the normal renal and respiratory system responses, as discussed above. Compensation may be complete or partial and may be respiratory or renal. Respiratory compensation occurs within minutes and reaches maximum efficiency within a few hours, whereas renal compensation starts within minutes but is slower and can take days to cause a beneficial effect.

Micturition or Urination

Micturition is the term used for the evacuation of urine from the bladder. The urine produced in the kidneys in the collecting tubules is transferred to the renal pelvis where it enters the ureter and is carried to the bladder. The bladder acts as a storage vessel for urine.

Micturition is a reflex activity stimulated by the fullness of the bladder itself. The bladder adjusts to the gradual inflow of urine from the ureters until the pressure becomes too high and reflex centres in the spinal cord are stimulated. This causes contraction of the muscles in the bladder wall and evacuation of the urine. Horses tend to urinate (stale) at rest when on grass or bedding. Many horses will wait to urinate (if the bladder is not too full) until they are brought into the stable, particularly when the bedding is clean and deep.

Horses adopt a typical posture when urinating, with the hind legs separated, the horse leaning slightly forward. There is contraction of the muscles of the abdominal wall and the tail is raised. Often they will grunt and groan when urinating. Horses produce about 5–15 litres of urine per day (depending upon water intake and diet) and will urinate approximately 4–6 times in that period.

Summary Points

1) The urinary system is primarily involved in the extraction and removal of waste products from the blood. It is also closely involved with the water, acid–base and salt balances of the horse.
2) Most domestic animals have bean-shaped kidneys similar to humans, but the horse has two different-shaped kidneys: the left is bean-shaped and the right is heart-shaped. In the adult horse each kidney weighs approximately 700g and measures 15–18 cm in length.
3) The horse has approximately 2.5 million nephrons. Ultrafiltration of blood takes place in nephrons, where fluid is forced through the glomerulus capillaries, forming a filtrate similar to blood but lacking proteins and blood cells. The filtrate is then modified by absorption and secretion to add and remove ions, before urine is formed.
4) There are three ways the horse's body prevents the development of an abnormal pH: extracellular and intracellular chemical buffers; ventilatory control of plasma carbon dioxide; and urinary excretion of bicarbonate or an acid urine as needed.
5) Urea is manufactured in the liver in a cyclical chemical reaction, known as the ornithine cycle, from ammonia.

Q + A

Q How does the horse's kidney differ from the human kidney?

A In horses the renal cortex lacks the divisions into individual lobes as seen in the human kidney. This is the same in goats and sheep. In all these animals, the renal papillae are actually fused to make the longitudinal renal crest.

Q What is unusual about the circulation within the glomerular capillaries?

A This renal microcirculation is a unique anatomical anomaly in that the glomerular capillaries are between two arterioles rather than an arteriole and a venule. The afferent arterioles go into the glomerulus and the efferent arterioles leave it.

Q Why is it important to maintain blood pH within a narrow range?

A Keeping the hydrogen ions (pH) level in the horse's body is of critical importance, as the three-dimensional shape of all body proteins is very sensitive to changes in pH. They will lead to a failure in enzymic reactions as all enzymes are proteins.

Q What are the three methods by which the horse's body regulates the acid–base balance?

A The protein buffer system, carbonic acid–bicarbonate buffer system and the phosphate buffer system.

Q What is the difference between metabolic and respiratory acidosis?

A Metabolic acidosis refers to when the body produces too much acid or the kidneys are not removing enough acid from the body. Respiratory acidosis refers to acid–base imbalances that come about as a result of primary or initial changes in carbon dioxide levels.

15

The Immune System

Health Versus Disease

A healthy horse is often described as one that is free from disease, but actually it should describe a horse that is in complete physical and mental health. Disease, on the other hand, is associated with specific symptoms that the horse may show which help to diagnose the disease. The term disease describes a condition whereby part or all of the horse's normal physiological functions are upset. All conditions in horses (apart from those that affect mental health) may be classified as physical in that they cause permanent or temporary damage to the horse's body. Physical diseases can be grouped into:

- infectious – caused by a pathogen
- non-infectious – for example, nutrient deficiency, degeneration (arthritis), inherited diseases (e.g. polysaccharide storage myopathy (PSSM)) and obesity.

Throughout the horse's lifetime, it will be continually challenged by disease-causing organisms (pathogens) of one sort or another. An example of a pathogen is *Clostridium botulinum*, and examples of pathogenic diseases are strangles, equine influenza and equine herpes virus (EHV) 1–4. Most pathogens (but not all) are microbes and fall into one of five categories:

- bacteria – for example, rickettsiae and mycoplasmas (bacteria without a cell wall)
- viruses

- fungi
- protozoans
- multicellular parasites – worms, ticks, and so on.

Horses may be susceptible to some pathogens but not to others. This is because many are species-specific (horses, for example, cannot catch 'influenza virus' from humans). Some pathogens can cause severe reactions and symptoms leading to acute infections; others may produce a slow reaction of the defence mechanisms and the horse will be slow to overcome the chronic infection that has resulted.

Microbes

Microbes are organisms that are too small for visual detection, that is, they are microscopic. All animals are surrounded by microbes and there are thousands upon thousands of species, with a huge diversity.

Microbes include all bacteria, archaea and most protozoa but not viruses. Bacteria and viruses vary in size and the largest viruses are only as large as the tiniest bacteria and bacteria have a much more complex structure compared to viruses. A bacterium contains all of the genetic information needed to make copies of itself in its DNA and may also have other smaller bits of DNA called plasmids in the cytoplasm. Bacteria also have ribosomes to copy DNA so they can reproduce.

Equine Science, Third Edition. Zoe Davies and Sarah Pilliner.
© 2018 Zoe Davies and Sarah Pilliner. Published 2018 by John Wiley & Sons Ltd.

Bacteria live everywhere – in the soil, air, food that horses eat and water that they drink. They can live within horses in huge numbers without causing disease (e.g. The Digestive System, see Chapter 5), for example, on the skin and in the anus, reproductive tract and upper respiratory tract. Species found in the horse's normal flora are shown in Table 15.1. In other words, this is the normal state for horses and the majority of bacteria are not harmful and in many cases help to suppress pathogenic species that live among them. There are many types of bacteria in the horse's mouth too; some of them form biofilms or plaque on the teeth. Bacteria in the gut will change according to the food eaten. Stomach acidity helps to reduce bacterial numbers and potential pathogenic activity, as few can survive the acidic conditions. However, food is not held in the stomach for long and therefore some bacteria will enter the small intestine and some species are able to thrive. The types of bacteria obtained from the gastric mucosa of horses include Firmicutes, Proteobacteria and Bacteroidetes and these are the dominant bacterial species; smaller numbers of *Lactobacillus* are also present. These are native microbiota that live in the stomach under normal conditions.

Disease Transmission Routes

The main transmission routes for potential pathogens are as follows:

- through droplets in the air from mucus or saliva (e.g. equine influenza, EHV)
- contaminated feed or water (e.g. *Clostridium botulinum*)
- during sexual reproduction (e.g. contagious equine metritis (CEM))
- through a break in the skin – caused by injury or a bite from an external parasite (e.g. tetanus, West Nile virus, eastern equine encephalitis (EEE)) or following surgery.

Cuts and grazes can allow the entry of harmful bacteria, such as *Clostridium tetani* which causes tetanus, affecting the nervous system. *C. tetani* is common in the soil and can enter the horse's body through punctures of the skin or animal/fly bites. Parasites are organisms that live on or within the horse, causing damage. Parasites that affect horses are numerous and include worms, ticks and lice. Ticks and lice feed on the skin by puncturing it and this can allow transmission of bacteria and viruses directly into the blood.

Table 15.1 Species of bacteria found in the horse's normal flora.

Digestive tract	Respiratory tract	Genital tract
Clostridium	*Bacillus*	*Micrococcus*
Enterobacter	*Streptococcus*	*Staphylococcus*
Escherichia coli	*Acinetobacter*	*Streptococcus*
Klebsiella	*Staphylococcus*	*Micrococcus*
Proteus	*Micrococcus*	*Staphylococcus*
Pseudomonas	*Pasteurella*	*Streptococcus*
Corynebacterium	*Veillonella*	
Bacterioides	*Fusobacterium*	
Streptococcus		
Lactobacillus		
Ruminococcus		
Fibrobacter		
Veillonella		
Megasphaera		

Infection

Disease impairs normal function and may be infectious, non-infectious, or acute or chronic. Infection may be localised (within a particular area or tissue) or systemic (if spread throughout the body); for example, entry of pathogens from the soil into wounds or during surgery can introduce localised infection, which could if the horse's immune system is weak become systemic. Pathogens vary in their ability to invade and multiply, and this capacity is known as virulence. Sometimes organisms may spread from a part of the body where they are normally harmless to another part where they become harmful. An example of this occurs when there is leakage from the gut into the surrounding abdominal space, resulting in infection of the gut lining (or peritoneum) known as peritonitis.

Non-infectious diseases may be caused by nutritional deficiencies, genetic defects or environmental factors. Examples include recurrent airway obstruction (RAO), laminitis, insulin resistance (IR), pituitary pars intermedia dysfunction (PPID), exertional myopathies and some forms of colic.

Infection is not the same as the horse having the disease. Before the disease develops there is an incubation period. This is the time in which the pathogen multiplies in the horse's cells, beginning a cycle of reproduction and colonisation which leads to infection. The horse's complex immune system, if working effectively, will try to prevent this occurring. If a horse breathes in droplets from another horse with equine influenza, for example, the virus particles are inhaled and attach to the epithelial cells of the mucous membranes. The cell surface membranes of the mucous membranes have protein molecules (see Chapter 1). The type of protein will depend upon the cell and genetics of the individual horse. The virus attaches only if the correct protein is present on the cell surface membrane of the respiratory tract of that horse. If it is, then the virus can enter the cell and begin the cycle of colonisation and infection. The horse's immune system will try to prevent this.

In addition, autoimmune disorders may occur where some of the horse's own cells or antigens are perceived as foreign and therefore elicit an immune response. The ability of the immune system to recognise body cells or antigens and differentiate between them and foreign cells is very important. The horse's own cells may have changed and therefore become recognised as foreign. An example of this is pemphigus foliaceus (PF), an autoimmune disorder in which the affected horse makes antibodies against its own skin. The immune system is therefore able to identify and eliminate the horse's own body cells that have changed and that therefore may become harmful. The identification and elimination of these altered cells is protection against the development of cancers. The horse responds to these changes with autoantibodies. Autoantibodies are produced by the horse's immune system and directed against its own tissues.

Biofilms

Microbes do not tend to exist on their own but rather as part of a complex community, members of which interact with each other. Many of these communities are associated with surfaces and are known as biofilms. They are found in thin layers on these surfaces, such as plaque on teeth and slime found in water troughs, pipes and so on. Most microbes do not like dry conditions. Bacteria in soil tend to be found in biofilms which help retain water on the soil particle surface.

Biofilm-associated cells generate an extracellular polymeric substance (EPS) matrix and have reduced growth rates. Attachment is a complex process regulated by characteristics of the surface. An established biofilm structure comprises microbial cells and EPS, has a defined architecture and provides an optimal environment for the exchange of genetic material between cells.

Biofilms can also form elsewhere within the horse's body, especially on plastic, for example, where inserted for various purposes, such as intravenous catheters, even though they were sterile when originally placed.

Symptoms of Disease

The horse's reaction to the presence of infection produces the symptoms of the disease. The symptoms are therefore caused in part by microbes damaging cells and tissues, releasing toxins and drawing on the horse's nutrient supply. Symptoms are also caused by the horse's own defences, including the immune system which destroys the offending microbes. The outcome will depend on whether the microbes or the horse's defence system gain the advantage. The strength of the immune system is often a reflection of the general health and well-being of the horse and will strongly influence this outcome.

Diagnosis

Apart from diseases in which the symptoms and signs are easily recognisable, such as tetanus and strangles, diagnosis often relies upon isolation of the causative agent. Testing may involve microscopic examination of a specimen of infected tissue or body fluid, culture techniques or detection of antibodies (proteins manufactured by the horse to defend against a particular organism) in a blood sample. A problem in detecting infectious diseases is that there is always a time gap between their entry and the appearance of symptoms, that is, the incubation period, which may be as little as a few days or as long as several months. Furthermore, symptoms may never develop in some infected horses, but these horses nevertheless continue to carry the disease-causing organisms and

unwittingly spread them to other horses. As a result of this, an epidemic can be well established before it is recognised and before control measures can be introduced. Early recognition of symptoms is therefore important if treatment and prevention of further spread is going to be effective.

Pathogenic Organisms

Disease-causing organisms are relatively simple organisms which can multiply in the horse's tissues, particularly when the horse's immune defences are low. Colonisation by internal parasites and insects tends to be called an infestation rather than an infection. Internal and external parasites include single-celled parasites known as protozoa, worms and insects.

Bacteria (Prokaryotes)

Bacteria are a group of single-celled microorganisms called prokaryotes which may cause disease. Each bacterial cell consists of cytoplasm enclosed by a surface membrane and a cell wall. They do not have cell organelles bound by cell membranes such as found in eukaryotic cells (see Chapter 2). Their basic structure is shown in Figure 15.1.

Bacteria have been recognised as a cause of disease for hundreds of years, even though the number of pathogenic bacteria is relatively low. They are naturally abundant in

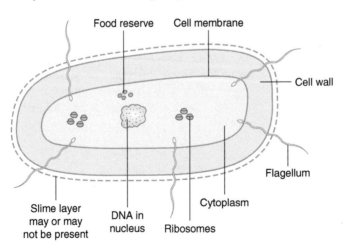

Figure 15.1 A generalised bacteria cell.

Food reserve Cell membrane

Cell wall

Flagellum

Slime layer may or may not be present

DNA in nucleus

Ribosomes

Cytoplasm

the air, soil and water, and most are therefore harmless to horses. When they invade horses and cause ill health they are called pathogenic. Bacteria may be categorised by their cell walls and features such as arrangement, motility, oxygen and requirements (anaerobic or aerobic). Mycoplasmas, for example, do not have a cell wall at all. Bacteria are also often classified on the basis of their shape into three main groups:

- cocci (spherical)
- bacilli (rod-shaped)
- spirochetes or spirilla (spiral-shaped).

Some bacterial infectious diseases are shown in Table 15.2. Diseases caused by cocci include pneumonia and strangles, while tetanus and botulism are caused by bacilli. Botulism, also known as grass sickness or equine dysautonomia, is a disease of horses, ponies and donkeys which is manifest by impaired activity of the gut due to damage to the autonomic (involuntary) nervous

Table 15.2 Some equine bacterial infectious diseases.

Disease	Bacterium
Tetanus	*Clostridium tetani*
Strangles	*Streptococcus equi*
Botulism, grass sickness	*Clostridium botulinum*
Summer pneumonia in foals (may spread to humans who are immunosuppressed)	*Rhodococcus equi*
Ulcerative lymphangitis	*Corynebacterium pseudotuberculosis*
Leptospirosis	*Leptospira interrogans* serovars
Glanders	*Burkholderia mallei*
Contagious equine metritis	*Taylorella equigenitalis*
Pseudomonas metritis	*Pseudomonas aeruginosa*
Salmonellosis	*Salmonella* species
Lawsonia – affects weanlings	*Lawsonia intracellularis*

system. The cause is not proven, but recent evidence strongly implicates the involvement of *Clostridium botulinum*.

Invasive Properties

Pathogenic bacteria can be grouped into three categories on the basis of their invasive properties of the horse's cells:

- extracellular bacteria
- facultative intracellular bacteria
- obligate intracellular bacteria.

Extracellular Bacteria

Extracellular bacterial pathogens do not invade cells but proliferate instead in the extracellular fluid (ECF). Some may not penetrate body tissues (e.g. *Vibrio cholerae*) but adhere to epithelial surfaces instead and cause disease by secreting potent toxins. Although bacteria such as *Escherichia coli* and *Pseudomonas aeruginosa* are termed non-invasive, they frequently spread rapidly to various tissues once they gain access to the horse's body. Extracellular bacteria do not have the capacity to survive inside cells, that is, the intracellular environment. Some examples of predominantly extracellular bacteria are:

- *Bacillus anthracis*
- *Escherichia coli* (enterotoxigenic)
- *Mycoplasma* species
- *Pseudomonas aeruginosa*
- *Staphylococcus aureus*
- *Streptococcus pyogenes*.

Facultative Intracellular Bacteria

Intracellular bacteria commonly cause 'granulomatous lesions'. Facultative intracellular bacteria invade host cells of the animal. Bacteria that can enter and survive within the horse's cells are shielded from humoral antibodies and can be eliminated only by a cell-mediated immune response (see below). However, these bacteria possess highly specialised mechanisms to protect them from the harsh environment and the lysosomal enzymes encountered within the host cells.

Examples of facultative intracellular bacteria include *Listeria monocytogenes* and *Salmonella* species, which are very resistant to intracellular attack by phagocytic cells. There are many different species of bacteria belonging to the genus *Salmonella*. Only a few cause food poisoning known as salmonellosis. When contaminated food is eaten by the horse the bacteria pass to the intestine where they multiply, causing illness by release of toxins. *Salmonella* species are intrabacteria and actually enter the cell lining of the small intestine and multiply. As they multiply some die, releasing an endotoxin which irritates the lining of the intestine, causing diarrhoea and abdominal pain.

Obligate Intracellular Bacteria

The obligate intracellular group of bacteria cannot live outside the host cells. For example, chlamydial cells are unable to carry out energy metabolism and lack many biosynthetic pathways and are entirely dependent on the host cells to supply them with adenosine triphosphate (ATP) and other substances. Because of this dependency, Chlamydiae were originally thought to be viruses, as all viruses are obligate intracellular parasites. *Rickettsia* and *Chlamydia* can only live and grow within the host's cells as they are intracellular bacteria. *Rickettsia* is associated with lice, ticks, fleas and mites which are responsible for its spread. Horses appear relatively resistant to chlamydial infections, although there have been limited reports of chlamydial-associated equine disease of the respiratory tract and also in aborted foetuses.

Spread of Bacteria

Bacteria that invade the horse's body thrive in the warm, moist conditions. Some bacteria are described as aerobic, meaning that they require oxygen to grow and survive. They are therefore found in places such as the respiratory system or on the skin. Anaerobic bacteria, on the other hand, thrive in areas low in oxygen, such as deep in wounds or tissues. Some bacteria (both aerobic and

Table 15.3 Bacterial species that may be found in equine wounds.

Aerobes – require oxygen	Anaerobes – require low or no oxygen
Escherichia coli	*Clostridium perfringens*
Pseudomonas aeruginosa	*Clostridium tetani*
Staphylococcus aureus	*Clostridium septum*
Streptococcus zooepidemicus	

anaerobic) associated with wounds and abscesses are shown in Table 15.3.

Many bacteria are naturally static and only move around the horse's body in currents of fluid or air. Others are very mobile and have filamentous tails to help them move. Bacteria are able to reproduce by simply dividing into two cells; these in turn divide again into four cells, then eight and so on (Figure 15.2). Under some conditions and in some species this can take place every 20 minutes, such as *E. coli*. After only 6 hours a single bacterium may have multiplied to form a colony of over 250,000 bacteria; *E.coli* can actually divide more quickly than it can copy its own DNA, and this is because it begins the next round of replication before it divides, so that by the time of cell division, it is already part of the way through producing the copies of its DNA that will be needed for the next cell division. Cell division does not therefore provide the signal for the start of DNA replication.

As well as dividing, some bacteria may produce spores. A spore is a single new bacterium which is protected by an extremely tough outer coat that can survive high temperatures, dry conditions and lack of nutrients. Spores can remain in a dormant state for many years. When environmental conditions are optimal they will 'hatch' and try to invade the horse's body tissues. Spore-producing bacteria include Clostridia (responsible for tetanus and botulism) which are able to lie dormant within the soil for many years. When a horse has a wound (often

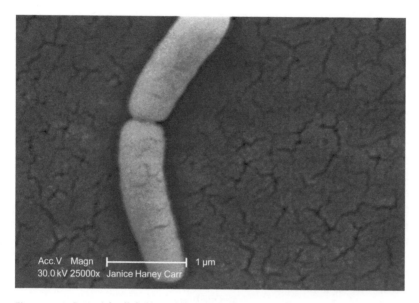

Figure 15.2 Bacterial cell division. Colourised electron micrograph of a *Salmonella* bacterium dividing. *Source:* Dale 2013. Reproduced with permission of John Wiley & Sons.

very minor) the tetanus-causing bacteria (*Clostridium tetani*) can enter the body through this route.

Mycoplasma Species

Mycoplasma species are the smallest bacterial cells that have been discovered. They lack a cell wall around their cell membrane and thus are unaffected by many common antibiotics such as penicillin and other beta-lactam antibiotics that target cell wall synthesis. *Mycoplasma* species can survive without oxygen and come in various shapes. They have been isolated from the respiratory tracts of horses and it is thought that they may be involved in mixed infections with other viruses or bacteria.

Antibiotics and Resistance

Antibiotics are drugs that kill or inhibit the growth of bacteria by interfering with the metabolic reactions that are crucial to the survival and multiplication of bacteria. There are two different types:

- bacteriocidal – kill bacteria, for example penicillin;

- bacteriostatic – prevent bacteria growing, for example tetracycline.

Viruses do not have their own enzymes or ribosomes but use those of the host cells, so antibiotics have no effect on them. However, bacteria have cell walls, unlike mammalian cells, and also have different proteins and enzymes. Some antibiotics inhibit enzymes that the bacteria need to make the chemical bonds in their cell walls. The bacteria then cannot grow and the cell wall weakens, allowing water to enter via osmosis from the surroundings, and the bacteria therefore bursts. Other antibiotics inhibit protein production by binding to ribosomes in the bacteria; this stops the bacteria making enzymes (all enzymes are proteins) and therefore the bacteria cannot survive.

Unfortunately, the overuse of antibiotics has led to increasing levels of resistance in many species of bacteria. Veterinary surgeons should not prescribe antibiotics for minor infections or wounds in horses or as a prevention. They should also rotate their use of different antibiotics.

Viruses

Viruses are specialised intracellular parasites and are responsible for many diseases of horses. It is difficult to know whether viruses are actually living organisms, as they do not respire and they do not feed. In fact, they are a collection of complex molecules which some scientists believe are based upon stray bits of DNA that have escaped from the genomes of higher plants and animals. While not inside an infected cell or in the process of infecting a cell, viruses exist in the form of independent particles. These viral particles are known as virions.

Viruses need living host cells in order to multiply. They use the host's cells to replicate more viral particles. The host range a particular virus will attack depends upon the presence of specific receptors on the host cell and the availability of the cellular factors required for viral multiplication. For animal viruses the receptor sites are on the plasma membranes of the host cells. Viruses cannot be killed when in an inert state. Immunisation is still the most effective method to control viral diseases at present. Viruses are grouped into families, some of which are shown in Table 15.4.

Viruses (as many pathogens can) gain entry to the horse's body through several possible routes. They may be inhaled in droplets or swallowed in food or water. They may be passed into the body through the saliva of biting insects, such as equine infectious anaemia, or they may enter the horse's body during covering or sexual reproduction. Many viruses, having entered the host's body, begin to replicate near the site of entry. Others may enter lymph vessels and spread to lymph nodes where many will be engulfed by leucocytes (white blood cells). Others may pass from the lymphatic system to the blood from where they can invade every part of the horse. They tend to have target organs such as the brain (rabies) or the respiratory tract (equine influenza). Equine influenza occurs globally and is caused by two main subtypes of influenza A (Table 15.5):

Table 15.4 Common virus families and examples of diseases they cause.

Family	Example of disease
Papillomaviruses (non-enveloped)	Warts
Adenoviruses (non-enveloped)	Respiratory and eye infections
Herpes viruses (*Herpes viridae*)	EHV 1 and subtypes, EHV 3 coital exanthema
Toga viruses (Togaviridae) (enveloped)	Equine arteritis (pinkeye)
Picorna viruses (Picornaviridae)	Equine rhinovirus 1, 2 and 3, stable picornavirus
Rhabdoviruses (Rhabdoviridae) (enveloped)	Rabies
Arbovirus – an acronym for ARthropod-BOrne virus	Viral encephalomyelitis
Tibovirus – an acronym for TIck-BOrne virus, sometimes used to describe viruses transmitted by ticks	Lyme disease
Orthomyxoviruses	Equine influenza

- equine-1 (H7N7) – also affects the heart muscle
- equine-2 (H3N8) – more systemic symptoms and more severe.

Viral infections vary from relatively minor problems such as warts to extremely serious diseases such as rabies. It is thought that some virus infections may lead to cancer. The sole aim of a virus is to invade the cells of other organisms which they then instruct to make more copies of themselves. Outside the living cell viruses are totally inactive. The number of different kinds of virus probably exceeds the number of types of all other organisms. Antibiotics have no effect on viruses, but several antiviral drugs have now been developed; for example, Aciclovir has now been proven effective in a study treating equine sarcoids via topical application.

Table 15.5 Influenza virus A – equine influenza.

Genus	Species	Subtype	Hosts
Influenza virus A	*Influenza A virus*	H1N1, H1N2, H2N2, H3N1, H3N2, H3N8, H5N1, H5N2, H5N3, H5N8, H5N9, H7N1, H7N2, H7N3, H7N4, H7N7, H7N9, H9N2, H10N7	Horse, human, pig, bird

Viruses can kill horses, such as West Nile virus which causes encephalomyelitis or inflammation in the brain and/or spinal cord. The virus was first found in North America in 1999. The disease is transmitted primarily by mosquitoes (Figure 15.3) and is characterised by central nervous system dysfunction. If the horse survives, continued symptoms can result in prolonged ill health. There has been a decline in this disease due to vaccination programmes, increased awareness of the need to control mosquito populations and increased immunity to the virus within wild bird populations (the reservoir hosts). All horses are susceptible to incidental infection if not vaccinated against the disease.

Structure

Viruses have a much simpler structure and a relatively uncomplicated method of multiplication compared to bacteria. A single virus particle is known as a virion and consists quite simply of a core of genetic material or nucleic acid. This is surrounded by a capsule or shell known as a capsid which is made of protein (Figure 15.4). These capsids may be surrounded by a viral envelope or membrane which again is made from protein

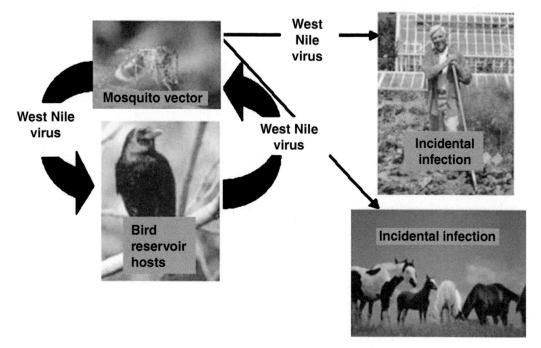

Figure 15.3 West Nile virus transmission cycle. *Source*: Centers for Disease Control and Prevention, https://commons.wikimedia.org/wiki/File:West_Nile_virus_transmission_cycle.jpg.

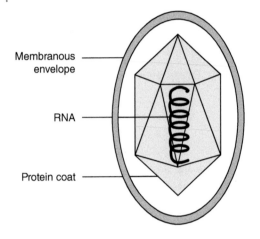

Figure 15.4 Structure of a simple virus.

and this envelope is usually lost when the virus invades the host cell. The central core of nucleic acid is known as the genome and consists of a string of genes that contain the code for making copies of that virus. Depending upon the type of virus, the nucleic acid may be either DNA or RNA. The DNA consists of a double strand in a double-helix formation, whereas the RNA is a single strand. Virions are minute infectious agents which are much smaller than bacteria (about one one-hundredth the size), though they vary in size. The diameter of the herpesvirus, for example, is around 250 nm.

Replication

Viruses do not reproduce in the usual way; instead they undergo a process known as replication (Figure 15.5). Basically, the virus invades the host cell and begins the process of making copies of itself from materials within the host cell. Viruses often have elaborate methods of replicating. Some are straightforward, as previously described, whereas others invade the nucleus and incorporate themselves into the cell's own genetic material before being able to replicate. Sometimes the viral genome may sit dormant within the nucleus, to become reactivated months later. The viral genome may also interfere with the host cell's chromosomes, causing

the transition of a healthy host cell to a tumour cell.

Eukaryotic Pathogens

Eukaryotic pathogens include fungi, protozoa and internal parasites (worms).

Fungi

Fungi are relatively simple parasites and include moulds, mildews, yeasts, mushrooms and toadstools. There are more than 100,000 species of fungi within the world. Most are actually harmless and may even be beneficial; for example, some moulds are used to make antibiotics.

Fungi are larger than bacteria. Some occur as colonies of individual cells, such as yeasts. Others form chains of tubes or filaments called hyphae which are formed into a complex network known as a mycelium. Many fungi form millions of tiny spores which can remain dormant until suitable conditions are available for them to grow. Fungal spores are found mainly in the soil. Spores can penetrate the tissue of the host. An example of this is *Aspergillus*, causing infection of the mucous membranes and guttural pouch of horses. Some yeasts which are present normally within the horse's gut may become a problem if the gut microflora are upset or disrupted by the use of antibiotics. They can then overgrow the bacterial population because antibiotics destroy bacteria but have no effect on fungi.

Probably the most common fungal infection of the horse is ringworm (Dermatophysis). Both *Trichophyton equinum* and *T. mentagrophytes* are primary causes of ringworm and Microsporum species have also been isolated. Antifungal drugs are used to treat ringworm. These work by damaging the cell walls of fungi, causing their eventual death. Also, some spores of fungi, particularly those found in mouldy hay, can cause damage when inhaled by horses, causing persistent allergic reactions in the lungs or recurrent airway obstruction (RAO). The principal culprits are *Micropolyspora faeni* and *Aspergillus fumigatus*.

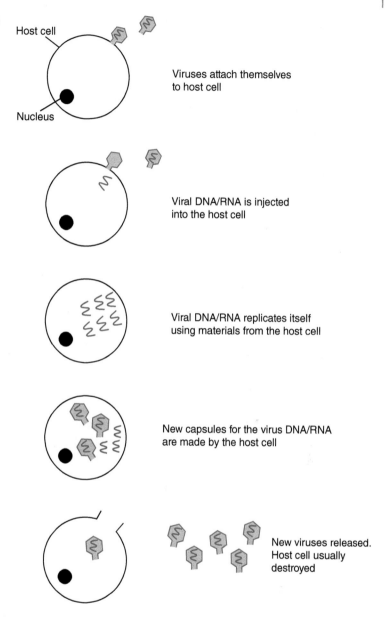

Figure 15.5 Viral replication within the host cell.

Host cell

Nucleus

Viruses attach themselves to host cell

Viral DNA/RNA is injected into the host cell

Viral DNA/RNA replicates itself using materials from the host cell

New capsules for the virus DNA/RNA are made by the host cell

New viruses released. Host cell usually destroyed

Mycotoxins

Fungi may cause disease in other ways. Certain fungi that infect cereal crops and conserved pasture produce dangerous toxins known as mycotoxins. Various mycotoxins cause significant health and performance issues in horses. These include aflatoxin, ochratoxin, deoxynivalenol, zearalenone, fumonisin, ergot and T2 toxin. The fungi *Aspergillus, Penicillium, Fusarium* species and *Claviceps* produce the toxins most harmful to horses. Poorly made haylage is particularly problematical as mycotoxins may be left behind following flare-ups of fungi during a slow fermentation or secondary fermentation. Haylage appears therefore to be more likely to contain mycotoxins than hay. Mycotoxins are more likely to be a problem when harvesting conditions for cereals are damp, that is, wet summers

Table 15.6 Common mycotoxins in equine feeds.

Mycotoxin	Fungi	Feed sources
Aflatoxin	*Aspergillus flavus*	Maize, hay, pasture
Ochratoxin A	*Aspergillus ochraeus*	Wheat, barley, maize, oats
	Penicillium verrucosum	
	Aspergillus carbonarius	
Tricoethenes	*Fusarium graminearum*	Maize, wheat, barley
Deoxynivalenol (DON)	*Fusarium culmorum*	
Zearalenone	*Fusarium graminearum*	Maize, wheat, barley, pasture
T2 toxin and 4,15-diacetoxyscirpenol (DAS)	*Fusarium sporotrichoides*	Maize, wheat, barley
Fumonisin	*Fusarium verticillioides*	Maize
Ergotoxin	*Claviceps purpurea*	Wheat, barley, maize, hay
Patulin PR toxin	*Penicillin roqueforti*	Haylage, pasture, cereals

where it is difficult to get crops off the field. Some sources of mycotoxins are shown in Table 15.6.

A fungus that infects cereals, particularly rye, produces a toxin known as ergot. Whereas ergot is highly toxic to humans, horses given 500 g of ergot showed only slight symptoms. More serious toxins are the aflatoxins. The horse seems more susceptible to aflatoxins than other domestic animals. Aflatoxins may be found in badly stored cereals or oil-seeds. Ryegrass staggers is caused by a neurotoxin present in perennial ryegrass (*Lolium perenne*). This condition affects grazing horses of all ages and occurs only in late spring, summer and autumn in pastures in which perennial ryegrass or hybrid ryegrass are the major species. It occurs sporadically in parts of North and South America, Europe and Australia. The neurotoxins involved are lolitrems, mainly lolitrem B. These are indole diterpene alkaloids and are produced in perennial and hybrid ryegrasses infected with the endophytic fungus *Neotyphodium lolii*.

Protozoa

Protozoa are simple, primitive, single-celled animals that belong to the kingdom Protoctista. They are microscopic but larger than bacteria. Among protozoans there are many differences in cell structure. Protozoa mostly inhabit water and soil habitats, but some are part of the natural microbiota of animals such as horses. Some species can therefore live on or inside horses. There are around 20,000 species of protozoans and most do not cause disease. Those that do are highly specialised intracellular parasites with complex lifestyles involving one or more hosts. Under certain conditions some protozoa may also create a protective capsule known as a cyst, allowing the protozoa to live inside during adverse conditions. The more advanced types are capable of respiration, reproduction and excretion. They move around by using a tail known as a flagellum. Some become parasites as part of their life cycle. A number of different protozoa affect horses. Babesia, trypanosomes, besnoitia and sarcocystis are examples.

Equine protozoal myeloencephalitis (EPM) is a common neurologic disease of horses in the Americas. Most cases of EPM are caused by an Apicomplexan protozoan, *Sarcocystis neurona*. Horses are infected by ingestion of *S. neurona* sporocysts in contaminated feed or water.

Internal Parasites

Internal parasites may cause extensive internal damage when horses are heavily infected. The effects of these internal parasites on a horse range from a dull haircoat and general unthriftiness to colic and death. Internal parasites lower the horse's resistance to infection, rob the horse of valuable nutrients and, in some cases, cause permanent damage to the internal organs. In terms of management priorities, establishing an effective parasite control program is vital.

There are more than 150 species of internal parasites that may infect horses. The most common are:

- small strongyles (cyathostomins)
- roundworms (ascarids)
- tapeworms
- large strongyles (bloodworms or redworms)
- pinworms
- bots
- threadworms.

The most important in terms of health risk to horses are small strongyles, roundworms and tapeworms.

The life cycle of most internal parasites involves eggs, larvae (immature worms) and adults (mature worms). Eggs or larvae are deposited on the ground in the manure of an infected horse. They are swallowed while the horse is grazing, and the larvae mature into adults within the horse's digestive tract (stomach or intestines). With some species of parasite, the larvae migrate out of the intestine, into other tissues or organs, before returning to the intestine and maturing into egg-laying adults.

The control of internal parasites is well researched and an important part of horse management, but is outside the scope of this book.

Protection from Disease

The immune system responds to potentially harmful pathogenic organisms which try to invade the horse's body. It is a highly complex, multi-response system – see Figure 15.6. Referring to this diagram will be helpful in understanding the horse's immune response to potential life-threatening pathogens.

It is very important that the immune system distinguishes between invading organisms and the horse's own body tissues. Occasionally the system can react against its own body tissues, causing autoimmune disease. The immune system is also responsible for allergic reactions and hypersensitivity, such as sweet itch.

Horses have many barriers to reduce the risk of invasion by harmful organisms; the three main ways they protect themselves are:

- external barriers – physical/mechanical and chemical (Figure 15.7)
- innate immunity – present from birth
- acquired or adaptive immunity – develops through either exposure of the horse to infectious organisms (after they have broken through the innate immune system) or through immunisation.

External Barriers

There are more bacteria living on the horse's skin than there are horses in the world, and most of these cause no harm. The skin helps prevents most micro-organisms entering the body, as microbes find it difficult to penetrate the outer layer of skin which consists of dead and dry cells made of keratin. Also the skin is continuously shedding, so many microbes fall off with the dead skin cells. Pathogenic microbes therefore are more likely to gain entry into the body via one of several routes including the eyes, mouth, nostrils (respiratory system) and genitals (urinary system).

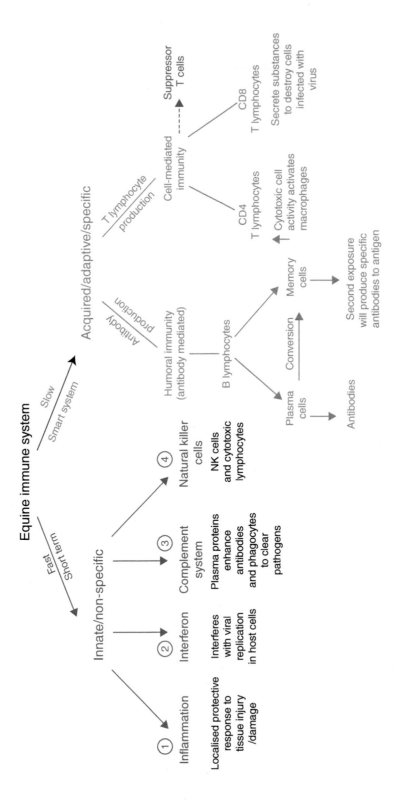

Figure 15.6 Summary of the equine immune system.

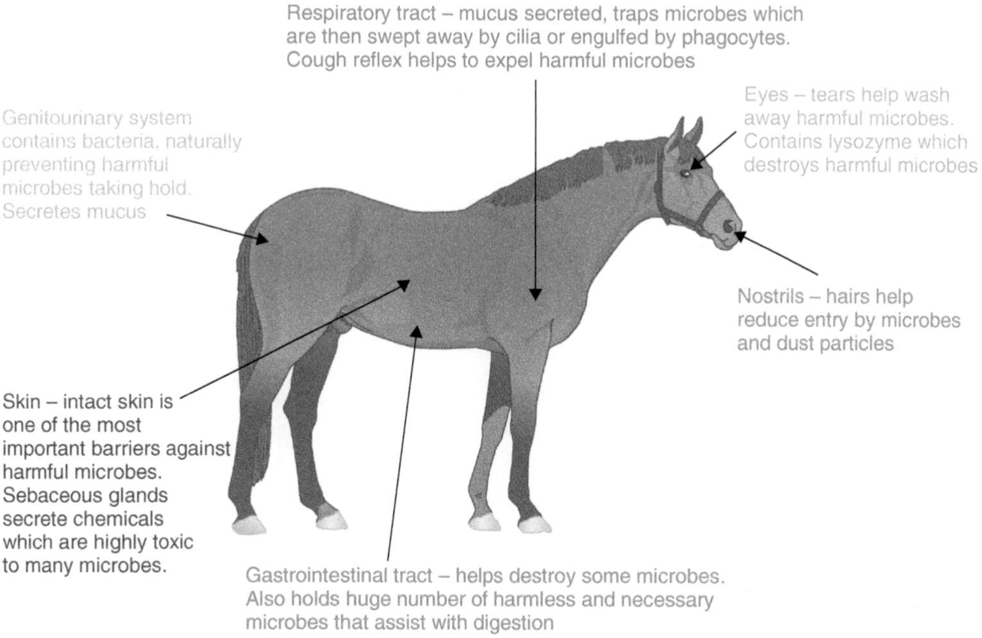

Respiratory tract – mucus secreted, traps microbes which are then swept away by cilia or engulfed by phagocytes. Cough reflex helps to expel harmful microbes

Eyes – tears help wash away harmful microbes. Contains lysozyme which destroys harmful microbes

Genitourinary system contains bacteria, naturally preventing harmful microbes taking hold. Secretes mucus

Nostrils – hairs help reduce entry by microbes and dust particles

Skin – intact skin is one of the most important barriers against harmful microbes. Sebaceous glands secrete chemicals which are highly toxic to many microbes.

Gastrointestinal tract – helps destroy some microbes. Also holds huge number of harmless and necessary microbes that assist with digestion

Figure 15.7 Summary of physical and chemical barriers against harmful organisms.

All these areas have mechanisms to try to reduce the possibility of pathogenic microbes taking hold.

Most of the horse's body is protected by skin or mucous membranes. The skin is particularly uninhabitable for microbes, as it often contains salt from sweat. Horses are unusual in that they produce a protein-rich sweat which helps in thermoregulation. A major component of this sweat is latherin, a non-glycosylated protein which acts as a wetting agent. It is known also to have antimicrobial properties. Sweat contains lysozymes which break down the cell walls of microbes. Equine antimicrobial peptides that have been found on the skin so far are lysozymes, cathelicidins, defensins, NK-lysin, psoriasin, hepcidin, granulins and equinins. In fact, equine antimicrobial peptides are found in many different tissues of the horse.

Innate Immunity

If a pathogenic microbe is able to penetrate the horse's external barriers, the innate immunity system of the horse will come into play. This consists of the physical barriers such as skin (fatty acids and normal skin microflora) and substances present in the mouth, urinary tract and eyes (lysosymes in tears) that kill bacteria, cilia lined with mucus in the respiratory system and cellular defences producing antibodies and immunoglobulins.

Innate immunity is non-specific. It is a rapid response system, allowing time for the acquired system to prepare. It includes neutrophils, eosoinophils, basophils, cytotoxic lymphocytes and monocytes (Figure 15.8). The innate response involves:

- inflammation
- interferons (IFNs)
- complement system
- natural killer (NK) cells.

Inflammation

Inflammation is a local protective response to tissue injury or microbial invasion. A summary of the inflammatory response is shown in Figure 15.9. The inflammatory response is aimed at removing debris and potential pathogens by bringing phagocytes to the affected area and preparing for

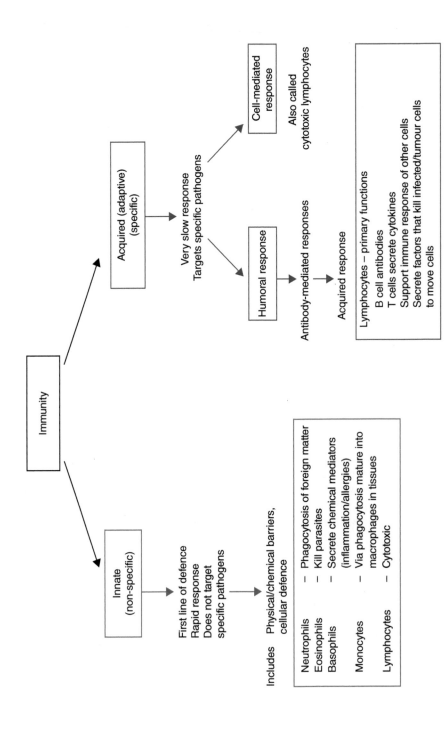

Figure 15.8 Comparison of innate and acquired immune responses.

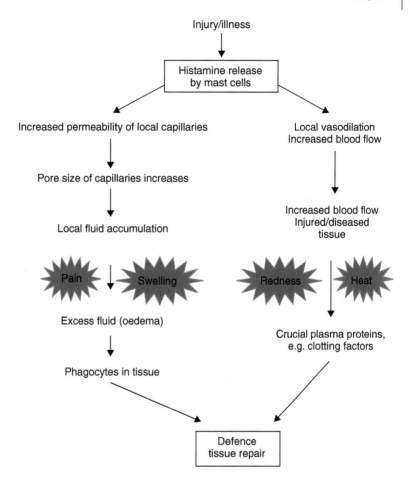

Figure 15.9 Summary of inflammation.

subsequent healing. Phagocytosis is a form of endocytosis. Vasodilation and increased permeability of local capillaries occurs, allowing immune system cells to reach the area, where they can then start to destroy the pathogen.

Interferons

IFNs are a group of signalling proteins made and released by host cells in response to the presence of several pathogens, such as viruses, bacteria, parasites and also tumour cells. Their function is to interfere with viral replication (Figure 15.10), enhance phagocytic activity of phagocytes, stimulate antibody production, enhance the killing power of NK cells and cytotoxic T cells, and slow cell division and tumour growth.

IFNs interfere with viral replication by the following steps:

- The body cell gets invaded by a virus.
- The invaded cell releases IFNs which leave the infected cell and go to neighbouring non-infected or healthy cells.
- At the neighbouring cells IFNs attach to receptors on the cell membranes, causing the cell to produce inactive enzymes in preparation for a possible invasion.
- When the neighbouring cell is invaded, the inactive enzymes are then activated and break down viral mRNA to inhibit viral protein synthesis, effectively killing the virus.

Certain symptoms of infections in horses, such as fever, muscle pain and flu-like

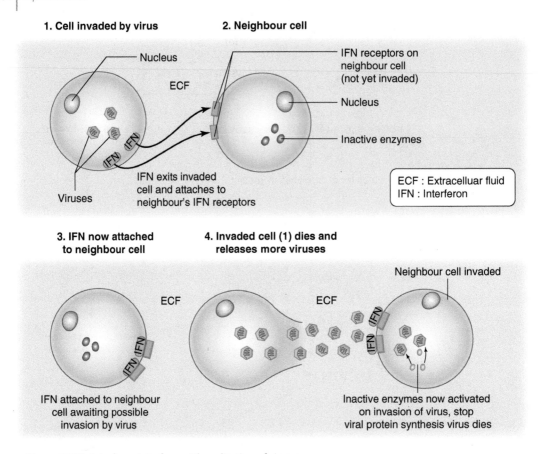

1. Cell invaded by virus

2. Neighbour cell

Nucleus

ECF

IFN receptors on
neighbour cell
(not yet invaded)

Nucleus

Inactive enzymes

IFN exits invaded
cell and attaches to
neighbour's IFN receptors

Viruses

ECF : Extracelluar fluid
IFN : Interferon

**3. IFN now attached
to neighbour cell**

**4. Invaded cell (1) dies and
releases more viruses**

ECF

ECF

Neighbour cell invaded

IFN attached to neighbour
cell awaiting possible
invasion by virus

Inactive enzymes now activated
on invasion of virus, stop
viral protein synthesis virus dies

Figure 15.10 Interferon interferes with replication of viruses.

symptoms, are caused by the production of IFNs and other cytokines. More than 20 distinct IFN genes and proteins have been identified in horses. They are typically divided among three classes: type I, type II and type III IFN. IFNs belonging to all three classes are important for fighting viral infections and for the regulation of the immune system.

Complement System

The complement system enhances (complements) the ability of antibodies and phagocytic cells to remove pathogens from the horse. It is activated by two different means, but only the first is part of the innate system:

- exposure to a carbohydrate chain on the surface of the invader;

- exposure to an antibody procured by the acquired immune system (acquired only).

The complement system consists of a number of small proteins found in the plasma which are made in the liver and normally circulate as inactive precursors (pro-proteins). If one of these proteins recognises a carbohydrate on, for example, a bacterial cell wall, it will bind to the bacterial cell and start a chain of events known as the membrane attack complex (MAC). This results in a pore or hole in the bacterial cell wall, allowing surrounding fluid to rush in and the bacterial cell will burst.

Natural Killer Cells

NK cells are cytotoxic lymphocytes which are very important to the innate immune system. NK cells are unique, however, as they have the ability to recognise stressed cells in the absence of antibodies and MHC, allowing for a much faster immune reaction. They are analogous (but not the same as) cytotoxic T cells in the adaptive immune response (see Figure 15.6). NK cells release perforins which attach to the infected cell membrane and perforate it, thereby making holes, allowing surrounding fluid to rush in and burst the cell, the same as MAC above. They target tumour- and viral-infected cells.

Adaptive/Acquired Immunity

Adaptive systems are based on recognition of the microbe or toxin before responding to it. Pathogens rely on being passed from one animal to another, as they mostly do not survive outside the body for long. Before the disease develops there is an incubation period in which the pathogen multiplies in the cells of the host, or horse. Infectious disease has two main effects:

- The pathogen directly damages the horse's cells.
- The pathogen releases substances that further injure the horse's body; for example, many bacteria produce exotoxins and endotoxins. Exotoxins are released by bacterial cells as they grow, whereas endotoxins are released by bacterial cells when

they die. Botulism is caused by the bacteria *Clostridium botulinum*, which releases a neurotoxin harming the horse's nervous system. Endotoxins may cause high temperature, bleeding and shock, whereas exotoxins account for the major damage caused by bacteria, such as tetanus.

The adaptive system, as the name implies, adapts its response to specifically fight each invading type of organism. It also retains a memory of this organism so that it will be prepared should the same organism attack the horse again. The horse is then said to have acquired immunity to the infection (Table 15.7).

Types of Adaptive/Acquired Immunity

Immunological memory is vital for the health of horses as it provides the basis for immunisation by vaccination against many diseases. When a horse is vaccinated, it receives a dose of killed or weakened microbes or parts thereof and the horse's T and B cells are activated. If the horse then encounters say equine influenza virus in the future, its body can initiate a secondary response; that is, the immune system has already encountered this pathogen and been primed. In many cases, boosters have to be given to maintain protection against specific pathogens, such as tetanus.

Table 15.7 Summary of adaptive/acquired immunity in horses.

Type of adaptive/acquired immunity	Method of acquisition
Naturally acquired active immunity	Following invasion by a microbe, B and T cells recognise the antigen and co-stimulation results; this leads to plasma cell-secreting antibodies and cytotoxic T cells plus B and T memory cells
Naturally acquired passive immunity	Transfer of IgG from dam to foetus via placenta or of IgA from dam to neonatal foal via colostrum
Artificially acquired active immunity	Vaccination introduces 'safe' pre-treated antigens which stimulate cell-mediated and humoral immune responses. This leads to production of memory cells
Artificially acquired passive immunity	Antibodies (Igs) are given to the horse via intravenous injection

The term 'live attenuated organisms' refers to strains of organisms that have been treated to render them harmless to the horse. Attenuation is achieved by artificially altering their genes or by infecting laboratory animals first, which reduces the ability of the organism to cause disease without reducing the ability to induce immunity. Other vaccines contain chemically modified bacterial toxins. There are numerous vaccines available depending upon the viral problems of individual areas of the world. For example, seven known mosquito-borne viruses affect horses worldwide, namely:

- West Nile virus (including Kunjin – an Australian strain)
- Japanese encephalitis virus
- Venezuelan equine encephalitis virus
- western equine encephalitis virus
- eastern equine encephalitis virus
- Murray Valley encephalitis virus
- Ross River virus.

Vaccines are now available to protect against a wide range of infectious diseases including equine influenza, tetanus, rabies, strangles, rhinopneumonitis/equine herpes virus (EHV-1), and eastern and western encephalomyelitis. Figure 15.11 shows equine eastern encephalitis (EEE) virions.

Adaptive immunity may take a few days or weeks – that is, it is slow in response. It targets specific pathogens (i.e. it is specific) and may be:

- humoral or antibody-mediated (B lymphocytes) – primary antibody-mediated immune response
- cell-mediated (T lymphocytes) – cell-mediated immune response.

Haematopoietic precursor or stem cells in the bone marrow produce B and T lymphocytes. B cells differentiate and mature in the red bone marrow (hence the name B cells, derived from bone marrow), before moving to the peripheral lymphoid tissues such as in lymph nodes, Peyer's patches and the spleen. They wait there until required following infection/invasion. If the body is invaded, B cells leave the peripheral lymphoid tissues and cause an antibody-mediated immune response.

The immature T cells (pre-T cells) are sent to the thymus (hence the name T cells, from thymus), where they are 'assessed' before they can leave and go to the peripheral lymphoid tissues (Figure 15.12). Two types of T cells eventually leave the thymus:

- Helper T cells (CD4 cells) – regulate, they do not kill; they secrete cytokines which enhance the activity of macrophages, NK cells, B cells (humoral activity), cytotoxic T cells, other helper T cells and suppressor T cells.
- Cytotoxic T cells (CD8 cells) – kill infected cells, tumour cells and transplant cells.

These have very different functions, as shown in Figure 15.12.

Suppressor T cells produce cytokines that suppress the activity of B cells, cytotoxic T cells and helper T cells; that is, they turn off the immune response. The hormone cortisol is produced by stress in horses and can suppress the training activity of the thymus and therefore reduce the immune response.

Humoral (Antibody-Mediated) Immunity

B cells are specific to certain antigens (bacteria, viruses, etc.) and respond to the antigen by transforming into plasma cells (white blood cells) which produce antibodies (specific proteins) to combine with the antigens. A given antibody can attach to and inactivate a given antigen. Humoral immunity works mainly against extracellular (i.e. outside the host's body cells) pathogens which include viruses, bacteria and fungi that have found their way into the fluids surrounding body cells. The word 'humors' refers to body fluids such as blood and lymph and refers to a very old medical term.

Helper T cells assist both cell-mediated and humoral immunity. Antibodies are all Y-shaped, with variable and constant polypeptide regions. When antibodies enter the blood they are known as globulins and immunoglobulins (Igs) and are glycoproteins:

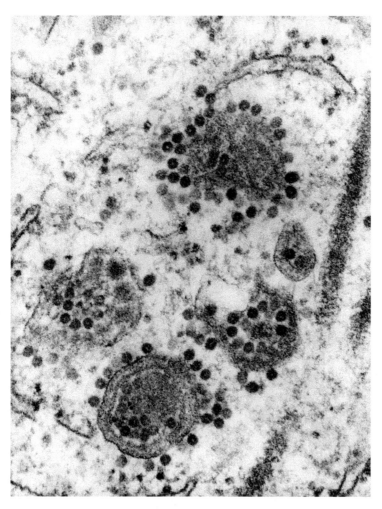

Figure 15.11 A 1975 transmission electron micrograph (TEM) revealing the presence of a number of eastern equine encephalitis (EEE) virus virions in a specimen of central nervous system tissue. *Source*: CDC/Dr Fred Murphy; Sylvia Whitfield, https://commons.wikimedia.org/wiki/File:EasternEquineEncephalitisVirus.jpg.

- IgM – 5–10% of all antibodies in plasma act as a B cell surface receptor for antigen attachment and are secreted in the early stages of the plasma cell response. Also found in lymph.
- IgG – the most abundant Ig in the horse's blood (80% of all antibodies in plasma) and produced in large amounts in response to some antigens. Also found in the lymph and intestines. IgG is the only class of antibody that crosses from dam to foetus via the placenta, providing the neonate with some immune protection.

- IgE – less than 1% of all antibodies in plasma, protects against parasites such as parasitic worms and is an antibody mediator in common allergic responses. Also found on basophils and mast cells.
- IgA – 10–15% of all antibodies in plasma. Found in secretions in the sweat, tears, mare's milk, saliva, mucus and the respiratory, digestive and urogenital systems.
- IgD – 0.2% of all antibodies in plasma and present on the cell surface of many B cells. IgD's function is to activate the B cell. Normally co-expressed with IgM.

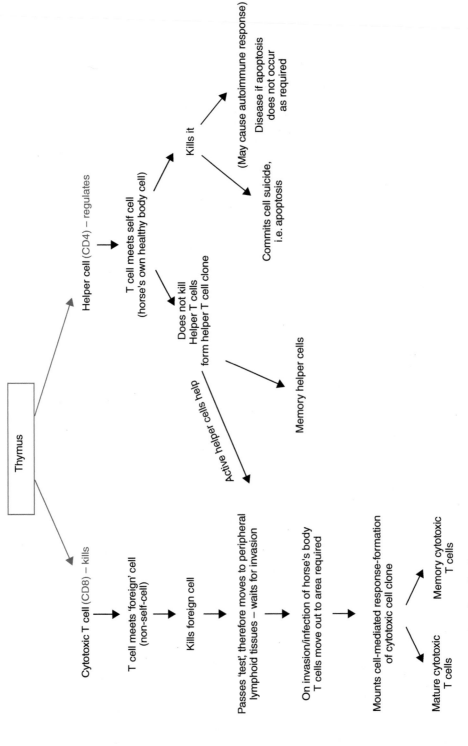

Figure 15.12 Training of T cells in the thymus.

B cells on first exposure to a specific antigen proliferate to become plasma cells which produce antibodies there and then and memory cells. This is quite a slow response and plasma cells are short lived, whereas memory cells are long lived. On second exposure to the same antigen at a later time, that is, another invasion by the same virus, the memory cells are also able to produce plasma cells and help with the immune response and this is much faster.

Cell-Mediated Immunity

Cytotoxic T cells directly attack antigens. Cell-mediated immunity is very effective against the following:

- intracellular pathogens; for example, viruses, bacteria and fungi inside cells (some fungi are small enough)
- tumour cells
- foreign tissue (such as transplants, cannulas).

Cell-mediated immunity involves cells attacking cells, hence the name. Each T cell or lymphocyte has a different receptor on its surface. When the receptor on the surface comes into contact with a complementary antigen it binds to it. Each T cell will therefore bind to a different antigen. This process activates the T cell and this is known as clonal selection.

Clonal Selection Clonal selection is a process whereby the T lymphocyte divides and differentiates in response to a specific antigen. This results in the production of a population of identical cells or a clone that is able to recognise the same specific antigen as the original T cell. A lymphocyte that has undergone clonal selection gives rise to two types of cells in the clone:

- Effector cells – include active helper T cells, active cytotoxic T cells and plasma cells which are part of a B cell clone. They mostly die following the end of the response. Thousands of effector cells effectively undertake the immune response against the specific antigen, eventually destroying the antigen.
- Memory cells – include memory helper T cells, memory cytotoxic T cells and memory B cells. They do not participate in the initial response to the antigen, but if there is a second invasion later in time, thousands of memory cells of a lymphocyte clone will be available, providing a much faster reaction to the invasion. They do not die at the end of a response but live a long time, waiting for the next invasion by a particular antigen.

Antigens and Antibodies

It is important to know the difference between an antigen and an antibody.

- Antigen – derived from the words *anti* body *gen*erator, antigens include viruses, bacteria, toxins and foreign material. An antigen will result in the production of antibodies if it invades the body.
- Antibody – an immunoglobulin, a specialised immune protein, produced as a result of the introduction of an antigen into the body.

Antibodies are able to destroy antigens via several methods:

- Neutralisation – many antibodies bind to the pathogen, blocking its activity.
- Agglutination – IgM and IgA clump antigens together so they can no longer work.
- Enhancement of phagocytosis or opsonisation – pathogens bound to antibodies are more efficiently engulfed by phagocytosis.
- Activation of the complement system – antibodies bound to pathogens activate the complement cascade, resulting in death or lysis of the pathogen.
- Stimulation of NK cells – abnormal body cells bound to antibodies are recognised by NK cells and subsequently destroyed using perforins.

Antigen Presentation

Prior to an adaptive immune response, B and T cells must recognise the foreign antigen. B cells are able to recognise and bind antigens in lymph, fluid between cells and plasma, but T cells only recognise cells that have the antigen–MHC complex inserted in the cell membrane of the antigen. This insertion is known as antigen presentation. In antigen processing, antigenic proteins are broken down into small fragments and combined with MHC molecules. These are then placed 'for presentation' in the cell membrane of a body cell of the horse, hence the phrase antigen presentation. Each horse has its own MHC molecules which are glycoproteins and help the horse's own immune system to recognise its own-self body cells. When an antigenic fragment from a self-protein comes into contact with a T cell, the T cell will ignore the antigen–MHC complex. However, if it comes into contact with an antigenic fragment from a foreign protein, it recognises this as foreign and an adaptive immune response follows.

Special cells know as antigen-presenting cells (APCs) are able to process and present antigens and these include:

- dendritic cells
- macrophages
- B cells.

APCs are strategically located in areas where invasion is more likely, such as the respiratory system, urogenital system, mucous membranes, lymph nodes, epidermis and digestive tract.

After processing an antigen, the APC migrates to the lymph tissue to present the antigen to T cells that have the correct antigen receptors that can recognise and bind to the antigen–MHC complex, resulting in a cell-mediated or humoral immune response. There are two classes of MHC molecules (class I and class II) with different properties (Table 15.8).

Ingestion of an Antigen – Mode of Action

- APCs phagocytose the antigen (bacteria, virus, tumour cell) where invasion has occurred in the horse's body.
- Within the APC, the antigen is broken down into short peptide fragments and packaged into vesicles.
- Simultaneously, MHC molecules are made and packaged into other vesicles in the APC.
- The vesicles containing both the antigen fragments and MHCs fuse.
- The newly formed antigen–MHC complex is taken to the APC's plasma membrane and inserted in it.
- The APC then migrates to lymphoid tissue to present the antigen–MHC complex to the T cells.
- A small number of T cells with the correct antigen receptors in the lymphoid tissue recognise the antigen–MHC complex on the surface of the APC and bind to the antigen–MHC complex, triggering

Table 15.8 Class I and II MHC glycoproteins have different properties.

Class I MHC glycoproteins	Class II MHC glycoproteins
Recognised **only** by cytotoxic T cells (CD8)	Recognised **only** by helper T cells (CD4)
Found on surface of **all** the horse's body cells	Found **only** on surface of special immune cells (B cells, cytotoxic T cells, macrophages and dendritic cells)
Response – will destroy body cells if invaded by foreign vital antigen	Response – helper T cell regulates immune response
Located in plasma membrane of every nucleotide cell in the horse	Enhances activities of the above cells when fighting antigens/invaders

a cell-mediated or humoral immune response.

T Cells and Cell-Mediated Immunity

Presentation of an antigen–MHC complex by APCs signals the T cells of the horse that invaders are in the body and a response is required. However, a second signal is also required and that is called co-stimulation. Interleukin 2 is a common co-stimulator, a cytokine, and is a chemical messenger travelling through interstitial fluid in the horse's body only. It is thought the need for two steps prevents overreaction of the immune system. Once the T cell has been activated it must first undergo clonal selection (see above), that is, lymphocyte proliferation and differentiation into more specialised cells in response to the specific antigen that has invaded. This results in a clone of cells recognising this specific antigen. Some of these become effector T cells and some become memory T cells. Note there are two types of mature T cells: helper T cells and cytotoxic T cells, as previously discussed.

Helper T Cell Activation

Helper T cell activation results in formation of a helper T cell and memory T cell clone. The memory T cells of this helper T cell clone are not active though, and only activate if the same invader returns to infect the horse's body sometime in the future, that is, a second time, when they will quickly respond by proliferating and differentiating into more active helper T cells, speeding up the response to the infection.

Active helper T cells help other cells of the adaptive immune system to fight invaders by enhancing activation and proliferation of B cells, T cells and NK cells. They also release interleukin 2 which acts as a co-stimulator (see above). Helper T cells are able to secrete B cell growth factor which enhances antibody secretion of the B cell clone. They can also secrete substances that attract neutrophils and macrophages to the invasion site and secrete a macrophage migration inhibition factor which prevents migrating macrophages from leaving the site. During parasitic invasions such as redworm, helper T cells activate eosinophils and promote IgE development.

Cytotoxic T Cells

A cytotoxic T cell clone results from activation of cytotoxic T cells. These attack and destroy infected body cells in the horse that are infected with the antigen. Memory T cells of the cytotoxic T cell clone are the same as those in the helper T cell clone, that is, they only activate if the same invader returns (see above).

Cytotoxic T cells are effectively an army doing battle with invaders in a cell-mediated response. They leave lymphoid tissue to travel to the site of invasion where they seek out and destroy infected cells and also tumour cells. They secrete gamma interferon which activates phagocytic cells and macrophage migration inhibition factor, similar to helper T cells, preventing migrating macrophages from leaving the site of invasion. They are also able to detach from one target cell and seek out another to destroy.

Cytotoxic T cells recognise and attack target cells in a similar way to NK cells. However, NK cells destroy a wide range of infected cells, whereas cytotoxic T cells only have receptors for a specific target antigen and have mainly two methods of action:

- They bind to infected cells and release two substances, namely perforin and granulysin. Perforin perforates the plasma membrane of the target cell, creating a hole, causing influx of extracellular fluid and the cell bursts. Granulysin makes holes in the plasma membranes of the invaded microbes.
- They have receptors on their surface which recognise target cells before binding to them and release protein-digesting enzymes called granzymes which trigger apoptosis or cell death of the invaded cell. The microbes released by the dying cell are killed by phagocytes.

Summary Points

1) Horses live around microbes and are continually exposed to them. Most of them are harmless and many live within the body, such as in the digestive tract. Only a few may become harmful.

2) If a pathogenic microbe is able to penetrate the horse's external barriers, which are the first line of defence, then innate immunity systems of the horse will come into play.

3) There are two types of immunity, namely innate and acquired or adaptive.

4) Innate immunity is present from birth.

5) Acquired immunity develops either through exposure of the horse to the infectious organisms (after they have broken through the innate immune system) or through immunisation.

6) Innate or non-specific immunity is fast and only lasts a short time, whereas acquired/adaptive immunity is specific, slower and more long term.

7) Acquired/adaptive response targets specific pathogens and may be humoral or cell-mediated.

8) B cells are able to recognise and bind antigens in lymph, fluid between cells and plasma, whereas T cells only recognise cells that have the antigen–MHC complex inserted in the cell membrane of the antigen.

9) Cytotoxic T cells are effectively an army doing battle with invaders in a cell-mediated response. They leave lymphoid tissue, to travel to the site of invasion where they seek out and destroy infected cells and also tumour cells.

10) When antibodies enter the blood they are known as globulins and immunoglobulins (Igs) and are glycoproteins.

Q + A

Q What is the difference between an antigen and an antibody?

A An antigen is derived from the words *anti*body *gen*erator and includes viruses, bacteria, toxins and foreign material. An antigen will result in production of antibodies if it invades the horse's body. An antibody is an immunoglobulin, a specialised immune protein, produced as a result of the introduction of an antigen into the body.

Q Briefly describe how interferon (IFN) affects the replication of viruses.

A A body cell gets invaded by a virus. The invaded cell releases IFNs which leave the infected cell and go to neighbouring non-infected or healthy cells. At the neighbouring cells IFNs attach to receptors on the cell membranes, causing the cell to produce inactive enzymes in preparation for a possible invasion. When the neighbouring cell is invaded, the inactive enzymes are activated and break down viral mRNA to inhibit viral protein synthesis, effectively killing the virus.

Q What is clonal selection?

A A process whereby the T lymphocyte divides and differentiates in response to a specific antigen, resulting in production of a population of identical cells or a clone that is able to recognise the same specific antigen as the original T cell.

Q What are APCs?

A APCs (antigen-presenting cells) are special cells able to process and present antigens. They include dendritic cells, macrophages and B cells.

Q Summarise the function of B cells in the immune response.

A B cells are specific to certain antigens (bacteria, viruses, etc.) and respond to the antigen by transforming into plasma cells (white blood cells) which produce antibodies (specific proteins) to combine with the antigens. A given antibody can attach to and inactivate a given antigen.

16

Exercise Physiology, Functional Anatomy and Conformation

Exercise Physiology

Exercise physiology is the study of the responses of the body to exercise. Human athletes have been breaking records year on year, but horses do not appear to have benefited as much from advances in science and technology; horse race records in terms of speed and times are rarely broken, for example (Figure 16.1). In humans, training can be tailored to suit the individual athlete's needs and muscle fibre types analysed to assess the correct balance and type of training for individuals. Nutritionists play a vital role in ensuring nutrients are available for maximum performance and physiotherapists help to assess the potential for injury, and change training schedules accordingly. This practice should be encouraged with equine athletes.

Fitness

Fitness refers to the horse's ability to perform consistently well in the field in which it is performing – whether racing, dressage or endurance. Strength, speed, suppleness and stamina are all important aspects of fitness. Fitness must be acquired, that is, built up over time with training. The level of fitness required is dictated by the intensity of the effort the horse must perform. Fitness training aims to gradually increase the horse's tolerance to work by slowly increasing workload and feed intake. Unfit horses soon sweat and breathe rapidly, while the heart rate goes up quickly.

Horses at Rest

Prior to exercise, horses at rest, even walking around grazing, have a low oxygen demand which is easily met by shallow breathing and low pulse rates. This metabolic state delivers oxygen and nutrients including glucose to the tissues to meet low requirements. At the same time, small amounts of waste products are also removed. Horses at rest are not sweating in normal moderate ambient temperatures.

Exercise

As soon as the horse starts to exercise, the metabolic rate of muscle tissue increases greatly by up to 20 times. To fuel this increase in activity, the body must quickly adapt. Cellular respiration is covered in Chapter 6. Different areas of equine physiology come into play when horses work, but cellular respiration is particularly important.

- Cellular respiration transfers energy for muscle contraction from glucose and lipids to adenosine triphosphate (ATP) for fuel. This takes place in the mitochondria.
- ATP splits into adenosine diphosphate (ADP) and inorganic phosphate (P) by hydrolysis to release energy to allow muscle fibres to slide over each other.
- Respiration then has to resynthesise ATP from ADP and inorganic P for further muscle movement to take place.

The splitting of ATP is a coupled reaction, that is, the hydrolysis of ATP is coupled with muscle contraction. When ATP is split

Equine Science, Third Edition. Zoe Davies and Sarah Pilliner.
© 2018 Zoe Davies and Sarah Pilliner. Published 2018 by John Wiley & Sons Ltd.

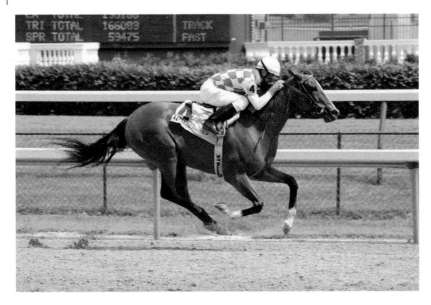

Figure 16.1 Racehorse at full gallop. *Source*: Kubina, https://commons.wikimedia.org/wiki/File:Horseracing_Churchill_Downs.jpg. CC BY-SA 2.0.

it is not entirely efficient and some energy is lost as heat. This is why hard-working horses may sweat profusely to try to lose this excessive heat.

At slow speeds the demand for energy is low and aerobic cellular respiration can meet the requirements for ATP synthesis. This is the primary pathway for regeneration of ATP during endurance-type exercise. Aerobic cellular respiration also contributes during short bursts of high-energy intense exercise, with anaerobic respiration making up the deficit.

Exercise and Energy

Muscle movement needs a continual supply of ATP. There are three sources of ATP:

- The ATP/creatine phosphate (CP) system – up to 10 seconds. Also known as the alactic anaerobic system, this uses ATP already present in cells from a period of relative rest, allowing movement to start on demand. When the horse is working fast, such as in a short sharp sprint, during maximum effort there is only enough ATP to last about 3 seconds. There is,

however, a back-up compound, CP, which can be used to quickly resynthesise ATP, allowing continued exercise for another 10 seconds. This is known as the ATP/CP system (Figure 16.2). Alactic means there is no build-up of lactate ions during this process. Oxygen is also not required for the ATP/CP system. All short sprints or bursts of speed rely on this system.

- ATP provided by glycolysis (see Chapter 6) – 10–60 seconds. This system is also known as the lactic anaerobic system or glycolytic pathway. Glycolysis provides 2 ATP molecules per glucose molecule during glycolysis. This is low compared to the 36 ATP molecules available from complete aerobic respiration (i.e. including the Krebs cycle). This source of ATP is small but fast and also does not require oxygen. This allows intense exercise to continue for up to 60 seconds. The disadvantage is that this process results in the production of lactate or lactic acid instead of pyruvate. This accumulates within the muscle cells, lowering the pH and making the cells more acidic. Fatigue follows.

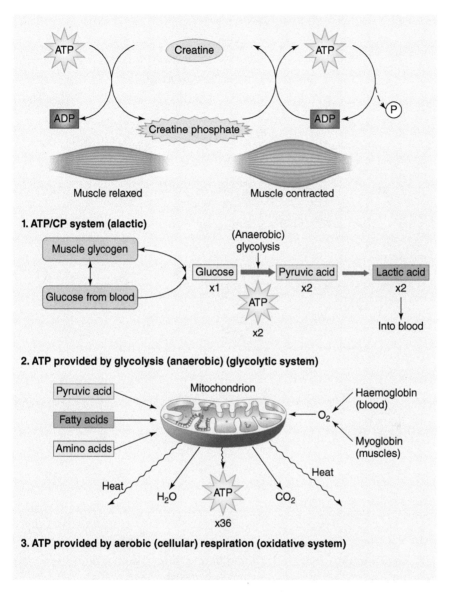

1. ATP/CP system (alactic)

2. ATP provided by glycolysis (anaerobic) (glycolytic system)

3. ATP provided by aerobic (cellular) respiration (oxidative system)

Figure 16.2 The ATP/CP system. (The energy continuum.)

- ATP provided by aerobic respiration – more than 60 seconds. This is energy from the complete breakdown of glucose in the presence of oxygen, when each glucose molecule results in 36 ATP molecules. This takes time and requires oxygen and if oxygen is available can fuel exercise for hours in horses.

All the above energy-providing processes blend seamlessly into one another and this is known as the energy continuum.

Fuels Available for Exercise

The process of cellular respiration releases energy from foods including carbohydrates, lipids and protein. All of these may provide

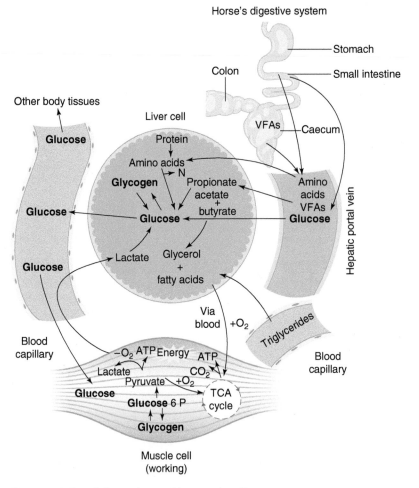

Figure 16.3 Use of glucose in a working muscle cell.

fuel if required (see Chapter 6). The main fuel for sprinting is glucose, whereas the main fuel for endurance work would be lipids. Glucose supplies normal every-day energy needs for horses that are not starving (Figure 16.3). Anaerobic exercise always depends on glucose, as lipids cannot be used to fuel glycolysis. Horses need to be trained to use lipids regularly and it takes longer to mobilise lipid stores, but once this process is in place the horse's body can use this fuel for as long as it lasts. Lipids are generally not used for short-term fast exercise, but they can be used to fuel longer slower aerobic exercise such as for endurance.

Protein provides a very small amount of energy for exercise, as low as 5%. This increases only during starvation, when there is no other fuel available. Table 16.1 shows the different energy-producing systems and timings of available energy for horses.

Immediate Response of the Horse's Body to Exercise

Exercise places great demands on the horse's body and greatly affects the homeostatic processes due to the physiological changes that occur during exercise (particularly maximum exercise).

Changes Occurring during Exercise

- Oxygen levels fall.
- Carbon dioxide levels increase.
- Lactate ions increase.

Table 16.1 Energy production systems available for horses and their timings.

	First	Second	Third
	ATP/CP system (alactic anaerobic system)	**Glycolytic system** (lactic anaerobic system)	**Aerobic system** (alactic aerobic system)
Energy derived from	ATP/CP already present in resting muscles	Glycolysis 2 ATP/glucose molecule	Complete cellular respiration 36 ATP/glucose molecule
Time of system	Up to 10 seconds	10 seconds to 60–120 seconds	Indefinitely
By-products	No lactate	Lactate	No lactate + CO_2
Type of activity	Fast explosive such as escaping danger, start of sprint	Longer sprints	Hacking, hunting, endurance, and so on.

- Body temperature increases.
- Blood glucose and glycogen levels fall.
- Fluid and electrolytes are lost via sweating.

As these changes take place during exercise, homeostatic mechanisms are required to return the body to some sort of balance as quickly as possible.

Homeostatic Mechanisms Involved during Exercise

- Increased breathing and heart rates – increased respiration within muscle cells results in increased CO_2 in the blood and this lowers pH (i.e. increases acidity, as CO_2 is an acidic gas). Specialised sensitive cells known as chemoreceptors detect these changes in the carotid and aortic bodies in major blood vessels. The chemoreceptors then send messages to the cardiovascular and respiratory control centres in the brain to increase heart and ventilation (breathing) rates. These changes result in increased gas exchange in the lungs and faster delivery of oxygen to the tissues. This also allows faster removal of CO_2.
- Heat loss – increased blood flow to the skin to remove excess heat produced during exercise from muscle respiration and contraction. Blood vessels dilate, a process known as peripheral vasodilation, pushing excessive heat to the skin surface.
- Increased sweating – sweat glands secrete a salty solution which then evaporates from the skin surface, taking heat with it. This, together with vasodilation, is quite efficient at removing excess heat from the body. However, too much sweating can result in dehydration and excessive loss of electrolytes and the horse's athletic performance will soon become compromised.
- Increased mobilisation of fuel – to maintain glucose availability for cellular respiration in muscles, stored glycogen must be mobilised from muscle and liver cells. Following prolonged exercise, horses must rest and this is when these glycogen stores are replenished from the horse's diet; this may take up to 48 hours.
- Production of lactic acid – during vigorous exercise, oxygen requirement exceeds supply from the respiratory system and muscle cells therefore produce lactic acid. Lactic acid then builds up in the muscle cells. Some of this diffuses out from the muscle cells and is transported to the liver where it is converted to glucose; this returns to the muscle cells, where it is further metabolised back to lactate. This is known as the Cori cycle (see 'Oxygen debt').

Lactate Threshold

As previously mentioned in Chapter 3, type I slow twitch muscle fibres produce less power but can work aerobically over periods, even up to a moderately fast pace. At a heart rate of up to 140 beats per minute (bpm) most endurance horses can meet all their oxygen needs. Above this heart rate, termed the lactate threshold, the muscles start working anaerobically, using faster produced but shorter lived fuel from glucose, and this results in the production of lactate. Excess lactate leads to fatigue. Endurance horses working below the lactate threshold will recover rapidly and can work for longer distances aerobically.

Over-training

Some horses can become over-trained, where the body does not have time to recover following training sessions and competitions. Over-training is particularly common in racing and can cause poor performance, muscle problems and result in chronic fatigue. This also negatively affects the immune system, leading to respiratory-type infections. This, combined with psychological stress in some horses that do not adapt well to particular training programmes, competing or travelling, may lead to increased-secretion of cortisol and adrenaline, both of which may further suppress the immune system. The skeletal system is also prone to damage from exercise – particularly joints, tendons and ligaments. In the long term, over-work may also result in the articular cartilage wearing away, causing pain and inflammation.

Over-training of young racehorses is particularly a problem because the skeleton and joints are still developing and maturing and more susceptible to injury.

Recovery

Following exercise the body must try to return to normal. This takes time, as the various systems take different amounts of time to do this. Fit horses take less time to recover following exercise or competition. Following exercise the heart rate slows quickly at first and then undertakes a slower return to normal.

Recovery Following Anaerobic Exercise

There are two aspects to immediate recovery that occur if the horse's body was not able to deliver enough oxygen to meet demand, that is, following anaerobic exercise:

- Recharging of the ATP/CP or alactic acid component of recovery – this may take about 2 minutes. However, if there was only a very short burst of exercise, such as a horse shying, then this may take only a few seconds to recover. The ATP/CP stores are replenished from aerobic respiration.
- Lactic acid component – that is, removal of lactate. This is the 'oxygen debt' and this will be repaid after completion of exercise.

Oxygen Debt Oxygen debt is removal of the lactate ions that accumulated during anaerobic exercise. Lactate ions make the blood more acidic and interfere with enzymes involved in normal cellular respiration. Lactate will soon build up in muscle tissue and also diffuse into the blood, making it more acidic (Figure 16.4). Eventually muscles become so painful that exercise must stop as the muscles are fatigued.

Horses should be gently cooled down following hard work as gentle exercise helps to reduce muscle soreness. Gentle exercise for up to 5 minutes keeps the capillaries in muscle fibres dilated which helps flush

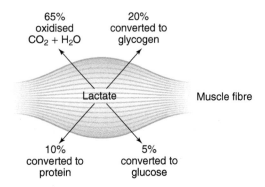

65% oxidised $CO_2 + H_2O$

20% converted to glycogen

Lactate

Muscle fibre

10% converted to protein

5% converted to glucose

Figure 16.4 Fate of lactate build-up in working muscles.

muscles with oxygen to reduce the oxygen debt.

Long-Term Responses of the Horse's Body to Exercise

The horse's body is highly adaptable to exercise and appropriate training can have remarkable effects on fitness and the ability to work and compete. Long-term adaptations depend upon the type of training but generally include changes within the heart, respiratory system and muscle tissue. These internal changes manifest themselves as a slower resting heart rate, a reduced rise in heart and respiratory rates for a given piece of exercise and improved recovery rates.

Training must slightly overload muscles before they can adapt and this should increase in intensity as training progresses. This is known as progressive resistance.

Changes to the Heart and Circulation

The heart is a muscle and therefore also adapts to appropriate training. Exercise with training slightly increases the size of the heart muscle or myocardium and this in turn increases the size of the heart chambers so more oxygen can be pumped to the working muscles. This increases stroke volume so that each beat of the heart now sends a higher volume of blood round the body. Once this ability occurs, it follows that at rest it can beat less often to pump the same amount of blood as pre training. This leads to a lower resting pulse rate in a fitter horse. The horse's resting heart rate normally lies between 36 and 42 bpm, but may be as low as 26 bpm in a fit horse, reaching a maximum of 240 bpm when galloping.

Both the red cell count (erythrocyte count) and packed cell volume (PCV) increase with training, improving the ability to carry oxygen. Erythrocyte turnover also increases. These cells have a limited life span and as horses work harder they simply wear out faster and need replacing, that is, the average age decreases. Younger erythrocytes have better oxygen-carrying capacity.

Changes to the Respiratory System

Training aims to improve oxygen intake so that blood-carrying capacity is maximised. The strength of muscles associated with breathing, namely the internal and external intercostal muscles and diaphragm, increases, allowing a greater volume of air to be breathed in and out. This helps increase ventilation rate. Vital capacity (total lung volume) and surface area of the alveoli also increase, leading to higher rates of gaseous exchange. Pulmonary capillaries that surround alveoli in the lungs respond to the increased demand for oxygen during repeated exercise by increasing in number. This, combined with the greater vital capacity described above, means that horses get more oxygen into the lungs and around the body to the muscles. These improvements to circulation and gas exchange systems result in a greater VO_2 max.

Changes to Skeletal Muscle

Changes to skeletal muscle depend upon the muscle fibre types involved and the nature of the exercise (sprinting or endurance). There is unlikely to be a significant change in the proportion of slow twitch to fast twitch fibres. The main changes relate to the metabolism of the fibres. Stamina training can increase the oxygen-using capacity of fast twitch fibres, thereby enhancing their ability to utilise oxygen. This in turn increases their oxidative capacity or capacity for cellular respiration. This is achieved by an increase in the number of mitochondria within muscle cells, increased enzymes associated with respiration and consequently an increased supply of ATP and CP. Increased exercise results in genes being switched on that make more mitochondria. Studies have shown that a single bout of exercise induces a rapid increase in production of mitochondria and this is mediated both by activation and increased expression of PGC-1 alpha. A variant of PGC-1 alpha was found to be absent before high levels of exercise, but was found immediately after 1 hour of aerobic exercise. This suggests that genes to make new mitochondria are switched on by exercise and with the help of transcription factors then produce components for mitochondrial synthesis. PGC-1 alpha docks on and coactivates transcription factors that regulate expression of genes in the nucleus that encode for mitochondrial proteins.

The ability of muscles to store glycogen, use lipids as an energy source and the amount of myoglobin in muscle cells also increases. The use of lipids as an energy source helps to reduce reliance upon glycogen and leaves more glycogen available in the energy 'reservoir'. The density of capillaries running through muscles increases in response to exercise. This process is known as capillarisation (Figure 16.5) and allows more efficient exchange between the blood and working muscle fibres.

Appropriate training also brings an improvement in performance due to improved coordination of motor units. For example, with dressage movements, which are repeated during training, there is an effect on antagonistic muscles. Active muscles work better, while antagonistic muscles will be suppressed so they do not interfere with the movement.

A muscle fibre can only adapt if given a suitable stimulus, so the training programme

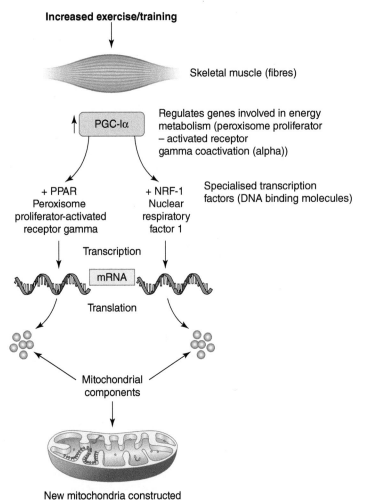

Increased exercise/training

Skeletal muscle (fibres)

PGC-Iα Regulates genes involved in energy metabolism (peroxisome proliferator – activated receptor gamma coactivation (alpha))

+ PPAR Peroxisome proliferator-activated receptor gamma

+ NRF-1 Nuclear respiratory factor 1

Specialised transcription factors (DNA binding molecules)

Transcription

mRNA

Translation

Mitochondrial components

New mitochondria constructed

Figure 16.5 Training causes increased capillarisation of muscle fibres. PPAR, Peroxisome proliferator-activated receptor gamma; NRF-1, nuclear respiratory factor 1.

must include work of similar intensity and type to that involved in the competitive area for which the horse is being trained. For speed, for example sprints, the training programme must include sprinting to recruit muscle fibres associated with power and acceleration, that is, fast twitch low oxidative fibres. For endurance work at varying speeds, prolonged exercise at similar levels is needed to increase the oxygen-carrying capacity of fast twitch high oxidative fibres and slow twitch fibres. Horses undertaking endurance work must also be trained to drink water and eat when required (Figure 16.6).

Fitness Training

The aim of a fitness programme is to produce a horse that is 'fit', in other words, in a state suitable for carrying out the work required without excessive stress. The level of fitness required is dictated by the intensity of the effort the horse has to perform. The basis of the fitness programme is to increase the horse's ability to tolerate work by gradually increasing its workload and energy intake. This slow, steady progression is fundamental to the physical and mental well-being of the horse.

Preliminary Work

Preliminary work is designed to exercise the horse slowly for increasing lengths of time to tone up the muscles, tendons and ligaments. The importance of initial walking and trotting work cannot be over-emphasised. Ideally, horses should be walked on the roads for up to 2 hours a day for 4 weeks and never less than 2 weeks.

After the initial walking work, trot can be introduced. Trotting can be alternated between the roads and grass or in the arena, but a certain amount of trotting on the road helps the horse's skeletal system cope with hard ground, but too much causes concussion and jarring. Initially, the trot should only be for a couple of minutes at a time, building up over the next few weeks to 15 minutes in total, split into three or four periods.

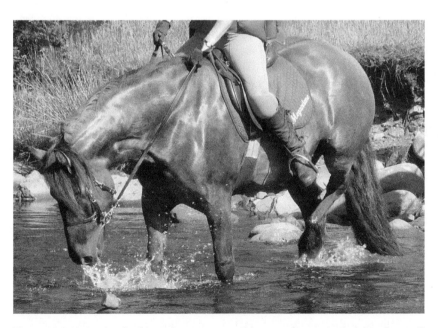

Figure 16.6 Horses involved in endurance competitions need extensive training. *Source*: Courtesy of Laureen Roberts.

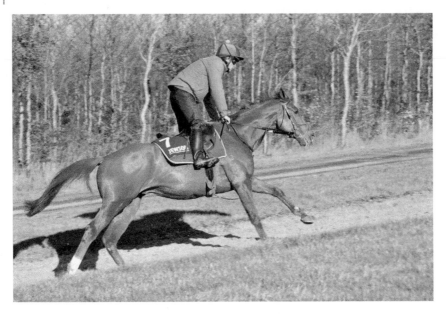

Figure 16.7 Training the racehorse. *Source*: Paul, https://www.flickr.com/photos/vegaseddie/11297384474/.CC BY 2.0.

Development Work

The horse should now be ready to progress to the next stage of training, with the introduction of canter work (see Figure 16.7) and suppling exercises. Development work will vary according to the discipline the horse is being prepared for, but the principle is to begin to work the horse harder so that the heart and lungs become accustomed to exercise, building up the horse's stamina while the muscles continue to strengthen and adapt to the work the horse is being given.

Fast Work

The third period of the fitness programme is even more specialised; the power and athleticism of the dressage horse and show jumper are developed further, while the racehorse and the event horse have fast work.

Interval Training

Interval training is a method of training of horses that involves both low- and high-intensity exercise training interspersed with rest or relief periods. The recovery periods involve lower intensity work. Interval training has been adapted for event horses and successfully used by top event riders and many other disciplines. It consists of giving a horse a period of specific work (canter), followed by a brief interval of semi-rest (walk) during which the horse is allowed to partially recover, before being asked to work again.

Aims of Interval Training

The aim is to increase the horse's capacity for using oxygen and performing aerobic work to the point at which the start of anaerobic work is delayed as much as possible. This delays lactic acid accumulation, enabling the horse to work for longer before fatigue sets in. The periods of work given during interval training develop and extend the horse's capacity for intensive work as the programme progresses, without a build-up of lactic acid. Lactic acid is a major factor contributing to fatigue; the walking periods between canters allow the blood to remove any lactic acid that may be building up in the muscle fibres. Interval training increases the horse's tolerance to stress, and the measurement of pulse, respiration and recovery rates means that the horse's reaction to the training programme can be closely monitored.

Monitoring Interval Training

An essential part of the interval training regime is monitoring the horse's temperature, pulse and respiration (TPR). To obtain 'normal' values, each of these measurements should be taken while the horse is calm and at rest. These values are then used as a baseline against which the values after exercise can be compared.

Beginning Interval Training

Interval training cannot cut corners and the following factors must be considered before starting a programme:

- The horse should be capable of 90 minutes' walk and trot over rolling terrain without distress. If conditioned slowly and carefully, the horse will stay in peak condition longer than one pushed too fast in the early stages.
- A notebook should be kept with a running record of the horse's response to work, allowing the programme to be adjusted accordingly. Hot weather can have a profound effect on how quickly the horse recovers from work – during hot and humid weather the horse will continue breathing fast for longer than expected because more rapid breathing is necessary to reduce body heat; so even though the pulse rate may drop to normal, the breathing may still be fast. Pulse is a more reliable gauge of the horse's recovery and how fit it is, and is the most important reading to take.

How to Use Interval Training

During interval training the horse is cantered at a pre-determined speed for a certain time. After this piece of work, the horse is pulled up and the pulse and/or respiration rates recorded immediately, the horse is walked for a set time and the rates recorded again. The difference between the two readings is the 'recovery rate'. The horse repeats these work-outs every 4 days, and the pulse and respiration rates are recorded at the same points; as the horse gets fitter, it will recover faster from the work. The pulse and respiration values will rarely return to the resting values obtained in the stable, due to excitement and the fact that the horse is recovering in walk, so a value for the horse's warmed-up pulse and respiration should be obtained and used as baseline values.

Fitness is gradually built up by slowly increasing the amount of work the horse is asked to do by increasing the speed and/or length of the work-out or using more demanding terrain. If the recovery rate is not good enough after a work-out, the work is adjusted so the horse is never over-stressed. This system is markedly different from the more traditional methods where horses are trotted and cantered for long distances with short sharp gallops later in the training programme and no repetition of fast work in each work-out.

During the first canter work-out the horse can be cantered for 3 minutes at 400 metres per minute (mpm). This is followed by 1 minute in trot and a recovery period in walk of 3–5 minutes. This is repeated twice, after which the horse is cooled down in walk for at least 20 minutes. The heart rate should be no more than 150 bpm at the end of each canter and no more than 100 bpm before the next canter commences. If the heart rate takes more than 5 minutes to drop below 100 bpm then either the canter was too long, the terrain too steep, the speed too fast or the initial work was not carried out correctly.

The canter work is gradually built up until the horse has reached the desired fitness. The flexibility of interval training means that it can be used to fitten horses as diverse as event horses and long-distance horses very effectively.

Points Regarding Interval Training

- Interval training must be monitored by pulse and respiration rate, not by time alone. It is the pulse rate immediately after the work that shows how much stress the horse has been subjected to, and the recovery rate that shows how fit it is. Without these records interval training is meaningless and can actually be harmful.

- If the horse is required to work anaerobically the pulse rate should exceed 200 bpm; this can be estimated by looking at the pulse 1 minute after pulling up. If the horse has been beneficially stressed the pulse will lie between 120 and 150 bpm 1 minute after stopping work. If greater than 150 bpm the horse has been overstressed, and below 120 bpm the horse has not worked hard enough.
- If pulse and respiration have not returned to normal within 20 minutes of completing the work-out the horse has been over-worked and the programme should be adapted accordingly.
- Respiration rate should not exceed the pulse rate. If it does, stop work and ask what has caused this – lack of fitness, environmental conditions or a problem with the horse's respiratory tract.
- Never finish the work if the horse is distressed, but, on the other hand, the horse must be slightly stressed to stimulate the body systems to become better adapted to exercise. The heart rate must be raised above 100 bpm after work.
- Always warm up and cool down thoroughly before cantering, particularly if the horse has to travel in a lorry or trailer to the work area.

Functional Anatomy

Functional anatomy of the horse's musculoskeletal system is an important area of exercise physiology, as horses are most commonly used for work as equine athletes. Equine biomechanics is an area of exercise physiology that is receiving much attention (see below).

The horse's forelimbs serve quite a different purpose than do the hindlimbs. The powerful hindquarter muscles are the engine for propulsion, whereas forelimbs have some propulsive capability, but their main function is more that of steering and support. Forelimbs also support the weight of the head and neck, creating a cantilever effect, with the head and neck projecting from a vertical support of the forelimbs which support 60–65% of the horse's weight. So, all horses are naturally on the forehand.

The more angular hindlimbs have a 'mechanical advantage' in terms of their ability to produce power and speed. The angles are the joints which can close or 'flex' on impact, absorbing shock, then deliver energy as they open during the next phase of the gait to propel the horse forward. This flexing allows the ligaments and tendons that support the joints to absorb shock, as without the flexion, the bones and cartilage themselves take the brunt of the impact.

Centre of Gravity

Unlike the greyhound, the horse has a large, bulky body and a relatively rigid spine; the horse is not a natural jumping animal. The centre of gravity is the point over which the horse's weight is balanced, and altering the centre of gravity plays an essential part in effectively propelling the horse at speed. The centre of gravity varies with the individual horse and depends on conformation and weight. In a stationary horse the position of the centre of gravity can be judged by dropping a line from the highest point of the withers and crossing it by a line from the point of the shoulder to the point of the buttock (Figure 16.8). This means that it lies nearer to the shoulder than the hips; this is why a standing horse can lift a hind foot off the ground and not lose its balance. The horse has a heavy head full of teeth, at the end of a long lever (the neck), and needs powerful muscles to support it. When the head is lifted the centre of gravity moves backwards, allowing the horse to lift its forehand off the ground; thus movement is preceded by a slight lifting of the head.

Unlike humans, the horse does not have a collar bone; no firm, bony union exists between the rib cage and forelimbs, there is

Figure 16.8 The horse's centre of gravity.

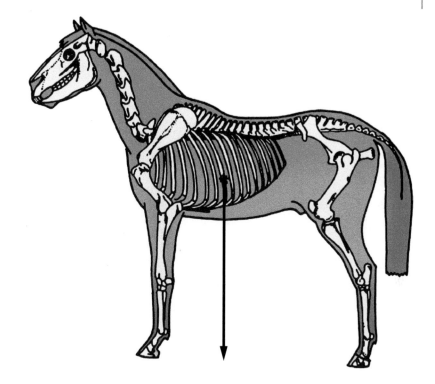

only muscle. The horse's body is slung in a cradle of muscle (serratus ventralis) between the two shoulder blades (Figure 16.9). These muscles allow the trunk to rise and fall or to lean a little to one side, and this enables the horse to keep its balance, particularly when cornering at speed – much like the suspension of a car. The following points affect the way the horse moves:

- The forelimbs are attached to the trunk only by muscles and ligaments.
- The forelimbs bear most of the weight and the concussion involved with movement.
- The head and neck act as a balancing weight and the neck gives muscle attachment to the muscles that extend the forelimb.
- The spinal column has only slight sideways and up and down movement between the neck and tail. Thus the trunk is almost rigid and its role in movement is to transfer the power from the hindquarters forward.
- The hindlimbs have a bony attachment to the spine to transfer the forces of movement directly to the spinal column.

Several conformational features ensure that the centre of gravity for the limb is in the upper part of the leg, close to its point of rotation. The large muscle masses are higher up the limbs, whereas lighter tendon and bone are lower. The largest muscles in the front limb are around the shoulder and elbow, with smaller muscles on the forearm. Below the knee there is virtually no muscle tissue. Long tendons transmit the forces from the muscles above to the lower limb. So, in fact, the front cannon, pastern and hoof account for less than 1% of the horse's weight. Evolution resulted in one toe – the hoof – which is lighter than the two hooves of cattle. So when applying protective boots or heavy shoes, more weight is added down on the leg, which makes the swing phase of the stride more energy-consuming.

Stay Apparatus

The stay apparatus is shown in Figure 16.10. Horses can rest for long periods of time in a standing position and this has the advantage of giving them a more distant horizon to spot

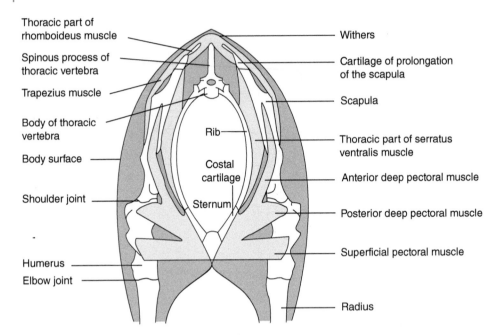

Thoracic part of rhomboideus muscle

Spinous process of thoracic vertebra

Trapezius muscle

Body of thoracic vertebra

Body surface

Shoulder joint

Humerus

Elbow joint

Withers

Cartilage of prolongation of the scapula

Scapula

Rib

Costal cartilage

Sternum

Thoracic part of serratus ventralis muscle

Anterior deep pectoral muscle

Posterior deep pectoral muscle

Superficial pectoral muscle

Radius

Figure 16.9 The horse's body is slung in a cradle of muscle known as the serratus ventralis.

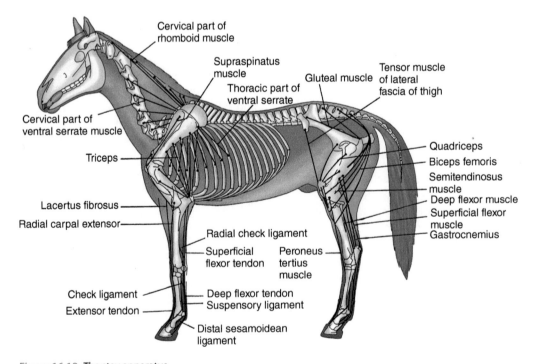

Cervical part of rhomboid muscle

Supraspinatus muscle

Thoracic part of ventral serrate

Gluteal muscle

Tensor muscle of lateral fascia of thigh

Cervical part of ventral serrate muscle

Triceps

Lacertus fibrosus

Radial carpal extensor

Quadriceps

Biceps femoris

Semitendinosus muscle

Deep flexor muscle

Superficial flexor muscle

Gastrocnemius

Radial check ligament

Superficial flexor tendon

Peroneus tertius muscle

Check ligament

Extensor tendon

Deep flexor tendon

Suspensory ligament

Distal sesamoidean ligament

Figure 16.10 The stay apparatus.

the approach of predators and also allows a faster getaway should predators surprise them. This is due to the stay apparatus – a system of muscles and ligaments that 'lock' the main joints into position without expending a lot of energy so that the muscles do not get fatigued. The arrangement is much the same in the fore- and hindlimbs; normally both the forelimbs are 'locked' but one hindlimb is relaxed or 'rested'.

The stay apparatus in the forelimbs is based on the suspensory apparatus, including:

- suspensory ligament
- deep digital flexor tendon with the deep digital flexor muscle (DDFT), running from the elbow to the back of the pedal bone
- carpal check ligament which joints the DDFT to the cannon bone
- superficial digital flexor tendon and muscle from the elbow to the short pastern bone
- radial check ligament.

The superficial digital flexor tendon of the forelimb has a check ligament which links to the radius of the forearm. The ligament stops the tendon being pulled too far down when the fetlock is weight-bearing and so helps prevent the fetlock collapsing onto the ground. The carpal check ligament of the deep flexor tendon links to the carpal bones of the knee. The suspensory ligament attaches to the top of the knee and runs down the back of the leg between the cannon bone and the flexor tendons. Just above the fetlock joint it divides into two; each branch attaches to one of the two sesamoid bones of the fetlock joint and then continues forward to join the extensor tendon at the front of the pastern. The suspensory ligament provides a link between the extensor and flexor systems, literally suspending the fetlock joint. As the bodyweight presses on the fetlock this joint moves down and the suspensory ligament tightens, followed by the superficial flexor and the deep flexor tendons. Higher in the forelimb the elbow is prevented from flexing, which in turn means that the biceps brachii, extending from the shoulder blade

to the forearm, can stop the shoulder from flexing. The knee is prevented from buckling forwards by the lacertus fibrosus tendon. The shoulder blade is balanced by two muscle groups:

- The ventral serrate (serratus ventralis) muscle acts horizontally, with the thoracic and cervical parts supporting in opposite directions. The muscle is interspersed with fibrous tissue to help take the weight.
- The supraspinatus muscle, biceps and triceps act vertically to balance the scapula with minimal fatigue.

The stay apparatus of the lower hindlimb is basically the same as that of the forelimb, but the superficial flexor tendon does not have an equivalent to the radial check ligament. The hindlimb stay apparatus has three essential elements. The first element, the stifle joint locking mechanism, allows the weight of the horse's rear of the body to rest, essentially, on the locked joint. The second element, the reciprocal mechanism, ensures that the stifle and hock joints will move in unison (Figure 16.11), and the leg will move in a

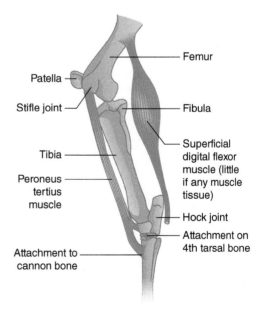

Figure 16.11 Reciprocal apparatus or mechanism of the hindlimb.

smooth, coordinated manner. The first and second elements work together. The third element involves other ligaments/tendons in the distal limb.

The patella or stifle plays a vital role; this bone has a 'hook' which can lock over the inner trochlear ridge of the femur in order to fix the whole hindlimb rigid. If one joint of the leg is locked the others will not move readily, so when the horse wants to move it contracts the tensor fascia muscle which attaches to the patella, so slightly lifting and freeing the bone. The stifle joint cannot be moved without moving the hock joint through the action of the gastrocnemius and the peroneus tertius. Finally, the horse can 'sit' in a hammock of hamstring muscles which run over the buttocks.

Moving the Front Legs

Moving off begins with an almost imperceptible transfer of weight; two-thirds of the horse's weight is carried by its forelimbs, so that it must shift its centre of gravity backwards to free the forehand. The front leg is moved forward by two main groups of muscles; some bend the elbow forwards, some actually pull the leg forward. The elbow-flexing muscles are the biceps (running from the shoulder blade to the radius) and the brachialis (humerus to radius). The limb is brought forwards by the action of the brachiocephalic and serratus ventralis muscle; the efficiency of this will depend on the position of the head and this is why a horse moves more freely in front when the neck is extended or carried high. Riding on a tight rein or fixing a horse's head with gadgets like a standing martingale can hamper movement. After the limb has moved forward sufficiently it is straightened again; the supraspinatus muscle straightens the shoulder joint, the triceps straightens the elbow, and the carpal and digital extensors straighten the lower leg. Once the foot is on the ground it acts as a fixed fulcrum with the body turning above it.

Backward movement of the leg starts with contraction of the pectoral muscles which lie between the lower chest wall and the leg, and the latissimus dorsi which stretches from the withers to the forearm. This pulls the humerus back; at the same time, various muscles pull the shoulder blade forward and the body rotates over the rigid leg. As the limb passes the vertical it no longer only supports weight but becomes a propulsive strut. The lower part of the leg is pulled backwards by the superficial and deep digital flexor muscles, acting on the foot via long tendons.

The amount of energy used to thrust off and swing the leg is important. At the middle of the swing phase, the hoof moves forward at a little more than double the horse's forward speed. For example, if the horse is galloping at 40 miles per hour the hoof may be moving at approximately 100 miles per hour during the swing phase. This includes the forward velocity of the horse's body. At a flat-out gallop, the horse may be taking around 2.5 strides per second, that is, 10 times per second one of the hooves is being accelerated and decelerated. The joints that are involved in swinging the leg are mainly the elbow in the forelimb and hip in the hindlimb.

Moving the Hind Legs

The muscles of a performance horse's hindquarters play an important role in generating power. The position of the superficial muscles can be traced through the skin: stretching down from the tuber coxae (hip bone) is the tensor fascia latae which attaches round the stifle; immediately above this is the superficial gluteal muscle. They both flex the hip joint, carrying the femur and a stifle forward. Behind the superficial gluteal is the biceps femoris, a curved muscle which appears to stretch from the spine to the stifle joint. This, with the semi-tendinosus at the back of the leg, extends the leg by moving the body forward when the foot is fixed on the ground. They also push the leg out behind when jumping and kicking.

The two muscles that can be seen at the front of the lower leg are the long digital extensor and the lateral digital extensor. Together with the tibialis anterior muscle these extend the leg forward. The muscles that flex the leg are not as evident, as they lie under the muscle of the thigh; they are the superficial and deep digital flexor muscles and their tendons. There is also the powerful gastrocnemius muscle which ends in the Achilles tendon.

The forward propulsive thrust of the limbs is quite small, so the speed of movement depends on the frequency with which the limbs operate; to move faster the hindlimbs must travel backwards faster than the speed at which the body is moving forwards at that moment. In order for a horse to gallop the muscles of the legs must pull the legs backwards as quickly as possible, even though they are bearing weight at the time; this calls for well-developed muscles. On the other hand, when the leg is pulled forwards it is not usually weight-bearing and so the muscles do not have to be so well developed, although they may still be quite sizable, like the brachiocephalic. All the muscles down the back of the hind leg, for example the hip extensors and hamstrings, are very important for pulling the hind legs back for thrust as the hind hooves are on the ground.

Forces reflect both the weight of the horse and the activity of muscles. The same horse generates higher forces if muscles are used to push harder against the ground surface. This will project the horse higher into the air, for example at trot, and also result in a heavier landing. The impact and concussion that occur immediately after the hooves hit the ground can also be affected by the horse's conformation and action, as well as things like speed and the type of surface it is working on (whether the horse is trotting on hard ground or pavement, or something softer like loose dirt or sand). Hard surfaces and higher speeds always have higher impact forces. The stride length increases with speed. That of a typical Thoroughbred (TB) is around 2 m at walk and 7 m at gallop.

Equine Biomechanics

Equine biomechanics is an area of exercise physiology that is receiving much attention. There are now many texts that cover this subject in detail and so only a brief summary is included here. Computer technology is now used to assess movement. Studying the mechanics of movement helps in the objective assessment of the way the horse moves, and hence the diagnosis of lameness and also assessment of youngsters for future athletic potential and therefore specific training programmes. Combined with a sound knowledge of anatomy and conformation, being able to assess the biomechanics of the horse can enable a specific training programme to be designed to also prolong the horse's working life by strengthening the weak areas and avoiding problems.

Some studies for biomechanics are carried out on treadmills, whereas others are carried out on the ground. Biomechanics may be divided into one of two areas:

- Kinematics – the study of movement of the limbs.
- Kinetics – the study of forces generated within movement.

Kinematics

For accurate gait study, computer equipment helps to slow down the timing so that it becomes visible with the naked eye. The use of modern video cameras is also very helpful for real-time and slow-motion studies. Gait analysis for horses using wearable sensors is now an inexpensive, convenient and efficient tool. Kinematics describes movement in a linear plane and angular movements of the limbs.

Kinetics

Kinetics involves using force plates, accelerometers, pressure-sensitive mats and force shoes to assess the impact of the hoof on the ground. These assessments are used to study the forces between the hoof and ground, known as the ground reaction forces (GRF), giving information on load bearing and propulsion/deceleration for each gait and phase of gait.

Conformation

Conformation is how the horse is 'put together' and consists of two aspects:

- the skeleton
- muscle and fat (known as 'topline').

Ideally horses should be skeletally correct with correctly developed muscles, adequate subcutaneous fat, and covered by healthy skin and a glossy coat. Minor skeletal imperfections can be disguised by well-developed muscle and a covering of fat. It is important to assess the skeletal conformation as this has a direct bearing on the horse's ability to withstand work and stay sound.

Assessment of conformation will also depend on the activity that the horse is to undertake. Each activity requires different levels of speed, strength, stamina and suppleness, perhaps indicating differences in conformation. Although opinion may vary depending on the discipline the horse is intended for, there is no doubt that equal proportions and symmetrical development are essential. The horse's centre of mass must be correctly placed: if it is too far forward the horse will be on the forehand; if it is too far back there will be strain on the lumbar region.

Before getting involved in a detailed assessment of conformation it is important to stand back and look at the overall impression the horse gives:

- Are the forehand and hindquarters balanced in relation to each other?
- Are the feet in proportion and balanced?
- Observe the length of the rib cage and loins.
- Observe the position and shape of the pelvis.

Ideal Conformation

Head

The head should be attractive and in proportion to the rest of the body. The eyes should be bold, large and set well apart; a good eye placement means that the horse has wide vision. The ears should be level and equally mobile. The mouth should be assessed for abnormalities and also suitability to take the bit. There must be ample room at the poll and jaw for the degree of flexion needed in dressage (Figure 16.12); the horse must not feel pain or discomfort from tissues being compressed. The horse's temperament and state of mind is expressed by ear, eye, nostril and head movements. Ideally the horse stands calmly, while showing a keen interest in its surroundings. A dull eye and unpricked ears may indicate an unhealthy, sour or ill horse. The head is very important in determining the weight distribution of the horse by altering the centre of gravity. If the head is raised the centre of gravity moves back, which helps the horse maintain its balance when landing over a fence, for example.

Topline

Horses should have a good topline running from between the ears, along the back and to the top of the tail. The head should be well set onto the neck and the withers, the withers should be defined but not prominent, the back should be fairly short and strong, the rump rounded and the tail well set on.

Neck

The head should be well set onto the neck so that the horse looks elegant at the poll. The neck should be long, elegant and well set onto a sloping shoulder. It should also flow smoothly into the chest, with the muscle under the neck not over-developed. The seven cervical vertebrae of the neck should give two equal curves (Figure 16.13); if the curve at the head end of the neck is too steep the horse will be 'peacocky', while a steep curve at the shoulder end gives 'ewe-necked' conformation. Both result in problems in bit

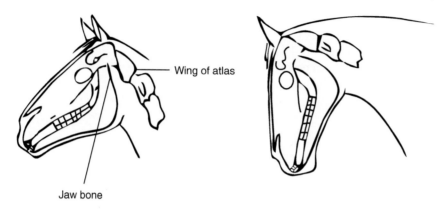

Wing of atlas

Jaw bone

It should be possible to lay two
fingers between the wing of atlas
and the jaw bone

Figure 16.12 There should be room at the poll and jaw for flexion.

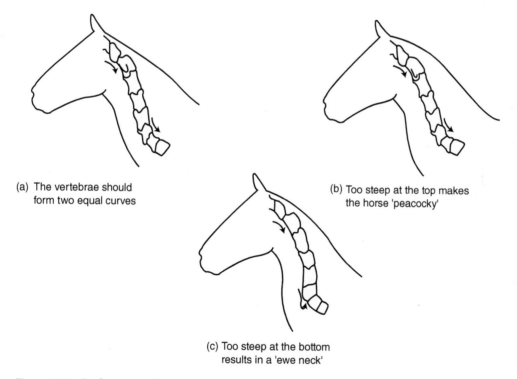

(a) The vertebrae should
form two equal curves

(b) Too steep at the top makes
the horse 'peacocky'

(c) Too steep at the bottom
results in a 'ewe neck'

Figure 16.13 Conformation of the neck.

communication and supporting self-carriage.
The length of the neck should be in proportion to the rest of the body; a long neck
may be weak and throw the horse onto its
forehand, while a short neck can shorten
the stride.

In general, the larger the head, the shorter
the neck needs to be. A weak neck can be
strengthened, but if it carries a heavy head
it may be difficult to lighten the forehand.
The way the neck is placed in relation to the
shoulders is very important; the dressage

horse needs an elevated set of the neck which will compensate to some extent for the weight and length of the head. Many TBs have a more horizontal neck set which makes it hard to develop the necessary lightness, although it is advantageous for the long stride needed for winning races.

Withers

The withers need to be well defined and to finish as far back as possible; there should be a continuous line to the neck with no dips. Well-defined withers allow plenty of room for muscle attachment and help keep the saddle in the correct position. If the withers are higher than the croup this will compensate for some limitations.

Chest

The horse needs plenty of depth of chest to allow for heart and lung room. The chest should not be too narrow with 'both legs coming out of the same hole', nor should it be too wide or too open in front, making the horse stable but slow.

Shoulder

Traditionally the ideal shoulder should have a 45° slope to the horizontal. The hoof pastern angle (HPA) should be the same as the shoulder (Figure 16.14) so that the concussive forces are absorbed equally by all the components of the limb. However, an HPA of 45° would tend to give a horse the long toe, low heel conformation associated with poor feet and soundness problems. As long as the shoulder is flat and long enough to ensure a good stride length it does not matter if it is a little upright. The angle of the humerus (shoulder joint to elbow joint) is also important and should be about 60° to the horizontal, which is fairly upright. The slope of the shoulder should balance the pelvis and hip articulation; it is to no advantage if the forehand can move excessively but the hindlimbs cannot match that movement. The gait will not be balanced and fluid, and the hindquarters will fatigue and suffer performance stress; eventually the horse will become unlevel due to long-term injuries caused by

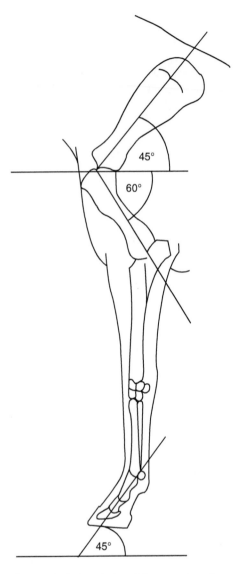

Figure 16.14 Angulation of the scapula and humerus.

over-use. At the walk the knee is usually carried as far forward as the point of the shoulder, at trot the knee reaches a line dropped from the poll, while at the gallop the point of the toe reaches a line dropped from the nose. If the point of the shoulder is less prominent it is possible that the walk stride may be shorter.

Elbow

The elbow should be 'free' and allow a fist between it and the ribs. A 'tied-in' elbow limits stride length. The point of the elbow should be in the same plane as the point of the shoulder, that is, it should not turn in or out. The measurement from the withers to the point of the elbow should be roughly the same as from the point of the elbow to the ground, ensuring adequate depth and 'heart and lung room'.

Forelimb

The forearm should be long and well muscled, and the cannon bone short with adequate good, flat bone. Seen from the side and front the forelimbs should be straight and not slope backwards, forwards or be angled in or out (Figure 16.15). From the front a plumb-line dropped from the point of the shoulder should bisect all the limb bones and the hoof. The space between the front feet when the horse is standing square should be enough to fit in another hoof. This shows that the bones are arranged in a column, directly on top of each other, giving strength and ensuring that the concussive forces are spread equally up the limb. The knee should be flat and broad at the front with a good depth.

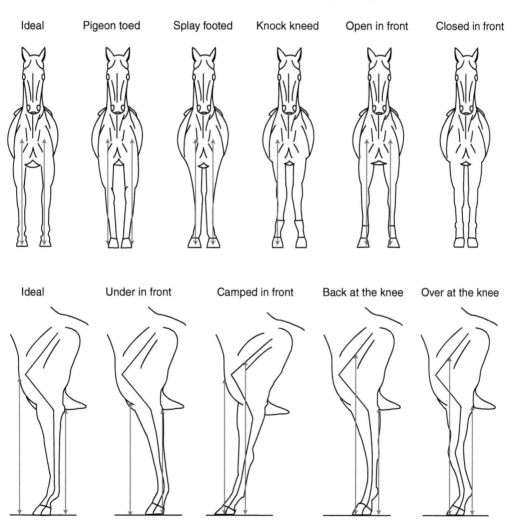

| Ideal | Pigeon toed | Splay footed | Knock kneed | Open in front | Closed in front |

| Ideal | Under in front | Camped in front | Back at the knee | Over at the knee |

* Over at the knee is when the horse stands as if the knee is slightly flexed

Figure 16.15 Forelimbs viewed from the front (above) and side (below).

Faults include:

- over at the knee – when the horse stands as if the knee is slightly flexed
- back at the knee – when the back of the knee appears pushed back and the front of the leg concave
- tied in below the knee – when the circumference of bone is smaller just below the knee than it is further down the cannon bone
- calf knees – which are shallow from front to back
- offset cannon bones – when the bones are not placed directly onto each other but are displaced to one side. The toe does not turn in or out.

The fetlock joints should be well defined and bony rather than round and puffy.

Feet

It is important that the feet should be a pair and a suitable size for the horse. The shape of the foot and the angles through the hoof and pastern should be as described for the balanced foot (see 'Assessment of Foot Balance', Chapter 4). The feet should not be boxy or flat, and the heel should be about half the height of the front of the foot. Always lift the foot and examine the underneath when assessing a horse's conformation and soundness; the wear on the shoe can tell you about the way the horse places its feet on the ground. Poor conformation and/or poor farriery can cause horses to be unsound (Figure 16.16).

Back

The back should be strong, of adequate length and in proportion to the forehand and hindquarters. There is considerable variation in the 'normal' conformation of the back: long-backed horses seem more prone to muscular injuries, while short-backed ones are more likely to suffer from the spines of the vertebrae rubbing together or impinging. The horse owner can judge whether his or her horse has a long or short back by using some well-proven measurements: first measure

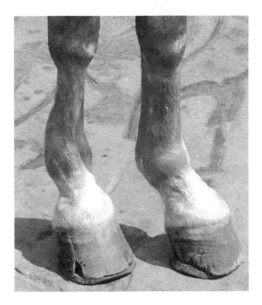

Figure 16.16 Poor conformation/farriery can cause horses to be unsound and more prone to injuries such as broken knees and bowed tendons. *Source*: Courtesy of Zoe Davies.

the head from the bottom of the nostril to the poll, just behind the ears – this is known as the 'standard' and the rest of the body should be in proportion to it (Figure 16.17). Some horses have very large or indeed very small heads and here the length of the back from just behind the shoulder blade to the point of the hip should be very similar to the standard. This measurement gives us some information about the weight-carrying ability of the horse; carrying weight for long periods of time causes stress, tires the horse and impairs performance. Remember that bending and rotation are minimal in front of the ninth thoracic vertebrae and maximal around the eleventh and twelfth; this is just beneath the saddle that you are sitting on.

If the back measurement is longer than the standard, stress will be put on the lumbosacral joint and the lumbar region. The lumbosacral joint is situated between the last loin vertebrae and the rump, and the ability of the horse to move freely is dependent on the full function of this joint. The lumbosacral joint is part of the spine and acts to transmit

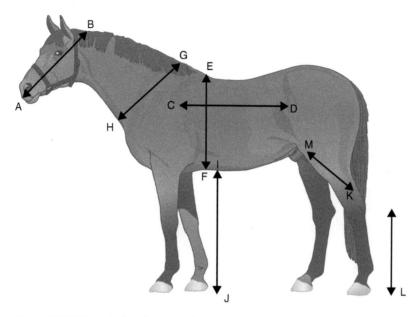

Figure 16.17 Using the head as a standard measurement.

the impulsion generated by the hindquarters to the forehand; its limited flexibility allows the pelvis and hindquarters to rotate forward when both hind legs move forwards, as when galloping and jumping. This should not be confused with the sacroiliac joint, which is the attachment of the sacrum to the pelvis. This area can be strengthened and supported with the correct muscle development.

Hindquarters

The hindquarters are the powerhouse of the horse and vital to successful performance, particularly for racing, jumping and dressage. The shape of the quarters and the angulation of the joints can indicate the horse's potential for speed, jumping and athleticism.

The hindquarters must be in proportion, with good articulation of the hip, stifle and hock. Seen from the side (Figure 16.18A) the rump should be rounded, with good length from the point of the hip to the point of the buttock and with a well-set tail. From behind (Figure 16.18B) the points of the hip should be level with each other, set well apart and lower than the croup, making a roof shape. Many horses have one hip that is slightly

dropped or uneven musculature that may indicate hind leg lameness.

The hock is one of the hardest working joints in the body and good conformation of the hind leg is essential for continued soundness. When a hind leg is well placed a vertical line could be drawn from the point of the buttock, down the back of the hock and lower leg to the fetlock. There should be plenty of length from the point of the hip to the hock – in which case the hocks are described as 'well let down'. The stifle joint should be close to the body but turned slightly outwards to allow free movement. The gaskin or second thigh should be well muscled. Viewed from behind there should be enough room between the horse's hind feet to accommodate another foot and the feet should face straight forwards. A horse that is 'too close behind' is probably also narrow through the trunk with front feet that are too close together. This horse is much more likely to brush or speedicut, that is, hit one leg with the other hoof either lower down (brushing) or higher up (speedicutting). Horses that are 'too open behind' tend to be stable, slow and powerful.

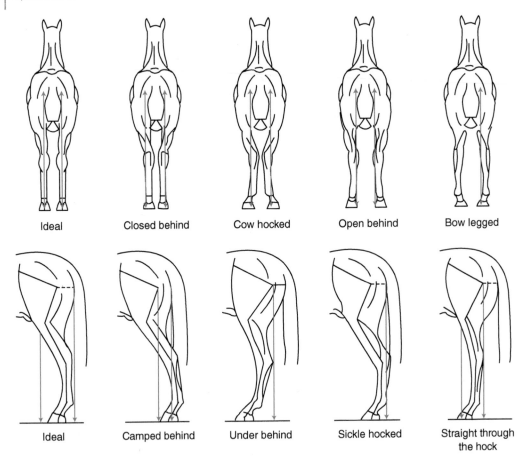

Figure 16.18 Hindquarters and leg viewed from behind (above) and side (below).

The hocks should be wide when seen from the side and well defined and they should not turn in or out. 'Cow hocks' turn in and are considered highly undesirable, as the increased strain on the hock may lead to spavins. A 'bow-legged' horse has hocks that turn out and a rope-walking action that places stress down the outside of the leg. A line dropped from the hip joint should pass through the tibia and middle of the hoof. The distance from this to a line dropped from the patella and a third line dropped from the point of the buttock parallel to the cannon should be equal.

A horse is said to be camped behind when its hind leg appears to be too long for it. These animals may look sickle hocked if made to stand up square, but will naturally stand with the hind leg out behind them, lengthening the base of support. While stable, this posture puts increased pressure on the muscles of the loins and back, and the horse may become 'sway-backed' (see Fig 3.12 in chapter 3). Horses that are camped behind tend to be slower, less able to engage the hindquarters and prone to backwards slipping. A horse that is under itself behind has a shortened base of support and less stability, making it prone to forging and slipping. These two faults in conformation will both affect the efficiency of the stay apparatus which is dependent on a vertical line running down the cannon bone. The hock itself may not be displaced by very much; it tends to be the angulation of the joints that is at fault.

A sickle-hocked horse has curved conformation of the hind leg due to excess angulation of the hock. This tends to increase

Table 16.2 Description of conformation.

Feature	Comment
Type	Thoroughbred/hunter/cob/lightweight/and so on
Condition	Feel the horse to assess subcutaneous fat
Sex	
Colour and markings	
Height	
Age	
Head	In proportion
	Eye
	Room for flexion
	Outlook
Neck	Length
	Muscle
	Way set onto shoulder
	How will it affect the way the horse goes?
Withers	Height
	Length
Shoulder	Angle and length of scapula and humerus
Forearm	Length and muscle
Knee	Flatness and breadth
	Back at? Tied in? Over at the knee?
Cannon bone	Length
	Amount of bone
	Tendons? Splints?
Fetlocks	Bony or puffy
Hoof pastern angle	Unbroken
	Same as shoulder (50–55°)
Feet	Pair
	Symmetrical
	Adequate heel
	Open and circular
Forearm as a whole	Straight, not tied in, and so on

Table 16.2 (Continued)

Feature	Comment
Chest	Adequate depth
	Straightness of limbs from in front
Rib cage	Depth
	Length
	'Well sprung'
Lumbar region	Strength and length
Hindquarters	Point of hip to point of buttock
	Croup high?
	Point of croup to hip
	Rounded
	Hocks well let down
	Tail well set on
	Adequate second thigh
	Plumb-line from point of buttock to ground
Hocks	Strong and bony
	Turn in or out? Curb? Spavins? Thoroughpin?
Cannon bone	Length
	Amount of bone
Fetlocks	Bony or puffy
	Windgalls?
Hoof pastern angle	Unbroken
Feet	Pair (i.e. similar in shape to each other, forefeet are a pair and hindfeet are a pair)
	Symmetrical
	Adequate heel
	Open
Hind leg as a whole	Plumb-line from hip joint
	Sickle or straight?
From behind	Level hip bones and even musculature

the wear and tear on the joint. The horse is described as straight through the hock when the tibia is more upright and the hock is placed in front of the vertical. This type of conformation tends to be quite common in TBs bred to race on the flat and is said to impart speed.

Before assessing the detailed aspects of conformation in a formal or examination situation, the type, condition, sex, colour markings, height and age of the horse should all be stated. The conformation may then be fully examined, feeling for heat, blemishes, sarcoids and so on, and then the conformation may be described methodically (Table 16.2).

Summary Points

1) Exercise places great metabolic demands upon the horse's body.
2) Homeostatic mechanisms have to cope with relatively rapid changes.
3) Horses lose significant amounts of water and salt through sweating.
4) The duration of the work/competition determines the type of energy system used.
5) The density of capillaries running through muscles increases in response to exercise. This process is known as capillarisation and allows more efficient exchange between the blood and working muscle fibres.
6) Functional anatomy of the horse's musculoskeletal system is an important area of exercise physiology, as horses are most commonly used for work as equine athletes.
7) The powerful hindquarter muscles are the horse's engine for propulsion, whereas forelimbs have some propulsive capability, but their function is more that of steering and support.
8) Unlike humans, the horse does not have a collar bone; no firm, bony union exists between the rib cage and forelimbs, there is only muscle.

Q + A

Q What effect does training have on the horse's circulation?

A Both the erythrocyte count and packed cell volume (PCV) increase with training, improving the ability to carry oxygen. Erythrocyte turnover also increases.

Q What is capillarisation?

A The density of capillaries running through muscles increases in response to exercise and allows more efficient exchange between the blood and working muscle fibres.

Q Which muscle fibre types should be trained for endurance work?

A For endurance work at varying speeds, prolonged exercise at similar levels is needed to increase the oxygen-carrying capacity of fast twitch high oxidative fibres and slow twitch fibres.

17

Teeth and Ageing

Equine Teeth

The horse has evolved a system of cutting and grinding teeth that is both effective and simple, allowing the horse to survive on its herbage diet. The horse's teeth (mandibular incisors) are also used to determine its age. It has two sets of teeth during its life:

- deciduous (milk, baby or temporary teeth)
- permanent.

Deciduous or milk teeth are smaller and whiter than permanent teeth and fall out as they are replaced by the permanent teeth; this is known as diphyodont. Horses will normally have 24 deciduous teeth, which emerge in pairs soon after birth. From the age of 2½ years the deciduous teeth are gradually replaced so that by the time the horse is 5 years old it has a full set of permanent teeth. Horses have no deciduous molar teeth. As the growing crowns meet at the grinding surface the teeth are known as 'coming into wear'. As teeth break the jaw surface they are known as 'erupting'. The times of eruption of equine teeth are very consistent, allowing accurate ageing of young animals. The age of older horses with a full set of permanent teeth is estimated mainly through examination of the wear patterns of the occlusal surfaces of the incisors.

Deciduous teeth are smaller, with a neck, and are covered in enamel, and therefore appear whiter than permanent teeth which are covered in cementum and appear more yellow than white. Permanent teeth have no neck, but a smooth tapering shape from root to crown.

Horses have more than one type of tooth, arranged in different positions in the upper and lower jaws (maxilla and mandible, respectively) in two dental arcades (Figure 17.1). There is a gap in each arch between the incisor and the molars/premolars known as the interdental space, and this is where the bit of the bridle sits (if correctly fitted). In fact, any gap between teeth, including molars and premolars, is known as a diastema. So this may be anatomically normal (as in between incisors and molars) or abnormal (as in between molars and/or premolars). The teeth are firmly anchored in a socket of bone known as the alveolus by the periodontal ligament and periodontal membrane in a dental-alveolar joint known as the gomphosis which binds the tooth to its bony socket.

Horses have different shaped teeth for different purposes and this is known as heterodontus.

- Incisors or biting teeth in the front of the mouth (Figure 17.2) – incisor teeth are called the centrals (the pair top and bottom in the centre), laterals (the teeth next to the centrals) and corners.
- Molars or grinding teeth lining each side of the jaw bone – the cheek teeth. These in turn can be divided into molars and premolars, with the molars at the back of the jaw. Unlike human teeth, the horse's premolars and molars are similar in shape.

Equine Science, Third Edition. Zoe Davies and Sarah Pilliner.
© 2018 Zoe Davies and Sarah Pilliner. Published 2018 by John Wiley & Sons Ltd.

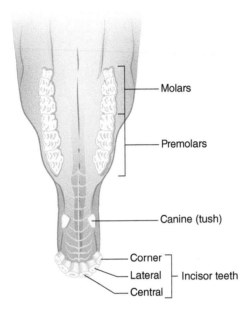

Figure 17.1 Dentition of the horse.

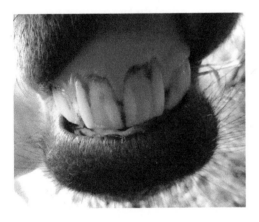

Figure 17.2 Incisors or biting teeth of a Mediterranean Miniature donkey. *Source*: Courtesy of Zoe Davies.

- Tushes or canine teeth – all stallions and geldings have canine teeth, two in the upper and two in the lower jaw. Only about a quarter of mares have canine teeth, which are much smaller in size and vary between one and four in quantity.
- Wolf teeth – up to a third of horses, split equally between male and female, also have wolf teeth (vestigial premolars).

These are more common on the upper jaw. Sometimes they interfere with the bit.

As the horse evolved, the structure of its teeth became different to that of carnivores and omnivores. Two major changes allowed the horse to cope with a diet of tough fibrous herbage without wearing its teeth down prematurely. First, the ancestral horse developed hypsodont dentition, each tooth having a high crown and a deep root (Figure 17.3). The crown is the part of the tooth above the gum line. Humans, for example, have low-crowned or brachydont dentition, the crown being above the gum and the root below the gum. The horse's diet of mainly silica-containing herbage wears the teeth down. In the horse, at any one time, only a small part of the crown protrudes above the gum, but the tooth grows continuously so that growth compensates for the wear occurring at the biting surface of the crown. As the teeth erupt the part of the crown embedded in the jaw becomes smaller and a distinct root begins to form. Second, the ancestral horse developed a third dental element in addition to dentine and enamel, called cementum, which acts to strengthen the teeth and protect them from breakage.

There are also differences between the horse's teeth and those of carnivores and omnivores in the way in which the teeth are organised within the jaw. The modern horse has fewer teeth than its ancestors, with gaps between the incisor and molar teeth. The ancestral horse had the dental formula making a total of 44 teeth: in both the upper and lower jaws three pairs of incisors, one pair of canines, four pairs of premolars and three pairs of molar teeth:

3.1.4.3   Dental formula of the ancestral

3.1.4.3   horse – total 44 teeth.

The modern horse has lost the first pair of premolar teeth. These can sometimes reappear in young horses, being known as wolf teeth. Thus male horses have the dental formula:

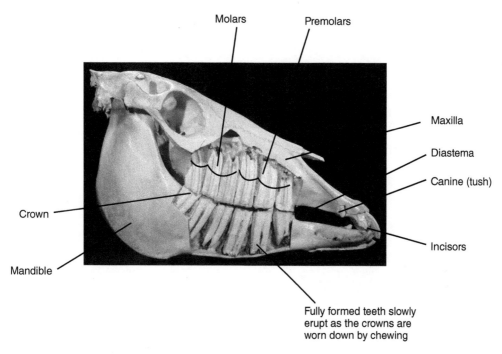

Figure 17.3 Hypsodont teeth. *Source*: Frandson 2009. Reproduced with permission of John Wiley & Sons.

Dental Formulae

3.1.3.3   Modern Male Horse – 40 teeth

3.1.3.3

3.0.3.3   Modern Mare – 36 teeth

3.0.3.3

Mares generally do not have the canine teeth or tushes.

The structure of the equine tooth is shown in Figures 17.4 and 17.5. Each tooth consists of three layers: dentine, enamel and cementum.

- Dentine (dentin) is a hard calcium-containing substance allied to bone making up most of the tooth. A cavity in the centre houses the blood vessels and nerves and is known as the dental pulp.
- Enamel is a porcelain-like covering of almost the entire hypsodont tooth and said to be the hardest substance in the body. It consists of inorganic crystals formed by specialised cells – ameloblasts – which

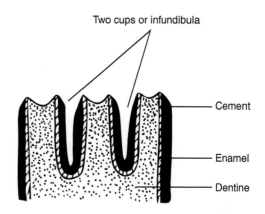

Figure 17.4 Vertical section through a molar tooth.

are lost after the tooth is formed. Enamel forms prominent folds on the crown of the molars and premolars to enable grinding of food.
- Cementum (cement) is a thin bone-like tissue which covers the hypsodont tooth and prevents it from being brittle.

The pulp and periodontal membrane (also known as the periodontal ligament) contain a

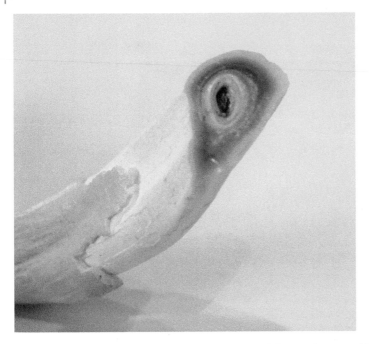

Figure 17.5 Incisor with part of the cementum removed. *Source:* Courtesy of Zoe Davies.

rich supply of blood vessels and can therefore bleed when damaged. Pulp fills the dental cavity and allows pain sensation to thermal, mechanical and chemical stimulants. The periodontal membrane serves as an anchor to the fibrous connective-tissue layer covering the cementum of the tooth and holding it in place in the jawbone.

In the newly erupted tooth the enamel is folded to make a funnel-like depression in the centre of the tooth called the infundibulum. This depression becomes filled with feed so that it looks like a black area on the grinding surface of the tooth and is known as the 'cup'. In cross-section it can be seen that the infundibulum gives rise to peripheral enamel and dentine on the outside of the tooth and central enamel and dentine on the inside of the tooth (Figure 17.6).

Wear and Tear

New permanent teeth have a large crown, much of which is below the gum. In the 5-year-old horse the last three or four molars in the upper jaw practically fill the maxillary sinus, reaching up above the facial crest (Figure 17.7). With use the tooth wears down, but growth of the root forces the crown up to compensate for this, so that by the time the horse is 12 years old the roots are distinct and closed up and the teeth occupy less of the jaw. As the horse grows older the teeth have less and less crown embedded in the jaw, and eventually very old horses will lose their teeth which often become wobbly as they approach the gum line. Old horses tend to run out of teeth by the age of 25–30 years.

As the biting surface of the tooth is worn away, the pattern on the tooth table changes. The cementum is worn off first, exposing the enamel, which is worn away to show the dentine. Soon after the tooth has come into wear the 'cup' or infundibulum is surrounded by five rings of cementum, enamel and dentine. The cementum and dentine wear away first, leaving the enamel standing proud. These ridges on the tooth surface give a highly effective grinding mechanism (Figure 17.8). Upper molars are slightly different to lower molars

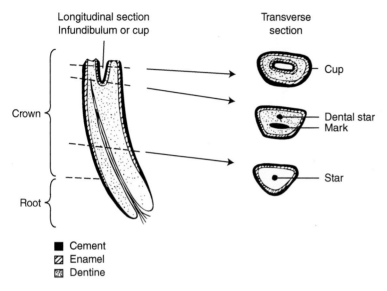

Longitudinal section
Infundibulum or cup

Transverse section

Cup

Dental star
Mark

Star

Crown

Root

■ Cement
▨ Enamel
▨ Dentine

Figure 17.6 Sections through an incisor tooth. As the tooth wears down, the pattern on the tooth table changes.

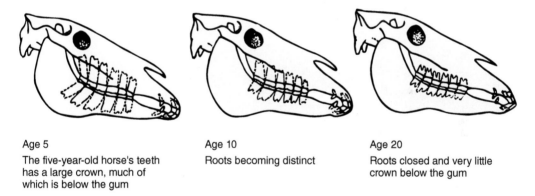

Age 5
The five-year-old horse's teeth has a large crown, much of which is below the gum

Age 10
Roots becoming distinct

Age 20
Roots closed and very little crown below the gum

Figure 17.7 Implantation and continual eruption of the teeth.

and have 'infundibulae' or cementum-filled enamel cones.

As the tooth table wears down so the infundibulum becomes more shallow, until all that remains is a 'mark' of enamel surrounding cementum. Initially the mark is a long oval shape which gradually becomes a smaller rounded spot of enamel. When the pulp cavity is reached it appears on the tooth table as the 'dental star'. For a short time both the mark and the dental star are visible, the star lying in front of the mark. The pulp cavity carries the blood and nerve supply of the tooth. As the tooth wears down, these

sensitive tissues are protected by a layer of secondary dentine, seen on the tooth table as the dental star. As the horse ages the dental star becomes more central and more rounded.

The general appearance of the teeth also changes, allowing the observer to estimate the horse's age. As the crown gradually emerges from the socket, the shape of the tooth table changes from oval to become 'rounded off' and thus more triangular. The angulation of the teeth also changes so that the incisor teeth protrude forwards (Figure 17.9).

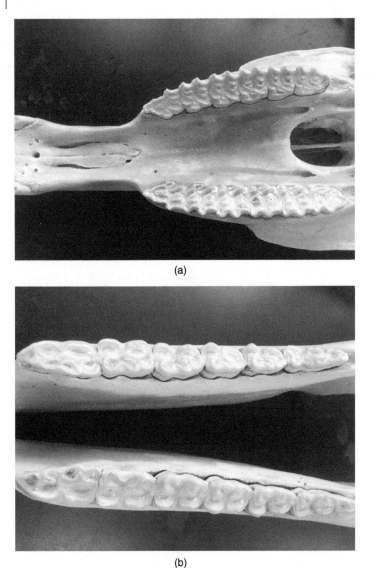

(a)

(b)

Figure 17.8 (a) Upper and (b) lower jaws, showing the wearing surface of molars.

Ageing

The changes in appearance of the teeth as the horse grows older can be used to age the horse (Figure 17.10). Generally, the lower incisor teeth are used, but it is useful to consider other factors such as the shape and angulation of the other teeth. There are clear differences in young horses between early and late foals, and the type and level of nutrition may affect the way in which the teeth wear. In general, from 5 to 9 years of age the tooth is wider than tall, from 9 to 10 years the tooth is square and at more than 11 years the tooth is taller than wide.

The practice of ageing horses falls into three areas:

• From birth to the age of 5 the eruption and wear of the temporary and permanent incisor teeth are used. The horse's age can be determined quite accurately, as the loss of the deciduous teeth and eruption of the

Figure 17.9 Incisor teeth sloping in an older horse.

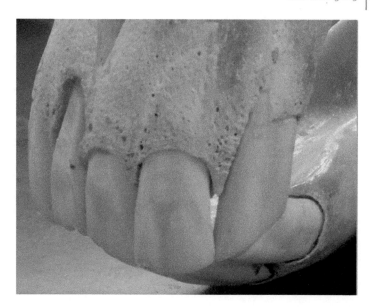

permanent teeth rarely vary by more than a couple of months.

- From 5 to 10 or 12 years old the pattern on the tooth table is used.
- After 12 years old the horse is described as 'aged' as the signs are much less reliable and general indications have to be taken into consideration.

The age of foals can be judged by their teeth but also by looking at the growth of their tail and the stage of development. Generally, the milk central incisor teeth erupt by the time the foal is 4 weeks old, the laterals erupt between 1 and 3 months and the corners erupt between 8 and 9 months of age (Table 17.1). By the time the foal is 12 months old it will have a full mouth of temporary incisor teeth. It takes 6 months from the time of eruption for an incisor tooth to grow to meet its partner and come into wear. This means that at 12 months the centrals and laterals are in wear but the corners do not yet meet.

The 2 year old has a full mouth of temporary incisor teeth that are all in wear. At about 2½ years the central incisor teeth are replaced so that a 3 year old has centrals that are up and in wear. These teeth will look large and yellow compared to the smaller and whiter temporary teeth. At about 3½ years

the lateral teeth are replaced so that by the time the horse is 4 years old both the centrals and laterals are in wear. At about 4½ years the corner teeth are replaced so that the 5 year old has a full set of permanent teeth, but the corner teeth only meet at the front. Between 4 and 5 years the tushes will erupt.

Although not as obvious, and therefore not used for ageing horses, the molars and premolars have been developing. The horse does not have any temporary molar teeth as the jaws are not big enough to accommodate them, but by the time the foal is 3 months old it will have three pairs of temporary premolars on each side of the jaw. The first permanent molar appears behind these at 9 months, so that the weanling can survive on a diet of herbage, and the second at 18 months of age. At 2½ years the first permanent premolar appears and the other two are replaced at 3½ years. The final molar tooth does not erupt until the horse is 4½ years old. These changes account for the lumpy appearance of the lower jaw of young horses and can lead to problems when teaching the young horse to accept the bit, as the premolars may be erupting at the same time, causing the horse's mouth to be sore.

Once the horse has a 'full mouth' the age is estimated by the changing patterns on the

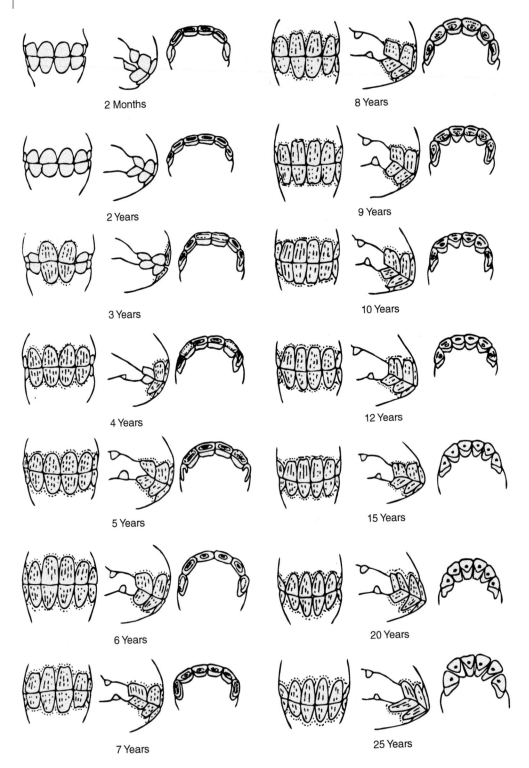

Figure 17.10 Ageing the horse.

Table 17.1 Eruption of the horse's teeth.

Age of eruption	Incisors			Premolars	Molars
	Centrals	Laterals	Corners		
0–1 month	*				
1–3 months	*	*			
9 months	*	*	*	**	●
18 months	*	*	*	***	●●
2.5 years	●	*	*	●●*	●●
3.5 years	●	●	*	●●●	●●
4.5 years	●	●	●○	●●●	●●●

* Milk teeth.
● Permanent teeth.
○ Tushes.

tooth table. It is useful to remember that the centrals are a year older than the laterals which are a year older than the corners, which means that any change taking place on the centrals will occur a year later in the laterals and a year after that in the corners.

The 6 year old will have a well-formed mouth with all the incisors in wear with level tables all showing a dark cup. In the 7 year old the 'cup' in the centrals will have worn out, leaving the 'mark' which is not as dark. The mark consists of an outline of enamel surrounding cement. The top teeth may overlap the bottom ones so that there may be a little 'hook' on the back of the corner incisors. The '7-year-old hook' is a useful guideline, but a hook can also develop at 9 years old.

By 8 years the cup will have worn out of the laterals, leaving a mark, and the centrals will have a dark line called the dental star near the front of the tooth. The hook will have disappeared. By 9 years the cup will have worn out of the corners, leaving a mark, and the dental star will be apparent on the laterals. There may be a small hook and the centrals will have rounded off, giving a triangular shape. Galvayne's groove appears as a dark groove on the upper corner teeth at between 9 and 10 years. The groove is found halfway down the crown, so that for the first years of the horse's life it is hidden in the socket and only appears as the tooth grows out of the gum.

The 10 year old will have stars and marks in all teeth and the marks will be more indistinct and the stars will be clearer. The laterals will have rounded off to be more triangular. Galvayne's groove gradually grows down the tooth. The 12 year old will only have dental stars in the centrals and the teeth are more triangular. The 15 year old will only have dental stars on the tooth tables and the teeth will have increased slope, while Galvayne's groove extends about halfway down the corner incisor. By the time the horse is 20 years old, Galvayne's groove will extend along the whole length of the tooth and the forward slope of the incisors will be pronounced.

Care of Equine Teeth

Teeth are sensitive with a good nerve supply and therefore can become painful. Dental disease and problems with tooth wear may cause the horse to have problems with chewing, such as 'quidding' where chewed food falls out of the mouth. The cheeks can be damaged by sharp edges caused by uneven tooth wear and this is often sore. Ulcers can also result. Horses may lose weight as chewing food is painful and tooth pain may also lead to problems such as head shaking, rearing and unwillingness to move forwards.

The horse's head is shaped so that the upper jaw is slightly wider than the bottom jaw. The molars overlap each other at the sides and this allows a sideways movement of the jaw that shears the food. As the jaw moves from side to side during chewing the molars grind against each other, but the lower ones do not reach the outer edge of the upper molars and the upper ones never reach the inner edge of the lower molars The more refined the shape of the head the more exaggerated this will be, resulting in sharp edges on the outside of the top molars and on the inner edge of the bottom molars (Figure 17.11). These can cut the tongue and cheeks, making eating painful.

Quidding or dropping half-chewed food out of the mouth is a sign of sharp molar teeth. Horses with sharp teeth may also

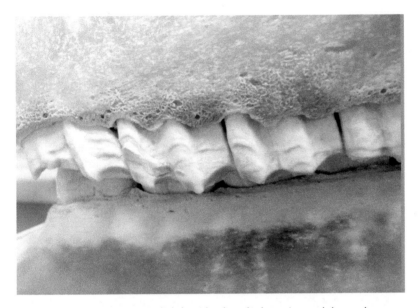

Figure 17.11 The upper jaw is slightly wider than the lower jaw and sharp edges may result.

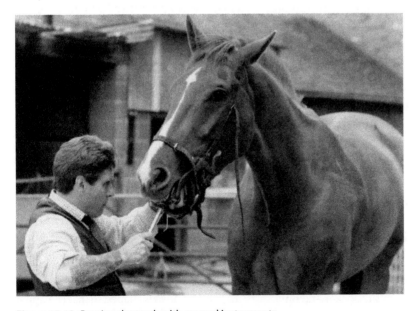

Figure 17.12 Rasping the teeth with manual instruments.

display discomfort when being ridden, as the bit, especially in combination with a tight noseband, can cause the horse pain. Any horse that is losing condition or not keeping its condition as well as expected should have its teeth checked by the vet or horse dentist and, if necessary, the rough edges can be rasped or floated. A horse's teeth should be routinely checked annually and rasped if required (Figure 17.12).

Overshot jaw or parrot mouth can lead to malocclusion where the molars of the upper jaw and lower jaw do not correctly meet at the grinding surface. This can lead to problems with tooth wear. In addition, these horses may find it difficult to graze, particularly on very short pastures. Horses can also suffer from dental decay or caries. Food can become trapped between abnormal gaps or diastema between molar and premolar teeth. Powered instruments for rasping teeth are now available and in the wrong hands these may cause severe and often permanent damage. Equine dentistry is a scientific process and should be undertaken by suitably qualified people. In the UK, Equine Dental Technicians (EDTs) are legally allowed to perform procedures that do not come under the Veterinary Surgeons Act (1966). This excludes all invasive procedures involving living tissues, and administration of veterinary drugs.

Summary Points

1) Horses' teeth are hypsodont, that is, high crowned.
2) Horses have more than one type of tooth, each of which has different functions (known as heterodonty), arranged in different positions within the skull.
3) Teeth are firmly anchored in a socket of bone known as the alveolus by the periodontal ligament and periodontal membrane in a dental-alveolar joint known as the gomphosis which binds the tooth to its bony socket.
4) Each tooth consists of three layers: dentine, enamel and cementum. Most of the tooth is made up of dentine (sometimes known as dentin), with a cavity in the centre housing the blood vessels and nerves and known as the dental pulp.
5) Teeth are sensitive with a good nerve supply and therefore can become painful when damaged or diseased.

Q + A

Q Give the dental formulae of ancestral and modern horses.

A
| 3.1.4.3 | Dental formula of the ancestral |
| 3.1.4.3 | horse – total 44 teeth. |

| 3.1.3.3 | Modern Male Horse – 40 teeth. |
| 3.1.3.3 | |

Q What is the difference between dentine and enamel?

A Dentine is a hard calcium-containing substance allied to bone, whereas enamel is a porcelain-like covering of almost the entire hypsodont tooth and said to be the hardest substance in the body.

Q How old is the foal when it has a full mouth of temporary or deciduous teeth?
A Twelve months old.

Q At what age does Galvayne's groove appear?
A It appears as a dark groove on the upper corner teeth at between 9 and 10 years.

Q What is quidding?
A This is when partially chewed food falls out of the mouth (often the side).

18

Evolution, Classification and Behaviour of the Horse

Evolutionary Time Period

Life has evolved on Earth over approximately 4 billion years. The Earth itself is thought to be 4.54 billion years old, according to the US Geological Survey 1997. Different life forms have appeared (and disappeared) over this time. A timeline is shown in Table 18.1.

The evolution of horses from ancestral *Hyracotherium* to the modern *Equus* is well documented in fossil records. The rich record includes many transitional fossils, enabling scientists to develop a robust model of horse phylogeny. Equine evolution is a complex tree-like lineage with many divergences, showing that a diverse array of horse species coexisted for some time over the 55-million-year period of horse evolution. The environmental transition from forest to grasslands drove many of the changes found in the fossil record, including reduction in the number of toes and size of cheek teeth, lengthening of the skull to accept bigger cheek teeth and increasing body size. Cooler climates prevailed in the Miocene period 923–925 million years ago (mya) and this bought about a reduction in forested areas, with grasslands becoming more abundant. The changing vegetation resulted in equids developing more durable teeth to cope with the harsher diet.

The majority of equine evolution took place in North America, although now-extinct species did migrate to other areas at various times. During the Late Pliocene (2.6 mya), *Equus* spread to the Old World and diversified into several species, including the modern zebra of Africa and the modern horse *Equus caballus*. Until approximately 1 mya, there were *Equus* species all over Africa, Asia, Europe, North America and South America. Wild horses were common throughout the Eurasian steppes from 35,000–10,000 years ago. Fossil records indicate that about 10,000 years ago, the wild horse population decreased sharply and by the Iron Age had almost disappeared.

The horse became extinct in the Americas about 11,000 years ago, but was reintroduced by Spanish explorers (see 'Mustangs'), followed by Columbus in 1493 in North America, and this continued into the sixteenth century. Escaped horses established a feral population that by the early 1800s had reached around 2 million in number. The population then declined with increased expansion of civilisation and exploitation by man. By 1959 there were only 15,000–30,000 feral horses remaining in the United States and 2000–4000 in Western Canada. Przewalski's horse is the last surviving subspecies of wild horse. Today around 1500 exist, with a large number living in zoos (Figure 18.1), though some are now also making up herds that have been reintroduced at several sites in Mongolia (Figure 18.2).

Classification

The taxonomy of the horse according to the Integrated Taxonomic Information System (ITIS) is as follows:

Equine Science, Third Edition. Zoe Davies and Sarah Pilliner.
© 2018 Zoe Davies and Sarah Pilliner. Published 2018 by John Wiley & Sons Ltd.

Table 18.1 Timeline of the appearance of different life forms.

Time	Life forms
4 billion years ago	Prokaryotes (simple cells)
3 billion years ago	Photosynthesis
2 billion years ago	Eukaryotes (complex cells)
1 billion years ago	Multicellular life forms
600 million years ago	Simple animals
570 million years ago	Arthropods (insects, etc.)
500 million years ago	Fish
475 million years ago	Plants on land
360 million years ago	Amphibians
300 million years ago	Reptiles
233 million years ago	Dinosaurs
200 million years ago	Mammals
150 million years ago	Birds
66 million years ago	Dinosaurs became extinct
52 million years ago	*Hyracotherium* (ancestor of the horse)
1.8 million years ago	*Equus caballus*
200,000 years ago	Recognisable humans

Kingdom: Animalia

Subkingdom: Bilateral

Infrakingdom: Deuterostomia

Phylum: Chordata

Subphylum: Vertebrate

Infraphylum: Gnathostomata

Superclass:Tetrapods

Class: Mammal

Subclass:Theria

Infraclass: Eutheria

Order: Perissodactyla

Family: Equidae

Genus: *Equus*

Members of the order Perissodactyla (odd-toed ungulates) have an odd number of toes on each foot, hooved feet, mobile lips and similar teeth structure. Within Perissodactyla there are three families: Equidae (horses, asses and zebras), Rhinocerotidae (rhinos) and Tapiridae (tapirs), divided into two suborders, Hippomorpha (horses, asses and zebras) and Ceratomorpha (rhinos and tapirs). Horses therefore share common ancestors with rhinoceroses and tapirs. Phenacodontidae is the earliest family in the order of condylarths believed to be the ancestor of Perissodactyla. The family lived from the Early Palaeocene to the Middle Eocene in Europe and was roughly the same size as sheep. Eocene refers to the Eocene epoch of the Tertiary period.

The first animal from the evolutionary pathway of the family Equidae is *Hyracotherium* (often referred to as eohippus or 'dawn horse'). Incidentally, the word eohippus should not be capitalised or in italics as it is not a valid scientific name; *Hyracotherium* (1840) is the older name and therefore takes precedence over, and includes, eohippus (1876). It was named *Hyracotherium* after a hyrax-like beast. The hyrax is a rodent related to elephants and manatees.

Species

Species of horses with their various common names are given below.

Equus caballus – modern horse

Equus przewalski – Przewalski's horse, Asiatic wild horse

Equus hemionus – Asiatic wild ass (Figure 18.3), includes the onager and kulan

Equus asinus – donkey

Equus kiang – Asian ass, with three subspecies

Equus grevyi – Grevy's zebra;

Equus hartmannae – Hartmann's zebra, Hartmann's mountain zebra

Equus zebra – Cape mountain zebra, mountain zebra

Equus quagga – common zebra, plains zebra.

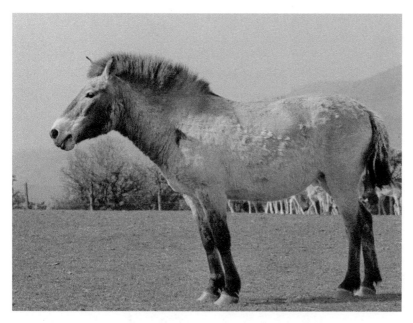

Figure 18.1 Przewalski's wild horse from Colwyn Bay Zoo. *Source*: Egan, https://commons.wikimedia.org/wiki/File:Przewalski_Wild_Horse.jpg. CC BY 2.0.

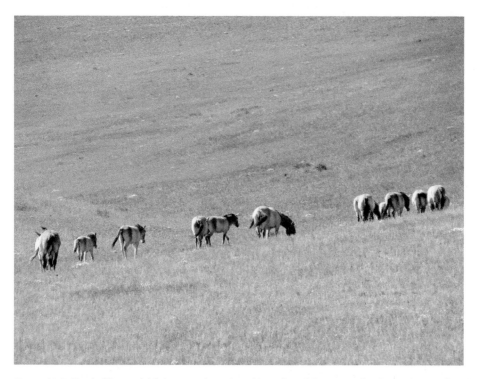

Figure 18.2 Herd of Przewalski's horses reintroduced into the wild in Mongolia. *Source*: Karamollaoglu, https://www.flickr.com/photos/okaramollaoglu/8367788369/. CC BY 2.0.

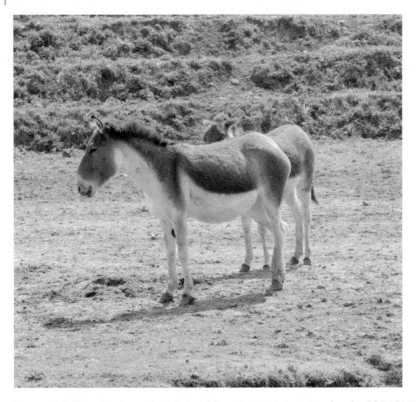

Figure 18.3 *Equus hemionus*, the Asiatic wild ass. *Source*: Agicart. Used under CC BY-SA 3.0, http://creativecommons.org/licenses/by-sa/3.0.

There are various subspecies of the plains zebra:

Equus quagga boehmi – Grant's zebra
Equus quagga borensis – Half-maned zebra
Equus quagga burchellii – Zululand zebra
                                 Damara zebra
                                 Burchell's zebra
                                 Bontequagga
Equus quagga chapmani – Chapman's zebra
Equus quagga crawshayi – Crawshay's zebra
Equus quagga quagga – Quagga (extinct).

Some like the domestic horse (*Equus caballus*) and donkey (*Equus asinus*) are entirely domesticated, with just scattered feral populations of escapees or releases. The significant wild Equidae today are the three species of zebra: most widespread is the common zebra (*Equus quagga*) and the other two, which are both much rarer and limited in range, are Grevy's zebra (*Equus grevyi*) (Figure 18.4) and the mountain zebra (*Equus zebra*), the latter found in southwestern Africa.

Research by the University of Oxford's wildlife conservation unit showed that only 2200 Grevy's zebra exist on the Horn of Africa in an area less than 10% of their original range and only 600 African wild ass remain on 2.5% of their natural range. Without intervention, these members of the equine family could disappear in their natural habitat.

The quagga lived in southeastern Africa but disappeared in the mid-1800s. It was the first extinct animal to have its DNA analysed in a 1984 study. This confirmed that it was more closely related to zebras than to horses. The quagga and mountain zebra shared an ancestor 3–4 mya ago; however, further research found the quagga to be closest to the plains zebra.

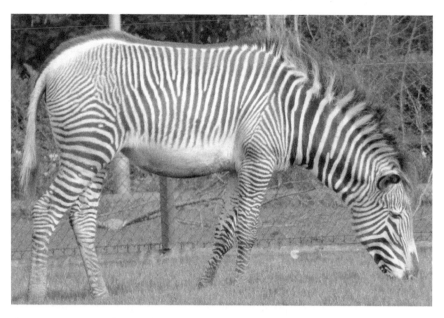

Figure 18.4 **Grevy's zebra.** *Source*: Courtesy of Rebecca Eastment.

Evolutionary Development

The evolutionary development of horses is shown in Figure 18.5. The horse evolved to roam grasslands, foraging on fibrous grasses, weeds and occasional browsing of small bushes. This was not a straight evolutionary line, but a sort of tree-shaped evolution, with many dead ends resulting from the loss of their previous particular ancestor . Thus, the modern horse was not the end result of the entire long lineage of equids, but rather the only genus of the many horse lineages to survive through time.

The environmental transition from forest to grassland drove the evolutionary changes seen in the equine fossil record. These include an increase in body size, reduction in the number of toes, increase in the size of molars and lengthening of the face to house them. The earliest ancestors of horses walked on several spread-out toes and lived in primeval forests. As grasslands evolved, their diets changed from browsing leaves and fruit and general foliage to grasses. This gave rise to larger more hard-wearing teeth. Over the following 50 million years and encompassing

several different climates including ice ages, many different descendant branches evolved as *Equus* ancestors. The horse's predecessors also had to outrun their predators on the open steppes and so the weight of the body was eventually taken off their multiple toes and onto the third longest toe to increase speed.

Grass contains silica, which is an extremely hard substance, and so equine ancestors evolved teeth capable of withstanding the grinding of herbage containing silica and also the frequent presence of soil particles attached to grass. The head became bigger in order to house the longer grinding teeth. The jaw increased in depth to house more powerful muscles for 'grinding'. The jaws became sideways moving, to more efficiently break down and tear the fibrous food. Teeth became coated with cement and became higher crowned or hypsodont. Eventually these teeth undertook continuous growth, that is, became hypsodont (see Chapter 17). The increasing size of the skull meant that the eyes became more laterally positioned, which was advantageous in increasing the field of vision to escape predators. The neck

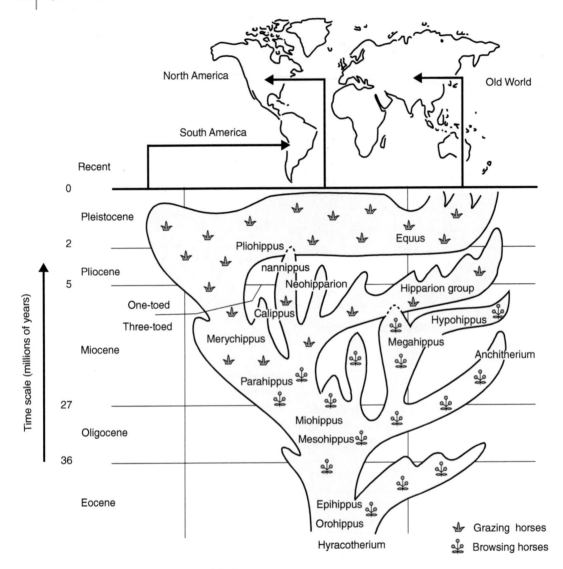

North America

South America

Old World

Recent

0

Pleistocene

2

Pliocene

5

Miocene

27

Oligocene

36

Eocene

Time scale (millions of years)

Pliohippus
nannippus
Neohipparion
Hipparion group
Equus
One-toed
Three-toed
Calippus
Hypohippus
Merychippus
Megahippus
Anchitherium
Parahippus
Miohippus
Mesohippus
Epihippus
Orohippus
Hyracotherium

Grazing horses
Browsing horses

Figure 18.5 Evolutionary pathway of the horse.

became longer to allow the animal to reach down and graze. The heavier head housing the longer teeth required a stronger neck and back muscles to support it.

The digestive system evolved in several ways to adapt to the grazing diet. In order to break down plant fibre (cellulose contained in plant cell walls), later ancestors of the horse adopted a symbiotic arrangement with millions of microbiota in their digestive tracts which produced an enzyme

called cellulase which broke down cellulose. The equine ancestors in turn provided a safe environment in which the microbiota lived in a specialised digestive area. Later ancestors further developed larger fermentation areas within the hind gut specifically in which millions of bacteria lived and fermented the ingested grasses anaerobically (i.e. in the absence of oxygen). Horses then were able to utilise many of the products of microbial fermentation.

The Evolutionary Family Tree

Hyracotherium appeared in the Early Eocene (roughly 52 mya). It was a fox-sized animal with a short neck and head and an arched back. It had 44 low crowned teeth. *Hyracotherium* was a scansorial (adapted for climbing) browser able to stand on its back legs to reach foliage above. It browsed on soft leaves and shrubs and fruit. It is thought to have had a small brain with especially small frontal lobes. The forelimbs had five toes. The feet were padded similar to dogs but with small hooves instead of claws at the end. *Hyracotherium* had four horn-covered toes on the fore feet and three on the hind feet.

Orohippus co-existed with *Hyracotherium* for a while about 2 million years after the first appearance of *Hyracotherium*, although *Orohippus* fossils are not as numerous or as geographically widespread as those of *Hyracotherium*. Fossils of *Orohippus* date from about 52–45 mya. *Orohippus* was still fox sized. The most significant change was seen in the dentition with teeth showing greater grinding ability due to a diet of tougher fibrous plant material. *Orohippus* had also lost the vestigial outer toes. It was followed by *Epihippus* in the Mid-Eocene around 47 mya. *Epihippus* was about 0.6 m (2 ft) tall and had five grinding low-crowned teeth with well-formed crests.

Figure 18.6 shows evolution of the horse from the Late Eocene to recent times. *Mesohippus* ('middle horse') lived around 37–32 mya. Many forests had turned into open flatlands where grasses thrived. In the Early Oligocene *Mesohippus* was quite widespread in North America. It had three toes on its fore and hind legs of which the third toe was stronger and carried more weight. It was more agile and slightly larger (45kg) than *Epihippus* with a less arched back and it had larger cerebral hemispheres.

Soon after, *Miohippus* ('lesser horse') evolved around 32–25 mya. It is thought that a *Miohippus* population split from the main *Mesohippus* group, coexisting with

them for around 4 million years and over time possibly replacing them. *Miohippus* had a larger head and body and continued to thrive. It diversified over time, branching into two groups, one of which adapted to life in the forests, whereas the other remained on the grasslands. Ancestors in the forest were known as *Miohippus intermedius* or *Kalobatippus*. Their second and fourth toes were long and well suited to soft ground found in forests. *Kalobatippus* possibly gave rise to *Ancitherium* which travelled across Asia and then on to Europe. In Eurasia and North America larger bodied animals evolved from *Ancitherium* such as *Megahippus* and *Hypohippus*. *Hypohippus* then became extinct in the Late Miocene period.

The ancestor of *Miohippus* that remained on the grassland is believed to be *Parahippus*, a pony-sized animal in North America. Parahippus lived around 24–17 mya. The skull structure resembled those of modern-day horses with the deep jaws. The third toes were stronger and longer, bearing the weight of the body. The upper incisors had a trace of a shallow crease marking the beginning of the cup (see Chapter 17).

In the middle of the Miocene *Merychippus* thrived from 17–11 mya. *Merychippus* retained the primitive character of three toes, and it was the first ancestor to look like a modern horse (although it was very small at 10 hands), with a long face. Its long legs allowed it to escape from predators and migrate long distances to feed. It had high-crowned cheek teeth, making it the first known grazing horse and the ancestor of all later horse lineages. Fossils of *Merychippus* are often found at many Late Miocene localities throughout the United States. The hind legs were relatively short and had side toes with small hooves which only touched the ground when running. *Merychippus* weighed around 100 kg and produced several additional grassland species, from which three lineages of Equidae are thought to have descended, namely *Hipparion*, *Protohippus* and *Pliohippus*.

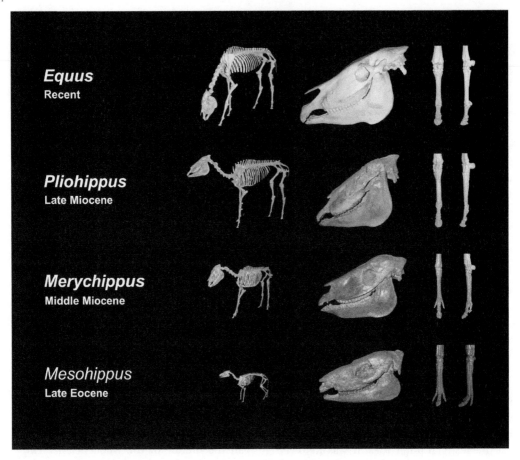

Figure 18.6 Equine evolution. Composed from skeletons of Staatliches Museum für Naturkunde Karlsruhe, Germany. From left to right: size development, biometrical changes in the cranium, reduction of toes (left forefoot). Highest point of the withers: *Equus* 1.5 m; *Pliohippus* 1.2 m; *Merychippus* 0.8 m; *Mesohippus* 0.5 m. *Source*: Zell, https://commons.wikimedia.org/wiki/File:Equine_evolution.jpg. Used under CC BY-SA 3.0, https://creativecommons.org/licenses/by-sa/3.0/deed.en.

As the climate changed and the swamps dried out, providing firmer ground, the four toes gradually became obsolete, until the first one-toed ancestor of the horse came into being from 12–6 mya. This was *Pliohippus*, often referred to as the grandfather of *Equus*. The ancestors of *Pliohippus* did not just lose toes, but gradually they shrank in size, becoming tiny dew hooves similar to the dew claws of a dog. Chestnuts present on the inside of a horse's leg just above the knee are visible reminders of the first toe lost during evolution and ergots on the back of the fetlock are small pieces of horn, remnants of the second and fourth toes. Splint bones

are the remains of the second metacarpal (fore leg) and metatarsal (hind leg) bones.

Figure 18.7 shows the significant changes to the forelimb through evolution which aided faster movement. *Pliohippus* arose from *Callipus* (which then died out). It is similar in appearance to *Equus*. It was fleet footed and a grazer. Its skull had deep facial depressions or fossae in the bones in front of its eyes, which are not present in *Equus*, and the teeth were curved, unlike modern horses which have relatively straight teeth.

Dinohippus (meaning 'powerful horse') was the most common species of Equidae in the Late Pleiocene in North America.

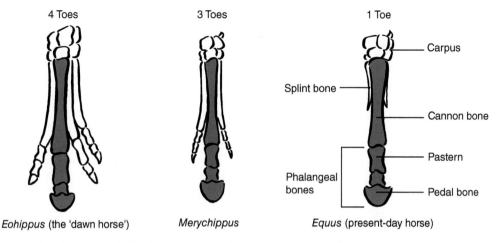

Figure 18.7 Changes to the forelimb through evolution.

Dinohippus is believed to be the closest relative to *Equus*. It lived from 13–5 mya and fossils have been found in North America at Upper Miocene localities. It was single hooved, although there appears to be some variation among individuals, and roamed grasslands. There are suggestions that some *Dinohippus* individuals had three toes, while others had only one.

Equus is now thought to have evolved from *Dinohippus* via the intermediate form *Plesihippus*. *Equus* has the distinctive passive 'stay apparatus,' formed by bones and tendons, to help conserve energy while standing for long periods. *Dinohippus* is the first horse ancestor to show a rudimentary form of the stay apparatus, providing additional evidence of the close relationship between *Dinohippus* and *Equus*.

The genus of all modern horses, the first *Equus*, was about 13.2 hands tall (pony size), with a rigid spine, long neck, legs and nose, and fused leg bones with no rotation. The brain was slightly larger than in early *Dinohippus*. Like *Dinohippus*, *Equus* was one-toed, with side ligaments that prevented twisting of the hoof. This species had high-crowned, straight, grazing teeth with strong crests lined with cementum, as seen in modern horses today. *Equus* evolved around 5 mya, surviving to the present day.

The modern-day species of *Equus* (horses, zebras and asses) are very different from the earliest known horse *Hyracotherium*. In recent years, new fossil skeletons have been discovered, challenging previously held theories regarding equine evolution. Fossils of *Equus* have been found on every continent except Australia and Antarctica. *Equus caballus* is the most recent ancestor of the horse. It evolved during the Pleistocene period (approximately 2 mya). It was well adapted to life on the open plains and capable of great speed, having long lower limbs with an absence of muscle but a highly muscled upper body. The foot pad of earlier ancestors is now the frog of modern horses.

A summary of the timeline of evolution of the main ancestors that developed into *Equus* is shown below.

- 55 mya: *Hyracotherium*
- 52–45 mya: *Orohippus*
- 37–32 mya: *Mesohippus*
- 32–25 mya: *Miohippus*
- 24–17 mya: *Parahippus*
- 17–11 mya: *Merychippus*
- 12–6 mya: *Pliohippus*
- 13–5 mya: *Dinohippus*
- 5 mya to present: *Equus*
- 2 mya: *Equus caballus*

Domestic Breeds and Types of Horses

It is thought horses started to be domesticated around 3000–5000 years ago, and remains of horses that not only were different from wild horses in their structure but also had some dental damage consistent with ancient biting became increasingly frequently found in archaeological sites in southern Ukraine and Kazakhstan.

Horses were domesticated at different times and places throughout the world. This has led to great variation in breeds and types and there are now over 200 breeds worldwide. Modern horses and ponies can have their origins traced back to one of four types. These types do not relate in any way to body temperature but to temperament and speed.

- Hotbloods – Thoroughbreds and Arabs.
- Warmbloods – carriage and sports horses.
- Cold bloods – heavy draught horses.
- Ponies – deeper bodies and shorter legs.

Donkeys

There are more than 40 million donkeys in the world today. Mostly used for working in poorer countries, they are often abused, having to carry overly heavy loads and/or travel many miles. Working donkeys in the poorest countries have a life expectancy of 12–15 years, but where kept as pets or not for working they may live to 30–50 years.

Donkeys vary considerably in size, depending on breed and management. There are Miniature donkeys (a separate breed of donkey originating from the islands of Sardinia and Sicily; see Figure 18.8) and much larger breeds such as the Baudet du Poitou (Figure 18.9). The height at the withers ranges from 7.3 to 15.3 hands.

Donkeys are mostly adapted to marginal desert lands, and unlike wild and feral horses, wild donkeys in dry areas tend to be solitary and do not form herds. The loud call or bray of the donkey, which typically lasts for 20 seconds, can be heard for over 3 km, helping them to keep in contact with other donkeys over the wide expanses of the desert. Donkeys are known for their large ears, which may pick up more distant sounds and may also help cool the blood and therefore body temperature.

Donkeys can interbreed with other members of the family Equidae and are commonly interbred with horses. The hybrid between a jack and a mare is a mule, valued as a working and riding animal in many countries. Some large donkey breeds such as the Asino di Martina Franca, the Baudet du Poitou and the Mammoth Jack are raised only for mule production. The hybrid between a stallion and a jenny is a hinny and is less common. Like other interspecies hybrids, mules and hinnies are usually sterile. Donkeys can also breed with zebras, in which the offspring is called a zonkey or a zeedonk (among other names).

Przewalski's Horse

First described scientifically in the late nineteenth century by Russian explorer N.M. Przewalski, Przewalski's horse (*Equus przewalskii*) once freely roamed the steppes along the Mongolia–China border. Exterminated from the wild in the late 1960s, they have since been kept and bred in captivity and reintroduced in Mongolia. Their extinction in the wild was brought about by hunting, loss of habitat and loss of water sources to domestic animals. Also known as the Asiatic wild horse, they are thought to be a sister species to the Tarpan, the European wild horse (*Equus ferus*), which gave rise to the domestic horse. Przewalski's horse is considered a wild subspecies because its ancestors were never domesticated. In fact, its extinction in the wild was due primarily to interbreeding with other domesticated horses.

Using material extracted from a leg bone found buried in permafrost in Canada's Yukon territory in June 2013, a group of

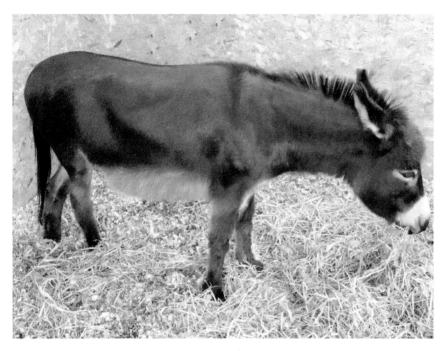

Figure 18.8 Mediterranean Miniature donkey. *Source*: Courtesy of Zoe Davies.

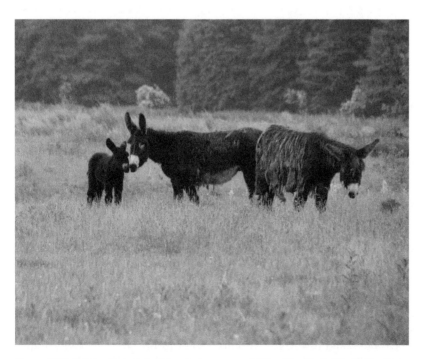

Figure 18.9 Poitou donkeys in the nature reserve of Olfen, Nordrhein Westfalen, Germany. Dreadlocks are a characteristic of this breed. *Source*: Laravalena, https://commons.wikimedia.org/wiki/File:Poitou-Esel_im_ Naturschutzgebiet_in_Olfen.JPG. CC BY-SA 3.0.

researchers sequenced the DNA of a 560,000 to 780,000 year-old horse. Prior to this, the oldest genome that had been success-fully sequenced was dated at 110,000 to 130,000 years ago. For comparison, the researchers also sequenced the genomes of a 43,000-year-old Pleistocene horse, a Prze-walski's horse, five modern horse breeds and a donkey. Analysis of the differences between these genomes suggested that the last com-mon ancestor of modern horses, donkeys and zebras existed 4–4.5 mya. The results also indicated that Przewalski's horse diverged from other modern types of horse about 43,000 years ago, and had never in its evolu-tionary history been domesticated – that is, it is a truly wild horse.

Mustangs

Mustangs are descendants of the Spanish horses that were brought to the Americas by Spanish explorers. The name is derived from the Spanish word *mustengo* which means 'ownerless beast' or 'stray horse.' These horses bred with other types of horses, including Quarter-horses and draft horses, to create the mustang we know today. Many people think that mustangs are simply wild horses rather than a specific breed.

Behaviour of the Modern Horse

Behaviour is defined as an organism's response to changes in its external envi-ronment. The influence of the social environ-ment is crucial for young horses; they must learn social skills as soon as possible to survive within a herd environment and the isolation of foals can cause long-term traumatic effects. Behaviour that involves members of the group interacting with each other is called social behaviour, and this has many advantages. Horses in a social group are more efficient at finding food as they can search a large area. There is a clear hierarchy which prevents energy wasted from fighting

as males already know their ranking in the group. Mares and foals are protected on the inside of the herd, keeping them safe. Adult horses within a herd will automatically and consistently deal with any unruly behaviour of young horses. Horses undertake grooming which helps to reinforce social bonds.

Innate Behaviour

Innate behaviour is instinctive behaviour that horses do without any thought. It is inherited from the sire and dam and so is genetically determined and not influenced by the envi-ronment. It is also stereotyped behaviour in that all horses do the same thing, such as grazing and sleeping patterns, fight or flight. There is an advantage to innate behaviour in that all horses respond in the same way in the herd environment and respond straight away as no learning is required. For example, foals will get up as soon as possible after birth and will suckle from the dam. Examples of innate behaviours include escape reflexes (mov-ing away from potential danger). Taxis and kinesis are both types of movement. Taxis is directed movement related to a stimulus whilst kinesis is random and without specific direction.

Horses have instincts that have evolved over many years to protect them in the wild. They have an excellent fight or flight response and can move sharply and quickly from a potential or perceived source of dan-ger. They are strongly motivated to seek out the companionship of other horses, partic-ularly those familiar to them, that is, family members. This behaviour can be seen in small groups when one horse is removed and some of those left behind will often run around and whinny frequently. Horses develop important social networks, allowing them to live more safely in herds, benefiting greatly from being with others in long-term groups (Figure 18.10).

Horses have evolved with a need to eat fre-quently. Wild horses spend most of their time grazing and eating small amounts often. This is known as trickle feeding and the equine

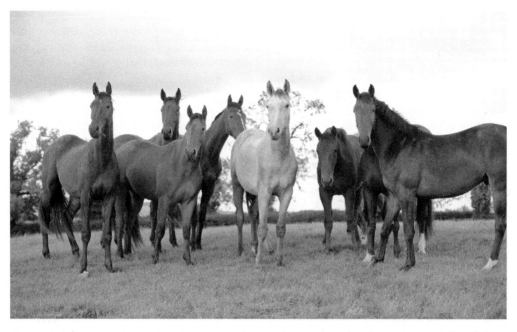

Figure 18.10 Youngstock turned out in groups are happier than on their own. *Source*: Courtesy of Harthill Stud.

digestive tract is specially adapted to this diet of high-fibre food. Horses do not naturally live in stables or very small enclosed areas. It is important to try to meet the natural needs of horses through correct management to stop them becoming depressed, sour or uncooperative. Horses should be allowed to follow their natural instincts as much as possible. If they are given the freedom to live as nature intended they will be healthier and less likely to be stressed.

Learned Behaviour

Learned behaviour is where a horse's behaviour has been modified due to its experience. Learned behaviour is influenced by the environment and allows horses to respond to changing conditions. For example, horses learn to generally not accept harmful food in their environment such as ragwort. Learned behaviour is vital for training horses to adapt to their new environments such as stabling, transport in horse boxes, competing, even hacking on roads and accepting the presence of moving vehicles.

The domestication of horses has led to them needing to be trained to undertake the work required of them. Some are better suited to learning than others, such as the acceptance of a saddle and bridle and rider, while others will need more time and patience. There are different types of learned behaviour:

- Habituation
- Classical conditioning
- Operant conditioning
- Latent learning
- Insight learning.

Habituation

Habituation is a reduced response to an unimportant stimulus after repeated exposure after time. An unimportant stimulus is a change that is not threatening or rewarding to the horse (such as a treat). Horses quickly learn to ignore these stimuli so they are not wasting time and more importantly energy responding to unimportant stimuli. Most quickly adapt to living in noisy environments, for example. Police horses are trained to ignore shouting and screaming crowds of people.

Classical Conditioning

Classical conditioning refers to horses learning to respond naturally to a stimulus that normally causes that response. In this type of learning the horse learns that 'this means that'. Examples include responding to certain voice commands and voice, whip and body cues: such as teaching horses to trot on the lunge by command (i.e. saying 'Trrrrrrrrot') and the horse learning the aids, for example moving away from the rider's leg when applied. The Pavlovian response in dogs is an example of classical conditioning.

Operant Conditioning

Operant conditioning is when animals learn to associate a particular response with a reward or punishment/correction: for example, rats pushing coloured levers, where one gives a treat and the other a small electric shock. This is positive and negative reinforcement of behaviour. Mistakes are often made at first, but soon the animal learns to press the correct lever for a reward. Overuse of negative reinforcement does not work with horses, as they appear much more adaptable to rewards for the required behaviour. Operant conditioning is the basis for clicker training in horses.

Operant conditioning is a form of 'cause and effect' learning, and so the horse realises and learns that 'when I do this, this happens'. Horses soon learn to keep away from an electric fence, which is an example of operant conditioning with punishment.

Latent Learning

Latent learning is hidden learning where the horse does not immediately show it has learned a behaviour. It involves learning through repeatedly doing the same thing. Foals naturally learn to make connections between different stimuli, that is, whether the stimulus is dangerous or risky or not. Foals need to familiarise themselves with the environment they are in, including, for example, noise, dogs, cars, horse boxes and even different surfaces. This is latent learning. What a horse has already seen as a foal under good circumstances and with positive experiences means that it will be less scared of as an adult.

Insight Learning

Insight learning involves solving a problem by using previous experience to work out a solution. This is quicker than trial and error because actions are planned and executed by the horse. This is when the horse is taught how to learn. This type of learning or training will require a strong relationship between horse and trainer.

Stereotypies

Stereotypies are typically learned behaviours that are repeated without any apparent or obvious purpose or function: for example, stable vices such as weaving, head banging and box walking, field walking, biting and kicking. Such behaviours involve a need-related drive that develops in an environment with inadequate opportunities for satisfying the need. Once established, a stereotypic behaviour may become a need in itself. Stereotypies are relatively invariant as horses repeat the sequence over and over.

Horses uniquely indulge in the oral-based stereotypy of cribbing or crib-biting, whereby the horse hooks the incisors onto an object, such as a fence rail, post, door, feeder or bucket. Grasping the surface with the teeth, the lower jaw is dropped and the throat opened. The horse then arches the neck, pulls backward and completes the act with a belch-like sound. In popular definitions, some cribbers are called windsuckers, because they appear to swallow air (aerophagia) with or without grabbing an object, but a recent study showed this to be incorrect and air is not swallowed into the stomach.

The exact causes remain unclear, although stereotypic behaviour seems associated with the time the horse spends in the stable.

Cribbing may start with gastric ulcers, that is, pain in the stomach. Poor stable management can increase these habits. Horses should never be stabled for long periods of time unless injuries prevent turn out. They are much better psychologically when turned out in a small group environment with long-term friends so they can undertake their social behaviour.

There is a genetic predisposition to showing stereotypic behaviour, with the sire, dam or half-siblings also showing signs of it. Thus most horses that show one kind of stall vice will have relatives that show it or another.

Imprinting

Imprint learning is a combination of a learned behaviour and an innate behaviour. For example, a foal does not have an innate instinct of what the dam looks like – this is learned very soon after it is born, allowing it to recognise its dam and instinctively follow her. Imprinting only occurs for a short time and this time is known as the critical period; in the first 24 hours of life, the hard disk of a foal is 'open' to record all the information needed. This is necessary because horses in the wild are prey animals and a foal should be able to immediately run with the herd after birth. Once learned, imprinting is fixed and irreversible. Horses use imprinting later in life to identify potential 'mates' in the wild situation.

The Dopamine Receptor D4

The horse's behaviour depends largely on the structure and function of its brain and involves neurotransmitters, synapses and receptors. Small differences in the brain appear to produce big changes in behaviour. The D4 receptor is a receptor in the brain for the neurotransmitter dopamine. Having too many D4 receptors has been linked with abnormal behaviour. D4 receptors are also involved in thinking, perception, memory and emotions.

It also appears that there are breed differences in horses in the dopamine receptor D4 gene (DRD4), which has been reported to affect the horse's personality.

Emotion

Recent research has found that horses have the ability to discriminate between positive and negative human facial expressions. This shows that horses are able to recognise emotional cues possibly following positive and negative experiences, but this is across species, that is, humans and horses in this case.

Summary Points

1) *Hyracotherium* (the ancestor of the horse) appeared roughly 55mya and *Equus caballus* (the modern horse) appeared 2.6 mya.
2) Today, Przewalski's horse remains as the last surviving subspecies of wild horse. Przewalski is considered a wild subspecies because its ancestors were never domesticated.
3) Grass contains silica, which is an extremely hard substance and so equine ancestors evolved teeth capable of withstanding the grinding of herbage containing silica and also the frequent presence of soil particles attached to grass.
4) *Equus* is one-toed, with side ligaments that prevent twisting of the hoof. This genus has high-crowned, straight, grazing teeth with strong crests lined with cementum, as seen in modern horses today.
5) Horses are highly social herd animals and their behaviours are very suited to their natural lives.
6) Innate behaviour is inherited from the sire and dam and so is genetically determined and not influenced by the horse's environment.

Q + A

Q Which order does *Equus* belong to?
A Perrisodactyla.

Q When were horses first thought to be domesticated?
A Around 3000–5000 years ago.

Q From which horses are mustangs descended?
A Mustangs are descendants of Spanish horses that were brought to the Americas by Spanish explorers.

Q How did the digestive system evolve to adapt to a grazing diet?

A In order to break down cellulose, later ancestors of horses adopted a symbiotic arrangement with millions of microbiota in their digestive tracts which produced an enzyme called cellulase which broke down cellulose. The equine ancestors in turn provided a safe environment in which the microbiota lived in a specialised digestive area.

Q What is the D4 receptor?
A It is a receptor in the brain for the neurotransmitter dopamine. Having too many D4 receptors has been linked with abnormal behaviour.

A

Anatomical Terms Based on the Median Plane

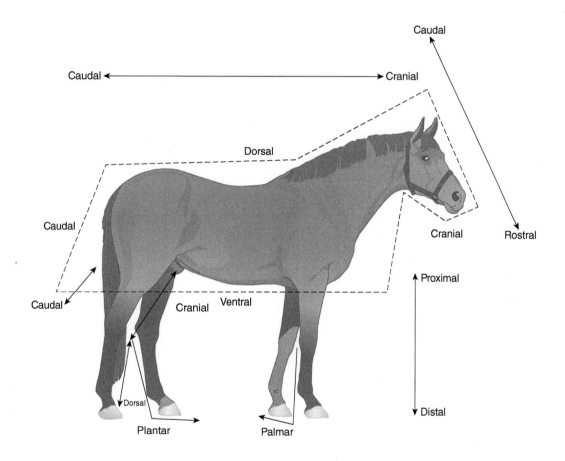

Equine Science, Third Edition. Zoe Davies and Sarah Pilliner.
© 2018 Zoe Davies and Sarah Pilliner. Published 2018 by John Wiley & Sons Ltd.

Caudal – (posterior) – nearer to the tail than; e.g. ribs are caudal to the head/neck

Cranial – (anterior) – nearer to the skull than; e.g. diaphragm is cranial to the stomach

Distal – further from the horse's body (only used on limbs); e.g. fetlock is distal to the knee

Dorsal – nearer the back of the horse than; e.g. spine is dorsal to the abdomen

Lateral – further from the midline than; e.g. ribs are lateral to the lungs

Medial – nearer to the midline than; e.g. bladder is medial to the hips

Palmar – below the proximal ends of the carpus (knee)

Plantar – below the proximal ends of the tarsus (hock)

Proximal – closer to the horse's body than (only used on limbs); e.g. shoulder is proximal to the elbow

Rostral – towards the muzzle/nose/mouth

Ventral – nearer the belly of the horse than; e.g. sternum is ventral to the heart

Sagittal plane – also known as lateral or median plane – divides horse's body into left and right parts

Frontal plane – also known as coronal plane – divides horse's body into anterior (front) or posterior (back)

Transverse plane – also known as axial or horizontal plane – divides horse's body into superior (upper) and inferior (lower) parts

B

Haematology and Plasma Biochemistry Tests

Table B.1 Haematology.

Blood test	Significance	Units	Normal range
Red blood cells (erythrocytes)	Oxygen-carrying capacity	$x10^{12}$/L	5.8–10.2
Haemoglobin	Low = anaemia	g/DL	9.8–17.0
Haematocrit (packed cell volume)	Proportion of cells to plasma Low = unfit or disease High = electrolyte imbalance or exhaustion	L/L	31.1–49.5
Mean corpuscular volume (MCV)	Size of erythrocytes. New ones are larger than older ones High = red worm damage	f/L	29–59
Mean corpuscular haemoglobin concentration (MCHC)	A guide to the oxygen-carrying capacity of blood Low = severe anaemia	g/dL	22–40
Total white blood cells (leucocytes)	Vary in response to disease Low = viral infection High = bacterial infection	$x10^9$/L	4.3–9.5
Percentage of neutrophils to total white blood cells	High = bacterial infection	%	60
Neutrophils	High = bacterial infection	$x10^9$/L	2.4–6.6
Lymphocytes	High = chronic bacterial/viral infection	$x10^9$/L	1.1–5.1
Monocytes	Seen in some viral infections	$x10^9$/L	<0.5
Eosinophils	Seen in allergic responses and parasitic infections	$x10^9$/L	<0.6
Basophils	A sign of inflammation	$x10^9$/L	<0.2
Platelets	If falls very low = increased chance of bleeding	$x10^9$/L	62–48

Equine Science, Third Edition. Zoe Davies and Sarah Pilliner.
© 2018 Zoe Davies and Sarah Pilliner. Published 2018 by John Wiley & Sons Ltd.

Table B.2 Plasma and enzyme biochemistry tests.

Blood test	Significance	Units	Normal range
Plasma tests			
Albumin	Shows nutritional status and gut function High = rhabdomyolysis Low = poor liver function, poor nutrition or intestinal disease	g/L	30–42
Globulin (antibodies)	Increases with infection	g/L	17–42
Plasma fibrinogen	Chronic infection, internal parasites	g/L	1.8–4.0
Calcium (Ca)	Vital for bone health and muscular function Low Ca = may be stress, laminitis, muscle problems	mmol/L	2.9–3.4
Phosphate (P)	Bone health	mmol/L	0.5–1.8
Urea	High = kidney problems	mmol/L	4.0–9.1
Bilirubin	Bile salt	µmol/L	<47
Enzymes – body function tests			
Aspartate aminotransferase/serum glutamic oxaloacetic transaminase (AST/SGOT)	High = rhabdomyolysis, liver problems	U/L	<420
Gamma glutamyl transferase (GGT)		U/L	<49
Alkaline phosphatase		U/L	<362
Creatine kinase/creatine phosphokinase (CK/CPK)	Muscle enzyme – increases with muscle breakdown, tying up	U/L	<678
Lactate dehydrogenase		U/L	<956
Creatinine		µmol/L	55–135
Copper		µmol/L	15–30
Selenium		µmol/L	1.2–3.2
Iron		µmol/L	18–35
Vitamin E (tocopherol)		µmol/L	>3.4
Glucose		mmol/L	2.4–6.8
Insulin (starved > 6 hours)		U/L	<20
Insulin (post 0.5 g/kg glucose)		U/L	<69
Insulin (post 1 g/kg glucose)		U/L	<81

C

Functions, Sources and Deficiencies of Vitamins and Minerals in Horses

Vitamin/mineral	Required for	Source	Deficiency signs
Fat-soluble vitamins			
A Beta carotene	Healthy eyes Immune system Growth and maintenance of body tissues	Grass Green forage	Lack of appetite Night blindness Poor growth Keratinisation of eyes Hoof and skin in poor condition Infertility
D 'Sunshine vitamin'	Aids absorption of calcium and phosphorus absorption in the gut Bone formation Joint integrity	Horses synthesise vitamin D in their skin in the presence of sunlight Sun-dried hay (stabled horses may need supplementing)	Bones fail to calcify, leading to rickets in young horses and osteomalacia in older ones Swollen joints Fractures
E Tocopherol	Muscle integrity Fat metabolism Acts with selenium as an antioxidant Reproduction	Alfalfa Green forage Cereals	Muscular disorders Infertility
K	Blood clotting	Produced by healthy hindgut microbes Leafy forage	True deficiency is rare Levels can be assessed by measuring blood clotting time

Equine Science, Third Edition. Zoe Davies and Sarah Pilliner.
© 2018 Zoe Davies and Sarah Pilliner. Published 2018 by John Wiley & Sons Ltd.

Vitamin/mineral	Required for	Source	Deficiency signs
Water-soluble vitamins			
C Ascorbic acid	Immune system Antioxidant Muscle and blood capillary integrity	Made in body tissues from glucose	Bleeding, ulcerated gums Internal bleeding Interacts with copper and iron
B_1 Thiamine	Fat and carbohydrate metabolism, particularly glucose	Produced by healthy hindgut microbial population	Deficiency may be caused by eating bracken Loss of appetite Incoordination Staggering
B_2 Riboflavin	Carbohydrate, protein and fat metabolism	Produced by healthy hindgut microbial population	Reduced growth rate Reduced utilisation of feed Possibly involved in periodic ophthalmia
B_6 Pyridoxine was known as vitamin H	Carbohydrate, protein and fat metabolism Enzyme systems	Grass Green forage	In absence of B_6, tryptophan and niacin cannot be utilised Poor growth, dermatitis Nerve degeneration
B_{12} Cyanocobalamin	Carbohydrate, fat and protein metabolism	Produced by healthy hindgut microbes, but requires cobalt to do this	Poor growth Infertility Poor appetite Rough coat
B_9 Folic acid Folacin	Maturation of red blood cells Interacts with vitamins B_2, B_{12} and C	Grass Green forage Synthesised in hindgut by healthy microbial population	Not described in horses
B_7 Biotin	Hoof horn production Carbohydrate, protein and fat metabolism	Maize, yeast, soya Green forage	Poor hoof condition, hoof crumbles at ground surface
B_3 Niacin Nicotinic acid	Enzyme systems in all body cells Cell integrity and metabolism Carbohydrate, protein and fat digestion	Can be synthesised from the amino acid tryptophan Cereals	Never been produced in the horse
B_5 Pantothenic acid Calcium pantothenate	Part of coenzymes Carbohydrate, fat and protein digestion	Synthesised in hindgut by healthy microbial population	No specific deficiency signs seen in horses

Vitamin/mineral	Required for	Source	Deficiency signs
Minerals			
Calcium (Ca)	99% of body Ca is found in skeleton and teeth Blood clotting Nerve and muscle function Lactation Bone Ca can be rapidly mobilised to maintain blood Ca levels	Alfalfa Limestone flour Green forage Sugar beet	Bone problems Rickets (young) Osteomalacia (old) Nutritional secondary hyperparathyroidism Enlarged joints Rhabdomyolysis Immobility such as stabling results in loss of Ca from bone
Phosphorus (P)	81% of body P is found in skeleton and teeth Energy production – ATP Enzyme systems Substantial P absorption from the hindgut	Cereals	Bone problems Rickets (young) Osteomalacia (old) Reduced or depraved appetite Decreased growth
Magnesium (Mg)	60% of body Mg is found in skeleton and teeth 32% in muscle tissue Enzyme systems Required for ATP, RNA, DNA, oxidative phosphorylation, protein synthesis Mg oxide poorly absorbed	Alfalfa Linseed Feeding average quality forage should meet Mg requirements	Weakness in limbs Muscular tremors Ataxia Sweating No scientific evidence for Mg as a calmer
Sodium (Na) Chloride (Cl) Potassium (K) (electrolytes)	Body fluid regulating Muscle and nerve function Acid–base balance Dietary cation–anion balance (DCAB) Osmotic homeostasis	Grass Hay Salt lick (NaCl only) Horses have specific central regulation of salt appetite	Sweating Dehydration Muscular weakness and fatigue Exhaustion Depraved appetite
Sulphur (S)	Found in all tissues mainly associated with amino acids methionine and cysteine Hoof and horn growth – keratin synthesis Enzyme systems Present in insulin	Grass	Poor hair and skin growth including hooves

Vitamin/mineral	Required for	Source	Deficiency signs
Trace minerals			
Iron (Fe)	Haemoglobin (Hb) synthesis	Most natural feeds	Anaemia
	60% of body Fe is found in Hb/myoglobin		Weakness
			Pale mucous membranes
	Small amount in enzymes		Fatigue
	Fe storage in ferritin and haemosiderin		Reduced growth
			Mares' milk is low in Fe
	Horses can maintain Fe levels by recycling red blood cells and Hb		
	Involved in immune defence		
Copper (Cu)	Keratin synthesis	Depends upon soil Cu content from which feed is grown	Developmental orthopaedic disease
	Haemoglobin synthesis		Intermittent diarrhoea
	Most Cu found in muscle, liver and blood	High Mo has not yet been shown to reduce Cu availability in horses	Loss of pigment in hair
	Pigmentation of hair		Poor performance
	Cartilage and elastin production		Reduced growth
	Bone development		
	Myelination of neurons		
	Interacts with S and Mo		
Zinc (Zn)	Skin health	Yeast	Hair loss
	Cell metabolism	Cereals	Skin lesions
	Enzyme activator including digestive enzymes		Reduced appetite
			Reduced growth
	High Zn interferes with Cu utilisation		
	Immune system		
Iodine (I)	Required for thyroxine hormone	Most feeds	Infertility
	Controls metabolic rate	Seaweed products	Goitre
	Deficiency and toxicity cause goitre		
	Do not feed extra to pregnant mares		
Selenium (Se)	Antioxidant – glutathione peroxidase (GSHPx)	Pasture	Muscle disease
		Soil content varies	Impaired cardiac function
	Interacts with vitamin E	Deficient areas are common	Respiratory problems
		USA has many areas where Se toxicity is common	Tying up

Vitamin/mineral	Required for	Source	Deficiency signs
Manganese (Mn)	Carbohydrate, protein and fat metabolism Bone formation Lactation	Bran Grass (depending upon soil content)	Bone abnormalities Poor feed utilisation
Cobalt (Co)	Required for synthesis of vitamin B_{12}	Trace levels present in most feeds	Anaemia Weight loss Reduced growth

Index

Equine Science, Third Edition. Zoe Davies and Sarah Pilliner.
© 2018 Zoe Davies and Sarah Pilliner. Published 2018 by John Wiley & Sons Ltd.